Fundamentals of
SMALL ANIMAL SURGERY

Fundamentals of

SMALL ANIMAL SURGERY

Fred Anthony Mann

Gheorghe M. Constantinescu

Hun-Young Yoon

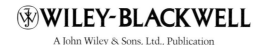

A John Wiley & Sons, Ltd., Publication

This edition first published 2011 © 2011 by Blackwell Publishing Ltd.

Blackwell Publishing was acquired by John Wiley & Sons in February 2007. Blackwell's publishing program has been merged with Wiley's global Scientific, Technical and Medical business to form Wiley-Blackwell.

Registered office: John Wiley & Sons Ltd, The Atrium, Southern Gate, Chichester, West Sussex, PO19 8SQ, UK

Editorial offices: 2121 State Avenue, Ames, Iowa 50014-8300, USA
The Atrium, Southern Gate, Chichester, West Sussex, PO19 8SQ, UK
9600 Garsington Road, Oxford, OX4 2DQ, UK

For details of our global editorial offices, for customer services and for information about how to apply for permission to reuse the copyright material in this book please see our website at www.wiley.com/wiley-blackwell.

Library of Congress Cataloging-in-Publication Data

Mann, Fred Anthony.
    Fundamentals of small animal surgery / Fred Anthony Mann, Gheorghe M. Constantinescu, Hun-Young Yoon.
        p. ; cm.
    Includes bibliographical references and index.
    Summary: "Fundamentals of Small Animal Surgery offers a thorough introduction to the surgical principles essential to good veterinary practice. With many high-quality line drawings and clinical photographs to complement the detailed descriptions, the book is a useful resource for building basic surgery skills. Covering topics ranging from assessment and surgical pack preparation to aseptic techniques and postoperative pain management, the book is a valuable reference for surgical procedure training in veterinary or veterinary technician schools, and serves as a refresher for veterinarians and technicians in practice." –Provided by publisher.
    ISBN 978-0-7817-6118-5 (pbk. : alk. paper)   1. Veterinary surgery.   2. Pet medicine.   I. Constantinescu, Gheorghe M., 1932- II. Yoon, Hun-Young. III. Title.
    [DNLM: 1. Animal Diseases–surgery.   2. Animals, Domestic–surgery.   3. Surgical Procedures, Operative–veterinary.   SF 911]
    SF981.M257 2011
    636.089'7–dc22

                                                                            2010042173

A catalogue record for this book is available from the British Library.

Set in 10/12 pt New Baskerville by Aptara® Inc., New Delhi, India
Printed and bound in Malaysia by Vivar Printing Sdn Bhd

2   2011

DEDICATIONS

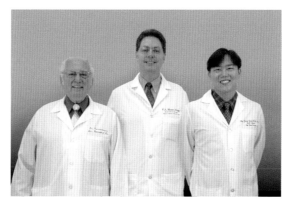

Left to right, Gheorghe M. Constantinescu, Fred Anthony Mann, and Hun-Young Yoon.

We, the authors, dedicate this textbook to all of the students who we have had the pleasure of training in the art and science of small animal surgery and to all of those companion animals who have benefitted from their surgical skills. The authors also state the following individual dedications.

I dedicate this textbook to my loving wife, Dr. Colette Wagner-Mann, my son, Lucas Mann, and my daughter, Danielle Mann. I thank them for their love, understanding, and patience as I have dedicated enormous amounts of time to veterinary student education, including the production of this textbook.

Fred Anthony Mann

My contribution to this book as an anatomist and medical illustrator started long ago and was encouraged by my wife, Dr. Ileana Constantinescu, whom I thank warmly for her unlimited support, understanding, and sacrifice. I dedicate this book to her, to my son Dr. Răzvan Constantinescu and daughter Adina Klima, and their families.

Gheorghe M. Constantinescu

I would like to thank my wonderful family, my wife, Kyunghwa Kim, and my son, Dongbin Yoon, for their support and encouragement during production of this textbook.

CONTENTS*

* All pencil drawings (see Chapters 5 through 14, 16, 17, and 20) are original and are illustrated by Dr. Gheorghe M. Constantinescu.

CONTRIBUTORS

Gheorghe M. Constantinescu, DVM, PhD, mult Drhc
Professor of Veterinary Anatomy and Medical Illustrator
Department of Biomedical Sciences
College of Veterinary Medicine
University of Missouri
Columbia, Missouri

John R. Dodam, DVM, MS, PhD, Diplomate ACVA
Associate Professor
Chairman
Department of Veterinary Medicine and Surgery
Veterinary Medical Teaching Hospital
College of Veterinary Medicine
University of Missouri
Columbia, Missouri

Fred Anthony Mann, DVM, MS, Diplomate ACVS, Diplomate ACVECC
Director of Small Animal Emergency and Critical Care Services
Small Animal Soft Tissue Surgery Service Chief

Professor
Department of Veterinary Medicine and Surgery
Veterinary Medical Teaching Hospital
College of Veterinary Medicine
University of Missouri
Columbia, Missouri

John P. Punke, DVM
Small Animal Surgery Resident
Department of Veterinary Medicine and Surgery
Veterinary Medical Teaching Hospital
College of Veterinary Medicine
University of Missouri
Columbia, Missouri

Carlos H. de M. Souza, DVM, MS, Diplomate ACVIM (Oncology)
Assistant Professor of Small Animal Surgery
Department of Veterinary Medicine and Surgery
Veterinary Medical Teaching Hospital
College of Veterinary Medicine
University of Missouri
Columbia, Missouri

Elizabeth A. Swanson, DVM
Small Animal Surgery Resident
Department of Veterinary Clinical Sciences
Veterinary Teaching Hospital
School of Veterinary Medicine
Purdue University
West Lafayette, Indiana

Hun-Young Yoon, DVM, MS, PhD
Research Professor
College of Veterinary Medicine
Veterinary Science Research Institute
Konkuk University
Seoul, South Korea

PREFACE

Today, owners of dogs and cats typically consider their pets to be members of the family. As such, the pet-owning public expects access to the same level of medical and surgical care that is available to human beings. Further, the general public expects veterinarians to have a certain level of surgical competence immediately upon graduation from veterinary school. To that end, veterinary educators are charged with preparing veterinary students to be competent surgeons. Competent surgery begins with a thorough knowledge of surgical principles and proficiency in basic surgical techniques. This textbook is intended to facilitate the initial stages of surgical training and to serve as a refresher to those in the profession who may have had little surgical experience since veterinary or veterinary technician schooling. It is the authors' hope that those studying to be veterinarians and veterinary technicians will find this textbook to be a helpful complement to their instruction and that graduate veterinarians and veterinary technicians will find this textbook to be valuable in postgraduate in-service training for veterinary staff.

ACKNOWLEDGMENTS

We thank the following individuals for assistance with photography, artwork, and portions of some chapters:

Mr. Howard Wilson
Senior Multimedia Specialist
College of Veterinary Medicine
University of Missouri
Columbia, Missouri
[Photographic and artistic assistance]

Mr. Donald L. Connor
Senior Multimedia Specialist
College of Veterinary Medicine
University of Missouri
Columbia, Missouri
[Artistic assistance]

Linda M. Berent, DVM, PhD, Diplomate ACVP (Clinical and Anatomic Pathology)
Clinical Assistant Professor
Department of Veterinary Pathobiology
College of Veterinary Medicine
University of Missouri
Columbia, Missouri
[Assistance in assuring accuracy in the first section of Chapter 16]

Eric A. Rowe, DVM
Small Animal Surgery Resident
Department of Clinical Sciences
Veterinary Teaching Hospital
College of Veterinary Medicine
North Carolina State University
Raleigh, North Carolina
[Assistance with portions of Chapters 3, 7, and 17 while employed as a Small Animal Soft Tissue Research/Teaching Intern at the University of Missouri, Columbia, Missouri]

Last, but not least, we extend our thanks and appreciation to Nancy Turner, Development Editor for Health Sciences, Wiley-Blackwell, Ames, Iowa, for her patience with the authors, assistance in attention to details, guidance through the publication process, and dedication to making this work the best it can be. We also thank the staff of Wiley-Blackwell for making this book a reality.

Fundamentals of
SMALL ANIMAL SURGERY

Chapter 1

PREOPERATIVE PATIENT ASSESSMENT

Elizabeth A. Swanson and Fred Anthony Mann

In general practice, the veterinarian often already knows the patient being presented for surgery. Even so, the veterinarian should take this opportunity to instill a sense of confidence and firmly establish a solid veterinarian-client–patient relationship. To that end, a complete history and physical examination are paramount in the surgeon's toolbox of information about the patient. The history and physical examination will determine whether a patient is a good candidate for surgery, will determine what further tests are necessary prior to anesthesia, and will allow the veterinarian to give the owner an accurate assessment of what to expect. The information gained also helps to guide decision-making regarding anesthetic protocol, type of procedure to be performed, pain management, and postoperative care. In short, nothing can replace a thorough history and physical examination in establishing a base of information about the patient that can be used for perioperative decision making.

Fundamentals of Small Animal Surgery, 1st edition.
By Fred Anthony Mann, Gheorghe M. Constantinescu and Hun-Young Yoon.
© 2011 Blackwell Publishing Ltd.

HISTORY

Even when the patient is known to the surgeon, a current and detailed patient history should be obtained from the owner at the time of presentation. The presenting complaint is ascertained and details recorded on the duration of the problem, what clinical signs have been observed, and whether the owner feels the problem is better, worse, or the same as when it was first noticed. Such historical information may not be pertinent for a healthy dog or cat being presented for elective ovariohysterectomy or orchiectomy; however, it is necessary to make certain that there have been no changes in the patient's health status prior to surgery. In addition, for dogs and cats presenting for ovariohysterectomy, it is important to always ask about when the animal was last in heat and if there is a possibility that the animal is pregnant.

Other information gathered when taking the history includes environment, diet, patient lifestyle, any current or previous medical conditions, previous surgeries, current medications (including over-the-counter medications, supplements, and heartworm and flea/tick preventatives), and adverse reactions to medication. Appetite, drinking, urination, defecation, and occurrences of coughing, sneezing, vomiting and/or diarrhea are also noted.

Medical information may lead the veterinarian to identify previously undiagnosed disorders, such as hyperthyroidism in a geriatric cat presented for dental prophylaxis with increased appetite and concurrent weight loss. Patient lifestyle can play a huge role in determining which procedure should be performed. For example, external fixation of a tibial fracture in a free-roaming farm dog may not be the best option for healing and management of that fracture.

In the case of an emergency, basic information should include signalment, the presenting complaint, major concurrent medical conditions, current medications, and drug sensitivities. The remainder of the history may be obtained at the first available opportunity.

PHYSICAL EXAMINATION

The physical examination may commence once the history has been taken. A more experienced practitioner will be able to begin the physical examination while still taking the history, a practice that can be most beneficial for triaging emergency cases. The importance of a good physical examination cannot be overly stressed. A thorough physical examination can identify both major and subtle changes in a patient's condition that may affect what is done for that patient. The finding of a swollen vulva in an intact female dog presented for ovariohysterectomy may lead the veterinarian to discuss with the owner the increased risk of hemorrhage and, potentially, the recommendation to postpone the surgery.

A consistent, systematic approach is recommended for physical examination. Important developments may be missed when the examiner makes the mistake of focusing only on the presenting problem. A full examination consists of close inspection of the head and neck (eyes, ears, nose, oral cavity), lymph nodes, cardiovascular system, respiratory system, digestive tract, urogenital system, integument, musculoskeletal system, and neural system. The precise order of the examination is not dictated, but to ensure that no system is missed, the examiner should establish an order and remain consistent from one patient to the next.

LABORATORY DATA

Findings during the history and physical examination will help determine which laboratory data are necessary. For a young, healthy animal less than five years of age that is presented for elective surgery, a laboratory baseline of packed cell volume (PCV), total protein (TP), blood urea nitrogen (BUN) or creatinine, blood glucose, and urine specific gravity will typically suffice. Full laboratory work-up, including complete blood cell count (CBC), serum chemistries, electrolytes, and urinalysis, are in order for patients older than five years and any sick or debilitated patient. A recent heartworm test should be required for patients who have lived or traveled in endemic areas. All cats should be tested for feline leukemia and feline immunodeficiency virus if they have not previously been tested. Cats that have access to the outside or that come in regular contact with an outdoor cat should be tested annually. Additional tests may be run in patients with specific medical conditions.

Advanced laboratory tests may be indicated in certain conditions. Breeds that have a high incidence of von Willebrand's Disease, such as Doberman pinschers, should have a buccal mucosal bleeding time (BMBT) performed as part of the preoperative work-up before any surgery, elective or otherwise, is performed, even if there is no history of abnormal bleeding tendencies. A prolonged BMBT (>5 minutes) indicates further testing, such as for von Willebrand's factor (vWF). An elective procedure may be postponed pending further information. If surgery is required and the patient is suspected to have Type I (low concentration of vWF) von Willebrand's disease, the animal may be pretreated with desmopressin acetate (1-deamino-8-D-arginine vasopression, also called DDAVP) or administered cryoprecipitate. Fresh whole blood, fresh frozen plasma, or cryoprecipitate may be necessary if significant hemorrhage occurs or in dogs with Type II (low concentration of large multimers of vWF) or Type III (complete absence or only trace amounts of vWF) von Willebrand's disease. If time allows, desmopressin can also be administered to a blood donor 30–120 minutes prior to blood collection. The BMBT is also indicated to assess the bleeding tendency of patients with suspected thrombocytopathia, such as dogs that have been treated with aspirin.

Platelet counts and coagulation panels are necessary for any patient showing signs of easy bruising, ecchymoses, or petechia pre- or postoperatively. Platelet counts and coagulation panels should also be run for patients undergoing procedures where significant hemorrhage is possible and adequate hemostasis may not be directly achieved, such as for liver biopsies obtained via laparoscopy or ultrasound-guided needle biopsy. If a coagulopathy is diagnosed, fresh frozen plasma should be administered to provide coagulation factors. Also, transfusion of fresh whole blood may be necessary to stabilize a patient with thrombocytopenia. It is important to realize that whole blood, platelet-rich plasma, and platelets do not significantly raise the platelet count.

Arterial blood gas analysis and acid–base status should be evaluated in patients with suspected hypoxia or hypoventilation, such as patients with pulmonary disease (i.e., aspiration pneumonia, pulmonary edema, thromboembolism), pneumothorax, pleural effusion, and in critical patients that are in shock, are septic, or are showing signs of systemic inflammatory response syndrome. The arterial partial pressure of oxygen (PaO_2), the arterial partial pressure of carbon dioxide ($PaCO_2$), pH, bicarbonate concentration ($[HCO_3^-]$), base excess (BE), anion gap, and electrolyte concentrations can be interpreted together to evaluate respiratory function and to determine the cause of acid–base imbalance. Blood gas analysis is used to help determine what, if any, supplemental therapy is necessary and to help monitor the response to treatment.

Critical patients, especially those with effusive disease processes, such as peritonitis, protein-losing enteropathy, generalized lymphangiectasia, and burns, may lose a large amount of protein into the effusion through leaky blood vessels. Loss of protein, especially albumin, causes movement of intravascular fluid into the interstitium (edema) or body cavities via osmosis. The pressure exerted within the blood vessels by albumin and other colloids is called colloid oncotic pressure (COP), which can be measured from a patient's whole blood sample. The measurement of COP is used to help direct fluid therapy, particularly the use of colloids, such as hetastarch, dextran, whole blood, and plasma.

DIAGNOSTIC IMAGING

Diagnostic imaging is not routinely performed prior to elective procedures in healthy animals. Other conditions, however, benefit from data obtained through radiography, ultrasonography, and more advanced imaging modalities, including computed tomography and magnetic resonance imaging (MRI). Patients undergoing surgery as therapy for neoplasia should be staged according to the suspected tumor type, and diagnostic imaging is part of the staging process. Minimal data obtained for oncological surgery patients should include CBC, serum chemistries, urinalysis, thoracic radiographs (right and left lateral views and ventrodorsal view), right lateral and ventrodorsal abdominal radiographs, and abdominal ultrasound. Computed tomography or MRI, whichever is more appropriate for the given situation, is used to map tumors and help plan surgical margins.

The minimal database for trauma patients should include PCV/TP, BUN, blood glucose, urine specific gravity, right lateral and ventrodorsal thoracic and abdominal radiographs, and sometimes abdominal ultrasound. Diaphragmatic continuity, body wall continuity, and the presence of a urinary bladder should be assessed, in addition to looking for pneumothorax, pleural and peritoneal effusion, and pulmonary contusions.

While orthogonal views are always preferred when interpreting radiographs, obtaining a right lateral radiograph of a critical, bloating dog will usually suffice in diagnosing gastric dilatation-volvulus (GDV). Right and left lateral and ventrodorsal thoracic radiographs should also be taken in geriatric dogs with GDV to evaluate for evidence of neoplasia, because the presence of neoplasia may influence owner decisions. Of course, the GDV patient must be stable enough to take additional radiographs prior to surgery.

Patients with a heart murmur or known cardiac disease should have right lateral and either ventrodorsal or dorsoventral thoracic radiographs taken and, if indicated, an echocardiogram performed prior to anesthesia. Right lateral and ventrodorsal thoracic radiographs are indicated for any vomiting or regurgitating patient to assess for aspiration pneumonia and for patients that develop an increased respiratory effort or respiratory distress during treatment.

Various forms of contrast radiography are used in the diagnosis of medical problems. Videofluoroscopy can be used to evaluate esophageal function and gastric emptying times. Oral administration of barium with sequential right lateral and ventrodorsal abdominal radiographs is used to evaluate gastrointestinal motility and to identify gastrointestinal obstruction, such as from a foreign object or tumor. Excretory urography is useful in evaluating renal function of the opposite kidney prior to nephrectomy if renal function is questionable. Evaluation of the urinary bladder and urethra for tumors, tears, and luminal filling

defects is performed, using positive-contrast cystourethrography.

Postoperative radiographs are indicated for any orthopedic procedure where metal implants are used or removed. Radiographs are also taken after cystotomy to document removal of uroliths from the urinary bladder. Proper nasogastric and esophageal feeding tube position and percutaneous chest tube placement should be checked radiographically with orthogonal thoracic views.

ASSESSMENT OF ANESTHETIC AND SURGICAL RISK

Once the full picture has been obtained, as appropriate for the patient and situation, the patient's anesthetic and surgical risk is assessed. In 1963, the American Society of Anesthesiologists developed a simple classification system by which to determine a patient's physical status and potential risk for complications. These same criteria have been adapted for use in veterinary medicine (Table 1.1).[1,2] In general, no adjustment to the anesthetic protocol is considered unless a patient is classified as Physical Status 3 or higher. In human medicine, a sixth level has been added to include brain-dead patients whose organs are being removed for donation. The letter *E* is used to denote an emergent case. For example, most cases of gastric dilatation-volvulus would be designated as physical status 4-E.

Clients should be alerted to the possible complications of the procedure to be performed and the relative likelihood of adverse events. Even routine, elective procedures carry risk, and it is wrong not to inform the client. For all patients, general anesthesia poses risk of death, albeit minor in healthy animals. Common risks, such as hemorrhage, incisional dehiscence, and postoperative infection of the surgical wound, should always be discussed, in addition to any complications specific to the procedure

Table 1.1　**Physical status classification system**[a]

Physical status	Patient condition	Examples
1	Normal, healthy patient	Elective ovariohysterectomy; elective orchiectomy
2	Patient with localized disease or mild systemic disease	Fractures; cranial cruciate ligament rupture; skin laceration; skin mass removal (*E: Open fracture*)
3	Patient with severe systemic disease	Renal failure; fever; hyperadrenocorticism; dehydration; anemia (*E: Gastrointestinal perforation*)
4	Patient with severe systemic disease that is a constant threat to life	Any condition prone to developing systemic inflammatory response; heart failure (*E: Gastric dilatation-volvulus*)
5	Moribund patient not expected to live with or without the operation	Systemic inflammatory response that is progressing toward multiple organ dysfunction; trauma with decompensatory shock (*E: Intestinal volvulus*)
6	Brain-dead patient whose organs may be removed for donation purposes	Currently no veterinary examples

Use "E" after the appropriate classification to denote an emergency operation

[a]Based on Classification of Physical Status. *ASA Relative Value Guide*. 2009. (www.asahq.org/clinical/physicalstatus.htm) of the American Society of Anesthesiologists. A copy of the full text can be obtained from ASA, 520 N. Northwest Highway, Park Ridge, Illinois 60068-2573.

performed. A well-informed client is in a better position to recognize and handle complications than one who is not.

REFERENCES

1. Muir WW. Considerations for general anesthesia. In: Tranquilli WJ, Thurmon JC, Grimm KA, eds. *Lumb & Jones Veterinary Anesthesia and Analgesia*, 4th ed. Ames, Iowa: Blackwell Professional Publishing, 2009:17.
2. Muir WW, Hubbell JAE, Bednarski RM, Skarda RT. Patient evaluation and preparation. In: Muir WW, Hubbell JAE, Bednarski RM, Skarda RT, eds. *Handbook of Veterinary Anesthesia*, 4th ed. St. Louis, Missouri: Mosby Elsevier, 2007:22.

ADDITIONAL RESOURCES

Additional information about preoperative patient assessment in small animal surgery can be found in the following textbook chapters:

1. Fossum TW. Preoperative and intraoperative care of the surgical patient. In: Fossum TW, ed. *Small Animal Surgery*, 3rd ed. St. Louis, Missouri: Mosby Elsevier, 2007:22–31.
2. Shmon C. Assessment and preparation of the surgical patient and operating team. In: Slatter D, ed. *Textbook of Small Animal Surgery*, 3rd ed. Philadelphia, Pennsylvania: Saunders, 2003;162–168.
3. Brooks M. von Willebrand Disease. In: Feldman BF, Zinkl JG, Jain NC, eds. *Schalm's Veterinary Hematology*, 5th ed. Baltimore, Maryland: Lippincott Williams & Wilkins, 2000:509–515.

Chapter 2

BASIC SMALL ANIMAL ANESTHESIA

John R. Dodam and Fred Anthony Mann

A single chapter cannot provide a comprehensive review of small animal anesthesia. Instead, this chapter will attempt to provide a procedural framework that can be expanded and modified to fit the needs and goals of the surgeon and anesthetist. The procedural framework will be based upon an anesthetic protocol that includes preoperative assessment of the patient; premedication with sedative, analgesic, and/or anticholinergic agents; induction of unconsciousness by intravenous injection of a hypnotic, sedative, or dissociative agent; maintenance of anesthesia with an inhalant anesthetic; and recovery of the patient.

DRUGS USED IN SMALL ANIMAL ANESTHESIA

The following is a summary of the classes of drugs used for premedication, induction, or maintenance of anesthesia. Please consult an appropriate resource for more detailed information concerning any of the listed agents, spe-

Fundamentals of Small Animal Surgery, 1st edition.
By Fred Anthony Mann, Gheorghe M. Constantinescu and Hun-Young Yoon.
© 2011 Blackwell Publishing Ltd.

cific drug combinations, or for appropriate dosing recommendations.

Drugs used in anesthesia premedication are usually given by intramuscular or subcutaneous injection 20–40 minutes prior to the induction of general anesthesia. Premedication of the patient is important from a logistical standpoint because the drugs may sedate or calm the patient, decrease the level of physical restraint required, and facilitate catheter placement. Importantly, anesthesia premedication drugs may improve the quality of anesthetic induction and/or recovery and decrease the requirement for induction or maintenance anesthetics. Premedication drugs may also be used to provide preemptive analgesia. Indeed, the administration of analgesic drugs prior to a surgical insult may improve the effectiveness of postoperative interventions aimed at treating a patient's postoperative pain. Premedication drugs may also be used to modify autonomic tone, stabilize or increase heart rate, or decrease salivary secretions.

Anticholinergics

Anticholinergic agents like atropine or glycopyrrolate interfere with the action of acetylcholine at muscarinic receptors of the autonomic nervous system. Thus, these agents are used to increase heart rate (or prevent bradycardia) and decrease salivary and respiratory secretions. They also increase gastric pH, decrease gastrointestinal motility, and evoke bronchodilation. Although many veterinarians use these agents routinely as part of premedication protocols, others prefer to use them only as needed to treat bradycardia. Both atropine and glycopyrrolate can cause tachycardia and/or ventricular dysrhythmias, but the risk is higher after intravenous injection than intramuscular or subcutaneous administration. Glycopyrrolate has a longer duration of action than atropine and does not cause central nervous system effects. Atropine has a shorter onset time than glycopyrrolate. For these reasons, glycopyrrolate is often preferred as part of an anesthesia premedication protocol, while atropine is preferred for emergency treatment of life-threatening bradycardia.

Phenothiazines

Acepromazine is a phenothiazine tranquilizer that produces mental calming without providing analgesia. It decreases histamine release, has antidysrhythmic properties, and has been reported to decrease mortality associated with anesthesia. However, acepromazine causes vasodilatation, hypotension, hypothermia, and decreased platelet function, and may decrease seizure threshold. Acepromazine is commonly used with opioids as part of premedication protocols, and because of its long duration of action, premedication with acepromazine may help to smooth postoperative recoveries.

Benzodiazepines

Benzodiazepine drugs (e.g., diazepam, midazolam, and zolazepam) are tranquilizers frequently paired with dissociative agents (e.g.,

ketamine and tiletamine) to induce anesthesia. Benzodiazepines are not typically given alone for preoperative sedation because they are relatively ineffective unless an animal is depressed, very young, or very old. Paradoxically, benzodiazepines can cause excitement in some animals when given alone. Moreover, diazepam is not absorbed predictably after intramuscular injection. When combined with induction agents, benzodiazepines decrease the required doses of those agents, provide for muscle relaxation, and have minor effects on the cardiovascular system. Benzodiazepines are also frequently used for their anticonvulsant properties. The actions of benzodiazepine drugs are reversible with administration of flumazenil, a specific antagonist.

Alpha-Two Agonists

Alpha-two agonists (e.g., xylazine and dexmedetomidine) decrease the release of norepinephrine in the central nervous system. This effect causes reliable sedation, analgesia, and muscle relaxation, and greatly decreases the requirements for other anesthetic agents. Alpha-two agonists cause cardiovascular changes that are characterized by bradycardia, biphasic blood pressure changes (hypertension followed by hypotension), and a significant decrease in cardiac output. These drugs also cause hyperglycemia, diuresis, and decreased gastrointestinal motility. Emesis is common when low doses of these drugs are given by the intramuscular or subcutaneous route. Xylazine is shorter-acting than dexmedetomidine and is more likely to be associated with cardiac dysrhythmias. The effects of alpha-two agonists can be reversed by specific antagonists. The effects of xylazine are typically reversed in small animal patients with yohimbine, while dexmedetomidine effects are reversed with atipamezole. Alpha-two agonists are frequently given in combination with opioid drugs to decrease the dose administered and to limit the cardiopulmonary effects of the alpha-two agonists.

Anticholinergic drugs may be given to limit alpha-two agonist-induced bradycardia, although the routine use of glycopyrrolate with dexmedetomidine is somewhat controversial.

Opioids

Opioids are commonly used for their analgesic activity and anesthetic sparing effects. In general, they cause mild to moderate sedation, but may be associated with excitation in some animals (especially in cats). Excitatory opioid effects are effectively eliminated when the agents are administered concurrently with tranquilizers or sedatives like acepromazine or xylazine. In general, full agonists (e.g., morphine, oxymorphone, hydromorphone, and fentanyl) are considered to be more efficacious than partial agonists or agonist/antagonists (butorphanol, buprenorphine, and nalbuphine). Side effects may also be more likely with the full agonist opioids. Respiratory depression, bradycardia, vomiting, decreased gastrointestinal propulsive motility, and urine retention are all potential side effects. Morphine may also evoke histamine release. Morphine, oxymorphone, and hydromorphone are commonly used as part of premedication protocols. Fentanyl may be given intramuscularly as part of a premedication protocol. However, fentanyl has a very short duration of action (less than an hour) and is frequently administered as a constant rate infusion when more prolonged analgesia is required. Partial agonists and agonist/antagonist drugs are generally used to treat mild to moderate pain. Butorphanol is frequently used to premedicate small animal patients. However, butorphanol's duration of action is short in the dog. Buprenorphine, because of its relatively long duration of action, is frequently used to provide postoperative pain relief in dogs and cats.

The effects of opioids are reversible. Naloxone is the most commonly used full antagonist used in small animal anesthesia today. Nalbuphine and butorphanol can also be used to reverse the effects of mu agonists (e.g., morphine and hydromorphone). The advantage of using nalbuphine and butorphanol is that, unlike naloxone, they will provide mild to moderate analgesia through their agonistic effects at the opioid kappa receptor.

Tramadol is an atypical opioid that is currently available in an oral formulation. Tramadol has effects on the opioid mu receptor and also works through other pathways in the central nervous system. Because an injectable formulation is not currently available in the United States, tramadol's use in the preoperative period is limited.

Nonsteroidal Anti-inflammatory Drugs (NSAIDs)

Nonsteroidal anti-inflammatory drugs decrease pain and inflammation by interfering with the production of prostaglandins and, in a few cases, leukotrienes. Newer agents like carprofen, deracoxib, meloxicam, and tepoxalin are markedly less toxic than older NSAIDs like aspirin, indomethacin, and phenylbutazone. Renal failure and gastrointestinal ulceration are the most significant toxic effects of NSAIDs, and anesthesia-induced hypotension can contribute to NSAID toxicity. Some NSAIDs also inhibit platelet function. Because of these potential side effects, and because NSAIDs do not alter anesthetic requirements, many veterinarians confine the use of NSAIDs to the postoperative period.

Dissociative Agents

Dissociative drugs like ketamine and tiletamine are N-methyl-D-aspartate receptor antagonists that may be administered intravenously or intramuscularly as part of premedication protocols or for the induction of anesthesia. Dissociative agents are not well suited to be given as a sole agent for premedication or induction of anesthesia because they provide poor muscle relaxation and are associated with patient movement. Ketamine is frequently given intravenously and concurrently with midazolam or diazepam to induce anesthesia, and tiletamine is available as a commercial preparation with zolazepam (Telazol, Fort Dodge Animal Health, Fort Dodge, IA) for intravenous or intramuscular administration in small animals. Dissociative agents provide effective somatic analgesia, but are poor visceral analgesics. Unlike most anesthetic drugs, dissociative agents generally maintain or increase blood pressure, heart rate, and cardiac output. They may also cause cerebral vasodilatation, an increase in cerebral metabolic rate, and an increase in cerebral blood flow.

Hypnotic Agents

Thiopental and propofol are two commonly used hypnotic/sedative drugs in small animal veterinary anesthesia. Both are used to induce unconsciousness by intravenous injection prior to inhalant anesthesia. Due to rapid clearance, propofol has a shorter duration of action than thiopental and may be used to maintain anesthesia by intermittent intravenous injection or constant rate infusion. Propofol causes as much, or greater, cardiovascular depression than thiopental, but is much less likely to be associated with cardiac dysrhythmias. Unlike thiopental, propofol does not cause perivascular damage and is not a controlled substance. Both drugs are respiratory depressants, but propofol is more likely to cause cyanosis and desaturation of hemoglobin. Whenever either drug is used, the practitioner should be prepared to orotracheally intubate the animal and provide for the administration of oxygen and ventilation. Propofol administration may be associated with pain and movement. Thiopental may be associated with transient excitatory behavior after injection. These drug effects can be minimized or eliminated by administration of a sedative, tranquilizer, or analgesic drug prior to induction of anesthesia. Moreover, the excitatory effects of thiopental can be minimized if approximately half of the calculated bolus is administered rapidly (the remaining drug should be given incrementally and to effect). Propofol administration is not typically associated with excitatory behavior, and side-effects like hypotension and apnea can be decreased by giving the drug slowly and to effect. Repeated daily administration of propofol may cause oxidative damage to feline red blood cells, but a single intravenous induction dose has not been shown to be problematic. Current preparations of propofol have a limited shelf life because the formulation promotes the growth of bacteria or yeast, and the contents of a bottle should be used within 6 hours of opening. Thiopental is associated with prolonged recoveries in sighthounds after a single induction dose, and in all animals after repeated administration for anesthesia maintenance.

STEP-BY-STEP APPROACH TO ANESTHETIZING THE SMALL ANIMAL PATIENT

The following outline details premedication, intravenous induction of anesthesia, and maintenance of anesthesia with an inhalant anesthetic. As one would expect, this outline should not be used as a substitute for methodical thought and practical adjustments for each individual patient, but it can serve as a checklist and training guide for performing small animal anesthesia.

1. A thorough history should be taken and physical examination performed prior to anesthetizing a canine or feline patient. Laboratory evaluations of hematocrit, plasma protein, serum urea nitrogen or creatinine, and urine specific gravity are also part of a routine preoperative workup.

Additional diagnostic tests may be necessary depending upon the condition of the patient and the procedure to be performed. Owners should be informed of the risks associated with anesthesia and should provide written permission to perform anesthesia. Owners should also be asked to express their wishes with regard to emergency management, should a catastrophic event occur during the animal's hospital stay.

2. The specific anesthetic protocol should be chosen based upon the history, physical examination, laboratory evaluation, and the procedure to be performed. The anesthetic protocol should also outline the strategy that will be used to control postoperative pain. A discussion of anesthesia for concurrent diseases or for specific diagnostic or therapeutic procedures is beyond the scope of this chapter.

   a. Consider the feasibility of local and/or regional analgesia techniques as a supplement to the general anesthetic protocol.

3. Calculate doses of drugs that will be used for premedication and induction of anesthesia. Label syringes for all drugs that will be used for premedication and induction. Make sure that all controlled substances are properly accounted.

4. Administer preanesthetic drugs (sedatives and analgesic drugs). An animal should be returned to its cage after premedication, and 20–30 minutes should be allowed before moving the animal for catheterization and induction. While waiting for the premedications to exert their effects, the animal should be observed to ensure its well-being, but should not be disturbed. Indeed, excessive stimulation may diminish the effectiveness of sedative drugs.

   a. Intramuscular sites for premedication are the quadriceps muscle (preferred), lumbar musculature, and semimembranosus/semitendinosus muscles.

5. Assemble supplies and equipment that will be used for anesthesia.

   a. Select the most appropriate endotracheal tube for the patient.

   b. Check the integrity of the endotracheal tube and cuff.

      i. Endotracheal tubes are used to maintain a patent airway, allow for controlled ventilation, protect the airway from contamination with foreign material, and to prevent exposure of personnel to waste anesthetic gas.

      ii. Examine the endotracheal tube for defects.

      iii. The endotracheal tube cuff system is checked using the following procedure:

         1. Attach an air-filled syringe to the inflating valve and fill the cuff with air until distended.

         2. Remove the syringe from the inflating valve.

         3. Allow the cuff to remain inflated for 5–15 minutes.

         4. Observe the cuff for deflation.

            a. If deflation occurs, the tube should be removed from service.

         5. If the cuff has remained inflated, withdraw all air from the cuff via the inflating valve using a syringe.

      iv. Keep the tube on a clean surface prior to use.

      v. The outside surface of the patient end of the endotracheal tube may be lubricated with a modest amount of water-soluble lubricating jelly prior to insertion into the airway.

   c. Check the integrity of the anesthetic circuit.

      i. Assemble the anesthetic circuit (y-piece and reservoir bag); attach the oxygen and evacuation sources, and perform a pressure check of the system.

ii. The patient circuit should be able to hold pressure (30 cm H_2O) for 15 seconds.

iii. Inspection and assessment of a non-rebreathing circuit depends upon the type of circuit being used. In general, a nonrebreathing circuit is used for patients less than 8-kg body weight. A circle system is used when the patient is greater than or equal to 8-kg body weight.

d. Check the level of inhalant anesthetic in the vaporizer. Fill as necessary.

e. Calculate the fresh gas flows for the anesthetic circuit.

i. To operate the system in a semi-closed fashion, the following guidelines should be applied:

1. Generally, oxygen flow rates of 22–44 mL/kg/min are considered to be acceptable maintenance flow rates for a semi-closed circle system. Alternatively, maintenance flow may be calculated based upon estimated oxygen consumption multiplied by three (i.e., 5–10 mL oxygen flow/kg/min × 3). Lower oxygen flow rates are used when a circle circuit is operated in a "closed" fashion.

2. Fresh gas flow is expected to be higher during anesthetic induction and recovery. In general, a fresh gas flow rate of 1–2 L/min is considered acceptable during induction, and 500 mL/min to 1 L/min is acceptable for the maintenance period of anesthesia when using a circle system.

3. The appropriate oxygen flow for a nonrebreathing system depends upon the system being used. In most cases, a flow that is calculated as 300 × body weight (kg) and expressed in ml/kg/min is appropriate for small patients on a Mapleson F nonrebreathing system.

6. Crystalloid intravenous replacement fluids (i.e., lactated Ringer's solution) are commonly used during general anesthesia.

a. Fluid rate and types may be altered depending upon the patient, the procedure being performed, and the duration of the procedure.

b. Calculate fluid administration rate prior to anesthesia. A rate of 10 mL/kg/h is calculated and administered for the first hour of anesthesia, 5 mL/kg/h thereafter.

c. Fluids may be administered by an electronically controlled fluid pump or by gravity flow. When calculating fluid rates using gravity flow, the size of the drip set is necessary to determine the administration rate (in drops/minute). Common sizes for drips sets are: 10, 15, and 60 drops/mL.

d. Insert a fluid administration set into the intravenous fluid bag and prime the tubing.

7. Once supplies and equipment are collected and prepared for use, the sedated animal should be placed on a table and restrained for catheter placement.

a. The animal should be restrained in a manner that minimizes stress for the animal and prevents injury to the handler or to the anesthetist.

8. The intravenous catheter site should be clipped and surgically prepared.

a. The cephalic/accessory cephalic and lateral saphenous veins are common sites of catheter placement in the dog.

b. The cephalic/accessory cephalic and medial saphenous veins are common sites for catheter placement in the cat.

9. An over-the-needle catheter is inserted into the vein, and a T-port is connected to the catheter.

a. Alternately, the fluid administration set may be attached directly to the intravenous catheter.

10. The catheter and attached T-port are taped into place and triple antibiotic ointment (or other nonirritating disinfectant/ antibiotic cream/gel/ointment) should be applied to the catheter site. Sterile gauze or a sterile band-aid may be used to cover the catheter site after the catheter is secured to the limb with tape.

11. Prior to injection of an induction agent, the catheter is assessed to ensure that it is placed into the lumen of the vein. Injection of sterile normal saline solution may be used for this purpose.

12. The animal should be assessed briefly prior to induction general anesthesia. Specifically, a final check of pulse rate, pulse quality, and mucous membrane color should be performed just prior to induction of anesthesia.

    a. Abnormalities in pulse rate, pulse regularity, or mucous membrane color should lead the anesthetist to investigate the cause of the abnormalities and reassess the plan of action.

13. Induction may be accomplished by administration of the selected induction agent.

14. The mouth of the animal should be held open by the assistant, and the tongue pulled forward using a gauze square.

    a. The tongue should be pulled rostrally and between the mandibular canines. The anesthetist should not place his/her fingers between the animal's teeth. Instead, the tongue should be moved outside the mouth, using the endotracheal tube or laryngoscope blade so that it may be safely grasped.

    b. If used, the laryngoscope blade should be pressed against the base of the tongue. This will pull down the epiglottis and expose the larynx.

    1. The laryngoscope blade may be used to gently depress the epiglottis, if necessary.

    2. In cats, lidocaine may be sprayed onto the larynx to decrease sensitivity and laryngospasm during endotracheal intubation.

    c. The endotracheal tube should be advanced into the mouth, through the larynx, and into the trachea.

    d. The length of the tube should be checked to ensure that the tip is located just cranial to the thoracic inlet.

    e. Endotracheal tubes have the potential to injure the patient. Cats are particularly prone to injury associated with endotracheal intubation. The following should be considered to prevent endotracheal tube problems:

    1. Proper inflation of the cuff

       a. Over inflation may damage the patient's airway.

       b. Under inflation will allow aspiration of foreign material into the airways and lungs.

       c. Once the cuff is inflated, the endotracheal tube should not be twisted, inserted, or removed without first deflating the cuff. [During dentistry procedures, temporarily detach the anesthetic tubing from the endotracheal tube before turning the animal from one side to the other, because twisting the inflated cuff can tear the trachea.]

    2. Proper placement of the tube

       a. Improper esophageal placement is not effective for delivering oxygen or anesthetic, does not protect the airway, and does not ensure airway patency.

       b. The tip of the endotracheal tube should be located in the trachea and just cranial to the thoracic inlet.

i. A tube inserted too far caudally may isolate a single mainstem bronchus and cause significant gas exchange abnormalities.

ii. A tube that is not inserted far enough into the trachea may be easier to dislodge. In addition, in this position, the cuff may be located in the larynx and inflation may traumatize the larynx.

iii. The length of insertion necessary may be estimated prior to induction of anesthesia by holding the tube next to the animal's head and neck.

iv. The length of insertion should be verified after placement by palpation of the tip of the tube in the trachea.

15. The animal should be placed in lateral recumbence, and the endotracheal tube should be connected to the anesthetic machine and the oxygen turned on (1–2 L/min).

16. The pulse and heart beat should be assessed.

17. The anesthetist should secure the endotracheal tube to the animal using roll gauze. The gauze should be tightly secured to the endotracheal tube with half of a square knot, and then tied over the animal's muzzle (dogs) or behind its head (dogs and cats) using a "bow" or other knot that can be untied easily and quickly. Other devices are commercially available to secure the endotracheal tube to the patient. Some practices use lengths of intravenous tubing for this purpose in place of roll gauze.

18. Check for a leak around the endotracheal tube by closing the pressure-relief valve on the anesthesia machine and squeezing the reservoir bag to a pressure of 20–25 cm H_2O. A leak can be heard in the oral cavity when positive pressure is being held in the circuit/patient.

a. Pressure should not be held in the system for more than 1–2 seconds.

b. If a leak is heard, the pressure-relief valve should be opened, and the cuff inflated with air. A volume of 1–3 mL is an appropriate volume for small animals.

c. The above steps should be repeated until a leak is no longer heard when a pressure of 20–25 cm H_2O is maintained in the circuit.

d. Open the pressure-relief valve when the cuff inflation procedure is complete.

19. The vaporizer may be initially set at 2–3% if isoflurane is the inhalant anesthetic that is being administered. If sevoflurane is used, the vaporizer may initially be set at 3–5%.

a. The actual vaporizer setting should be determined after evaluating depth of anesthesia and cardiovascular performance.

b. The initial vaporizer setting will be influenced by the drugs used for premedication and induction of anesthesia.

20. The animal's respirations, pulse rate, and depth of anesthesia should be monitored in a continuous fashion. Entries should be made onto the anesthesia record every 5 minutes.

21. The esophageal stethoscope is lubricated and advanced through the oral cavity and into the esophagus while simultaneously listening through the earpieces. Insert to the depth where cardiac sounds are most clearly heard.

22. Connect crystalloid fluids to the intravenous catheter aseptically. Begin administration at the calculated rate (see 6.b. above).

23. Lubricate the eyes with sterile ophthalmic ointment to decrease the risk for corneal ulceration.

24. The animal may now be prepared for surgery (positioning/clipping/skin preparation).

25. Anesthetic and oxygen flow should be adjusted to maintenance levels when an

appropriate and stable plane of anesthesia has been established (5–15 minutes after induction).

    a. Record observations, physiological parameters, and interventions on the anesthesia record.

    b. Adjust the vaporizer setting to maintain an appropriate depth of anesthesia.

26. Physical monitoring should be combined with device-based assessment to ensure patient well being. The following are frequently used to monitor anesthetized patients:

    a. Electrocardiography

    b. Capnography

    c. Pulse oximetry

    d. Noninvasive blood pressure monitoring (oscillometric or Doppler)

    e. Rectal or esophageal temperature measurement

        i. Temperature support is routinely required to prevent hypothermia during anesthesia and surgery.

27. When the diagnostic or therapeutic procedure is completed, the vaporizer may be shut off and oxygen flow continued until the patient begins to swallow. Based upon the procedure performed, the premedications used, and the incorporation of local and regional analgesia techniques, it may be necessary to administer additional analgesic drugs prior to recovery.

28. The endotracheal tube cuff should be deflated completely prior to removal.

    a. In some cases, partial deflation is utilized if there is suspicion that fluid or foreign material may have entered the trachea next to the endotracheal tube.

29. In general, fluid administration is discontinued when anesthetic administration is completed. The intravenous catheter is flushed with saline solution and left in place until the animal has recovered and can maintain homeostasis. In routine cases, the catheter is maintained until the animal can ambulate. Animals with excessive surgical blood loss, electrolyte disturbances, ongoing fluid losses, increased risk for seizures, abnormal cardiopulmonary function, or those exhibiting pain or dysphoria should not have their catheter removed immediately. These animals should be reassessed and the appropriate therapy instituted.

30. The animal should be monitored during the postoperative period. The following parameters are particularly important to assess:

    a. Respiratory and cardiovascular function

        i. Pulse rate and quality

        ii. Respiratory rate

        iii. Hemoglobin saturation (via pulse oximetry)

    b. Temperature

    c. Level of pain

    d. Mentation

ADDITIONAL RESOURCES

Additional information about small animal anesthesiology, analgesia, and perioperative medicine can be found in the following textbooks:

1. Tranquilli WJ, Thurmon JC, Grimm KA, eds. *Lumb & Jones Veterinary Anesthesia and Analgesia*, 4th ed. Ames, Iowa: Blackwell Professional Publishing, 2009.

2. Carroll GL, ed. *Small Animal Anesthesia and Analgesia*. Ames, Iowa: Blackwell Professional Publishing, 2008.

3. Muir WW, Hubbel JAE, Bednarski RM, Skarda RT. *Handbook of Veterinary Anesthesia*, 4th ed. St. Louis, Missouri: Mosby Elsevier, 2007.

Chapter 3

ASEPSIS IN SMALL ANIMAL SURGERY

Fred Anthony Mann

General principles of aseptic technique have been established to minimize the likelihood of wound contamination and subsequent wound infection. Thorough understanding of aseptic technique requires knowledge of the following five widely used terms:

- Asepsis: condition in which there are no viable pathogenic microorganisms present in the tissue.
- Sepsis: condition in which there are pathogenic microorganisms, or byproducts of the said microorganisms, present in the tissue.
- Antisepsis: safe application of an agent (antiseptic) with the purpose of removing or inactivating offending microorganisms. An antiseptic is a chemical substance that can be topically applied to living tissue.
- Disinfection: application of a chemical substance (disinfectant) with the purpose of destroying the vegetative forms of bacteria but not the spores. A disinfectant is a chemical

substance that can be applied to inanimate objects, such as certain surgical instruments or operating room furnishings.
- Sterilization: destruction of all microorganisms and spores on an object. Sterilization can be performed by application of heat (steam autoclave), ethylene oxide gas, vapor phase hydrogen peroxide, irradiation, and chemicals (glutaraldehyde). Sterilization is used for surgical instruments and any object that will have direct contact within or around open surgical wounds.

Prevention of bacterial contamination is of utmost importance in surgical wounds. Consequences of bacterial contamination and pursuant infection include systemic disease (peritonitis, sepsis, etc.), increased healing times, prolonged pain, delayed recovery, and altered cosmesis. Eliminating microorganisms from within or around a surgical wound would ultimately render it impossible for bacterial contamination and infection to occur. Therefore, it is important to know and be aware of the sources of bacterial contamination in the operating theater. These sources include: scrubbed and nonscrubbed personnel within the operating room, surgical equipment, operating

Fundamentals of Small Animal Surgery, 1st edition.
By Fred Anthony Mann, Gheorghe M. Constantinescu
and Hun-Young Yoon.
© 2011 Blackwell Publishing Ltd.

room equipment, and the patient, the latter being the most common source of bacteria for surgical wound infections. Aseptic techniques have been designed and implemented in order to minimize the risk of contamination. If these techniques are properly followed, wound infection is unlikely unless there is a gross breach in the established surgical barriers. Surgical barriers and specific techniques of aseptic patient preparation are discussed in Chapters 9, 10, and 11.

The air in the room acts as a vehicle for introduction of bacteria into the wound. Therefore, it is important to keep air turbulence to a minimum by limiting the number of unnecessary personnel, the amount of needless action, and the amount of talking while in the operating theater. This being said, there is no such thing as a sterile surgery and there is a level of contamination that is present in all wounds. There is a preponderance of evidence supporting that 10^5 organisms per gram of tissue or per milliliter of fluid constitutes an infection. In most cases, an immunocompetent individual would be able to clear pathogens in lower concentrations without intervention.

An infection may develop due to impaired host defenses and characteristics of the bacterial inoculums, and as a result of various local factors, such as tissue necrosis, dead space, reduced blood supply, and presence of foreign material. One goal of the surgical team must be to preoperatively address patient characteristics listed above as well as evaluate perioperative and intraoperative measures to ensure that contamination of the surgical wound is avoided at all costs. Perioperative measures include patient preparation, sterilization of surgical instruments, surgeon scrub, and donning of sterile barriers (on both surgeon and patient). Specifics of these perioperative measures and other practices designed to prevent surgical wound contamination are discussed in Chapters 6 through 11. The following is a list of rules commonly followed to minimize intraoperative contamination:

1. Scrubbed personnel are to stay inside and only touch objects located within the sterile field. The converse is equally true that non-scrubbed personnel are only allowed outside of the sterile field.
2. Talking and unnecessary movement must be kept to an absolute minimum.
3. Members of the surgical team should visualize the sterile field at all times. The reason is that direct visualization of sterile objects decreases the likelihood of contamination with nonsterile objects.
4. The patient table and instrument table, once donned with sterile barriers are only considered sterile at table height. The drapes and cords that hang off of the tables are out of the surgical team's sight and must be considered contaminated.
5. The drapes used to cover the patient, patient table, and instrument table(s) should be impermeable to moisture. This will ultimately lead to prevention of strikethrough contamination. (Strikethrough contamination is defined as the translocation of bacteria from the nonsterile side to the sterile side of a surgical barrier due to the material becoming saturated with either body fluid or irrigation fluid.)
6. Gowns, once donned, are considered sterile from just below the shoulders to the waist and from gloved finger tips to 2 inches above the elbow. Because of this, hands should be kept above the level of the waist, close to the body, and clasped together when not in use.
7. Scrubbed personnel that sit during a surgical procedure should remain seated until the procedure is completed.
8. Only use properly sterilized equipment that has sterility indicators both within the pack and on the outer wrapping. If sterility of an object is not known or is questioned for any reason, consider it contaminated.
9. If a sterile instrument, contained in a sterile pouch, touches the open edge of that

pouch while being opened, the instrument is considered contaminated and a new instrument must be opened. A surgical pack/pouch whose outside barrier has become damaged, wet, or compromised in any way must be considered contaminated and must not be used.

10. Pouring sterile liquid into a sterile bowl should be performed by a nonsterile person with the sterile person holding the bowl away from the sterile field. The nonsterile person should carefully pour the liquid without splashing or dripping onto the sterile field. The nonsterile fluid receptacle must not touch the sterile bowl.

These rules are mainstays of aseptic technique that when first introduced appear laborious and somewhat cumbersome; however, once practiced, most of the rules quickly become second nature.

There are several antiseptic solutions that are currently used in veterinary practice today. Examples of these include: aliphatic alcohols, iodophors, and chlorhexidine.

Aliphatic alcohols, such as 70% isopropyl alcohol, are effective against a wide range of bacteria and many viruses. Alcohols are rapid in action and work by denaturing bacterial cell walls and cell wall proteins. There is minimal residual action when used alone and side effects include skin irritation, desiccation, and tissue necrosis in open wounds. Alcohols are commonly used with other agents when preparing skin for surgical incision. However, since isopropyl alcohol may decrease the residual activity of chlorhexidine, it is recommended not to follow chlorhexidine application with an isopropyl alcohol rinse during skin preparation. Alcohol must also be avoided in preparation of patient skin for laser surgery to prevent the possibility of an intraoperative fire when the laser beam contacts the alcohol.

Iodophors, such as povidone-iodine solution, are effective against a wide range of bacteria, fungi, viruses, protozoa, and yeasts, and can also be effective against bacterial spores with prolonged contact times. Iodophors are rapid in action and work by penetrating the cell wall and replacing the intracellular molecules with free iodine that has been liberated by the iodophor solution. Dilute iodophor solutions are considered more efficacious due to the fact that more free iodine molecules are liberated in weaker solutions. There is minimal residual action (therefore, reapplication every 4 to 6 hours is warranted) and there is inactivation in the presence of organic material, such as red and white blood cells and necrotic tissue. Higher concentrations of iodophors have been shown to cause tissue necrosis; therefore, a 1% solution has been advocated (1:10 dilution of 10% stock solution). Side effects include cutaneous hypersensitivity reactions (up to 50% of canine patients). Care must be taken because iodine can be systemically absorbed across open wounds and mucous membranes and has been reported to cause increases in systemic iodine concentration and transient thyroid dysfunction. Systemic absorption of iodine is of concern especially in very young animals, patients with large open wounds, or patients that have severe burns. Metabolic acidosis has also been reported with repeat application. Iodine containing detergents are commonly used when preparing the patient's skin for surgical incision or the surgeon's skin prior to donning sterile surgical gloves.

Chlorhexidine is effective against a wide range of bacteria; however, it is minimally effective against fungi and viruses. It is rapid in action and works by disrupting the cell membrane and precipitating cellular components such as proteins. There is good residual action (up to two days) and chlorhexidine is not inactivated in the presence of organic material. The efficacy of chlorhexidine solution increases with repeated applications. Systemic absorption and hypersensitivity do not appear to be significant disadvantages with chlorhexidine as with the iodophors. However, one disadvantage of these solutions is otic and corneal toxicity. Care should be taken to avoid contact with the tympanic membrane and the cornea. A concentration of 0.05% chlorhexidine has been shown to be effective when used as an antiseptic solution (1:40 dilution of stock solution) in wounds. The gluconate and diacetate salts will precipitate when diluted using 0.9% sodium chloride or lactated Ringer's solution; therefore, sterile water is recommended as a diluent. However, this precipitation has not been associated with decrease in antibacterial activity of the compound or wound morbidity. Chlorhexidine containing detergents are commonly used when preparing the patient's skin for surgical incision or the surgeon's skin prior to donning sterile surgical gloves. Alternatively, waterless and scrubless hand antiseptics have become popular for preparing the surgeon's skin. One such product (Avagard™, 3M, St. Paul, MN) contains 1% chlorhexidine gluconate and 61% w/w ethyl alcohol and has been approved by the Food and Drug Administration for the preparation of skin prior to a surgical procedure. This scrubless

product is touted to provide a rapid antimicrobial kill of a broad spectrum of microorganisms with greater than 99% microbial kill in 15 seconds.

There are other products on the veterinary market intended for use in skin preparation prior to surgical procedures; however, the products listed above are by far the most commonly used agents.

ADDITIONAL RESOURCES

Additional information about asepsis in small animal surgery can be found in the following textbooks:

1. Fossum TW, ed. *Small Animal Surgery*, 3rd ed. St. Louis, Missouri: Mosby Elsevier, 2007.
2. Busch SJ, ed. *Small Animal Surgical Nursing Skills and Concepts.* St. Louis, Missouri: Mosby Elsevier, 2006.
3. Slatter D, ed. *Textbook of Small Animal Surgery*, 3rd ed. Philadelphia, Pennsylvania: Saunders, 2003.

Chapter 4

ANTIBIOTIC USE IN SMALL ANIMAL SURGERY

Elizabeth A. Swanson and Fred Anthony Mann

Proper aseptic technique during surgery minimizes the occurrence of surgical infections; however, when infection does occur, the consequences can be dire. Antibiotics are used in surgery to help prevent and treat infection, but lack of basic understanding of antibiotic use leads to misuse, overuse, improper application, and creation of super infections, all to patient detriment. The goals of this chapter are to introduce the basic concepts of perioperative antibiotic therapy and to offer guidance in developing an appropriate plan for antibiotic use in surgery.

With the development of methicillin-resistant *Staphylococcus* species and other multidrug-resistant bacteria, it is no longer considered acceptable to administer an antibiotic to every surgical patient. Furthermore, it has never been acceptable to use antibiotics to compensate for poor aseptic technique during surgery. Veterinarians must be diligent about when, where, and how antibiotics are being used in their patients.

Appropriate surgical antibiotic use revolves around two concepts: prophylaxis and therapy. Prophylactic antibiotic use is the administration of antibiotics before contamination occurs and only when there is high likelihood that infection could develop or when an infection would be catastrophic, should one develop. Therapeutic antibiosis is used when an infection is already present and is based on culture and susceptibility testing whenever possible. Empiric therapy may be started based on expected contaminants while waiting for culture and susceptibility results, but wise empirical selection is advised because poor responses to susceptible drugs may occur when the contaminant was not susceptible to the first antibiotic administered.

The decision to use perioperative prophylactic antibiotics to prevent infection is determined by an assessment of the risk of infection according to the length of the procedure, certain host factors, and the surgical wound environment. As mentioned above, prophylactic antibiotic use cannot offset poor surgical performance, such as excessive tissue trauma or faulty aseptic technique. After all, the mere presence of bacteria rarely causes infection. Alteration of local host defenses caused by the surgical trauma (i.e., local ischemia) is

Fundamentals of Small Animal Surgery, 1st edition.
By Fred Anthony Mann, Gheorghe M. Constantinescu and Hun-Young Yoon.
© 2011 Blackwell Publishing Ltd.

necessary for routine numbers of bacteria to establish a wound infection. Therefore, proper surgical technique in an immunocompetent patient undergoing a procedure anticipated to last for a reasonable duration forgoes the need for antibiotic therapy. See Chapter 3 for information on asepsis and prevention of wound infection.

Prophylactic antibiotics should be considered for any procedure expected to last longer than 90 minutes. Infection risk doubles for every 70 minutes the patient is in surgery.[1] Prophylactic antibiotics should also be administered in any case where an implant (e.g., bone plates, synthetic mesh, polymethylmethacrylate bone cement, nonabsorbable suture) is placed. Infection around an implant at the very least will delay healing and at the worst will cause surgical failure. Examples of catastrophic failure include the need to remove implants after a total hip arthroplasty or amputation of a limb due to intractable infection at the surgical site. Implants promote formation of a biofilm that harbors bacteria and inhibits natural host mechanisms and antibiotic effectiveness. The only way to assuredly eliminate a surgical infection where an implant is involved is to remove the implant.

Certain host factors, such as the presence of concurrent disease, very young or advanced age, or immunosuppressive therapy may also increase a patient's assessed risk and prompt the use of perioperative antibiotics. For example, patients with diabetes mellitus or hyperadrenocorticism have impaired immune systems and are, therefore, more prone to developing infection. Very young and geriatric patients have immature or impaired immune systems, respectively, that may increase the chance of developing a postoperative infection. Chemotherapy by its nature suppresses the immune system. Any patient currently undergoing chemotherapy or that has recently completed an immunosuppressive chemotherapeutic regimen should be considered at high risk for infection at the surgical site.

During surgery, care must be taken to minimize contamination of the surgical site and surrounding tissues to maximize the effect of prophylactic antibiotic administration. The environment around a surgical wound can have a profound impact on the risk of developing infection. Large hematomas or blood clots, necrotic tissue, and foreign objects (including surgical sponges) left at a surgical site inhibit host defense mechanisms and promote bacterial growth. Traumatized and devitalized tissues are unable to mount protective forces against infection and are often also hypoxic, thereby promoting both aerobic and anaerobic bacterial growth. Unless a wound has been made under controlled aseptic conditions, such as a planned surgical incision after antiseptic preparation, some contamination from the outside environment has likely occurred. Contaminated wounds can be converted into clean-contaminated wounds through careful debridement of devitalized tissues and copious lavage, which may negate the need for antibiotic therapy altogether. In contaminated wound surgery, antibiotic therapy should be limited to perioperative prophylaxis, if used at all. Obviously, infected wounds warrant antibiotic administration to be continued postoperatively with therapeutic intent, meaning a daily course of administration until the infection is resolved.

Most body lumens have a native flora. These bacteria often serve vital functions, such as aiding in digestion. However, these same organisms in the peritoneal cavity will lead to life-threatening illness. Controlled, surgical incisions into body lumens are considered clean-contaminated wounds; prophylactic antibiotics are not warranted unless anticipated surgical time is 90 minutes or longer. Careful surgical technique to prevent gross spillage of luminal contents into the body cavities is essential. If luminal contents spill into a body cavity, the surgical site becomes contaminated and should be treated by removal of the spillage and copious lavage. Such spillage is not a reason to continue antibiotics postoperatively. As with traumatic wounds, contaminated surgical sites can be converted to clean-contaminated ones through copious lavage. Antibiotic therapy beyond perioperative prophylaxis is not necessary and could even be detrimental by promoting development of resistant infection or by masking serious infection, such as peritonitis, thereby delaying prompt aggressive therapeutic management.

Selection of which prophylactic antibiotic to use is based on the expected bacteria in the targeted tissue. The most common bacterial source for surgical wound infections, especially in orthopedic and neurosurgical procedures, is from the skin. Skin bacteria are typically gram positive cocci, usually *Staphylococcus aureus* or *S. intermedius*. A second common source of infection is from fecal contamination. Feces contain colorectal organisms, such as enteric gram negative bacilli (*Escherichia coli*) and anaerobes (*Bacteroides* spp.). Whenever a body lumen is entered, prophylaxis should be centered on the typical flora of the lumen entered. Gastrointestinal organisms include gram-positive cocci, enteric gram-negative bacilli, and anaerobes. Airway organisms include gram-positive cocci (*Staphylococcus* spp.) and gram-negative bacilli (*E. coli*). Urogenital organisms include *E. coli* and S*treptococcus* spp., and are more likely found with urinary tract infection, pyometra, or prostatic abscess. Antibiotic prophylaxis is not recommended for routine, elective procedures involving the urogenital tract, such as ovariohysterectomy and orchiectomy. Normal flora of the liver include anaerobic organisms as well as gram-positive and gram-negative aerobic bacteria, but hepatobiliary procedures may be also be contaminated by organisms arising from the gastrointestinal tract.

The most commonly used perioperative prophylactic antibiotic is cefazolin because of its effectiveness against the most common perioperative contaminants and its ability to penetrate most tissues of the body.[2] Typical perioperative protocol is to administer cefazolin (22 mg/kg) intravenously at induction (ideally, 30 minutes prior to the skin incision) and repeat that dose every 90 minutes during surgery. Administration is terminated within 24 hours, preferably as soon as the surgery is finished, even if contamination occurs during the operation. All patients should be monitored for signs of infection (e.g., redness, heat, swelling, pain, purulent discharge, fever, poor doing, vomiting, anorexia, respiratory distress, body cavity effusions) in the postoperative period and treated accordingly. Table 4.1 lists commonly used prophylactic antibiotics with dosages and indications for use.

Colorectal surgeries carry perhaps the greatest risk of infection because of the high numbers of bacteria that live in this area. Preoperative preparation with oral antibiotics can help decrease the number of bacterial organisms within the colon. The most common oral antibiotic used for this purpose is neomycin started 24–72 hours before the planned procedure at a dosage of 20 mg/kg every 8 hours. Intravenous prophylaxis at the time of anesthetic induction is typically used as well (see Table 4.1). Mechanical bowel preparation with enemas and intestinal cathartic agents (i.e., GoLYTELY®, Braintree Laboratories, Inc., Braintree, MA) are not recommended because, although they will reduce the amount of fecal material present, they also liquefy remaining fecal material and increase the risk of contamination from spillage.

In order to work prophylactically, the antibiotic must be present at the potential site of infection before contamination occurs. For that reason, the selected antibiotic is administered intravenously 30–60 minutes prior to first incision (or roughly at the time of anesthetic induction) and then repeated based on the pharmacokinetics of the selected antibiotic. Prophylactic antibiotics are discontinued within 24 hours of wound closure, preferably at the end of the surgical procedure. Continuing antibiotics beyond 24 hours actually puts the patient at risk for infection. Animals with clean wounds that receive antibiotics other than a perioperative prophylactic protocol have higher infection rates than animals that do not receive

Table 4.1   Antibiotics used for perioperative prophylaxis in small animal surgery

Antibiotic	Dosage	Route	Frequency[a]	Indications
Cefazolin	22 mg/kg	IV	Every 90 minutes	Most commonly used prophylactic antibiotic; orthopedic procedures; most soft tissue procedures; neurosurgical procedures
Cefoxitin	22 mg/kg	IV	Every 90 minutes	Gastrointestinal surgery; hepatobiliary surgery
Ampicillin	20 mg/kg	IV	Once at induction	At risk urogenital procedures
Potassium Penicillin G	70,000 U/kg	IV	Every 90 minutes	Orthopedic procedures
Neomycin	20 mg/kg	PO	Every 8 hours[b]	Preoperative preparation for colorectal procedures
Erythromycin	10–20 mg/kg	PO	Every 8–12 hours[b]	Preoperative preparation for colorectal procedures
Metronidazole	20 mg/kg	IV	Once at induction	Preoperative preparation for colorectal procedures
Enrofloxacin	5 mg/kg	IV[c] or IM	Every 2 hours	At risk urogenital procedures

IV, intravenous; PO, oral; IM, intramuscular.

[a]All prophylactic antibiotics are given at the time of anesthetic induction, ideally 30 minutes prior to the skin incision, but no longer than 60 minutes prior to the skin incision. [Exception: When intraoperative culture samples are planned, antibiotic administration is typically withheld until the sample is obtained. Then, the first dose of antibiotic is given.]

[b]Oral antibiotics given for colorectal preparations are begun 24–72 hours prior to surgery. At the time of surgery (at anesthetic induction; 30 minutes prior to the skin incision), intravenous prophylaxis (such as cefoxitin or metronidazole) is also employed.

[c]Intravenous administration of enrofloxacin has been associated with anaphylactic reaction. If given intravenously, enrofloxacin should be diluted and given slowly.

antibiotics.[3] If infection is noted during surgery, or if sepsis is suspected, antibiotic treatment may be continued postoperatively pending culture and susceptibility results, when available, and adjusted according to patient response.

REFERENCES

1. Eugster S, Schawalder P, Gaschen F, et al. A prospective study of postoperative surgical site infections in dogs and cats. *Vet Surg* 2004;33:542–550.
2. Page CP, Bohnen JM, Fletcher JR, et al. Antimicrobial prophylaxis for surgical wounds: guidelines for clinical care. *Arch Surg* 1993;128:79–88.
3. Brown DC, Conzemius MG, Shofer F, Swann H. Epidemiologic evaluation of postoperative wound infections in dogs and cats. *J Am Vet Med Assoc* 1997;210:1302–1306.

ADDITIONAL RESOURCES

Additional information about antibiotic usage in small animal surgery can be found in the following textbooks:

1. Fossum TW, ed. *Small Animal Surgery*, 3rd ed. St. Louis, Missouri: Mosby Elsevier, 2007.
2. Slatter D, ed. *Textbook of Small Animal Surgery*, 3rd ed. Philadelphia, Pennsylvania: Saunders, 2003.

Chapter 5

BASIC SURGICAL INSTRUMENTS

Fred Anthony Mann

Successful accomplishment of small animal surgical procedures requires proper instrumentation. There are many specialized instruments for specific procedures, but there are certain basic instruments that are common to nearly all surgical procedures. These basic instruments are designed to secure surgical drapes; to cut, manipulate, and retract tissues; to suction surgical fields for maintaining visualization; to provide hemostasis; and to achieve wound closure.

Surgical drapes are secured to each other and to the patient's skin with towel forceps (also referred to as towel clamps or towel clips). The Backhaus towel forceps are the most common instrument used to secure sterile surgical drapes (Figure 5.1) (see also Chapter 11).

Basic surgical instruments for cutting are scalpels and scissors. The most common scalpel blade sizes used in small animal surgery are 10, 11, 12, and 15 (Figure 5.2a), and the most common handle to accommodate these blade sizes is the number 3 Bard-Parker scalpel handle (Figure 5.2b). The number 3L Bard-Parker scalpel handle (Figure 5.2c), a long version,

and the number 7 Bard-Parker scalpel handle (Figure 5.2d), a fine (thin) version, also accommodate the four blade sizes listed above. Scalpel blades should always be used on a handle, and a ratcheted instrument, such as a needle holder, should be used to manipulate the blade onto the handle. Using a blade without a handle or loading the blade onto the handle inappropriately puts the surgeon's valuable fingers at risk for accidental injury. The main use of the scalpel is for cutting skin, but it can be used for cutting other tissues. Scissors are cutting instruments for tissues other than skin. Because of the crushing effect of scissors, skin incision is reserved for scalpels. Subcutaneous tissues, fasciae, tendons, and other structures beyond the skin are often cut with scissors. Most scissors come in both straight and curved varieties. Curved tissue scissors are more versatile and nearly always preferred over straight scissors when available. There are numerous scissor types for specified procedures, but the three basic types are those for cutting delicate tissues (Metzenbaum scissors; Figure 5.3a), muscle fasciae and other tough tissues (Mayo scissors; Figure 5.3b), and sutures. Metzenbaum and Mayo scissors should not be used for cutting sutures because such will shorten the sharpness

Fundamentals of Small Animal Surgery, 1st edition.
By Fred Anthony Mann, Gheorghe M. Constantinescu and Hun-Young Yoon.

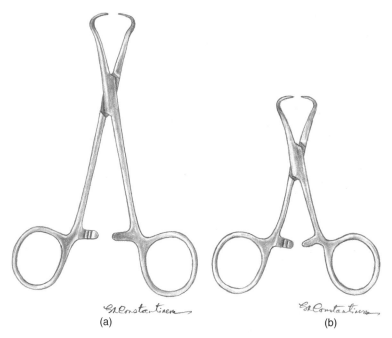

(a)
(b)

Figure 5.1   Backhaus towel forceps: (a) standard and (b) small sizes.

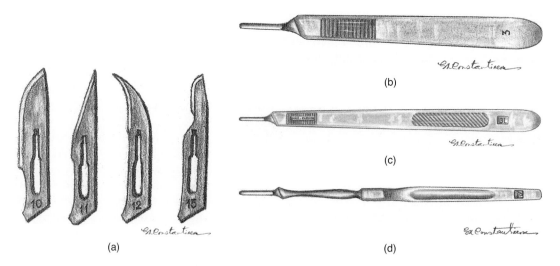

(a)
(b)
(c)
(d)

Figure 5.2   Common surgical scalpel blades and handles to accommodate them: (a) scalpel blade sizes 10, 11, 12, and 15, (b) number 3 Bard-Parker scalpel handle, (c) number 3L Bard-Parker scalpel handle, and (d) number 7 Bard-Parker scalpel handle.

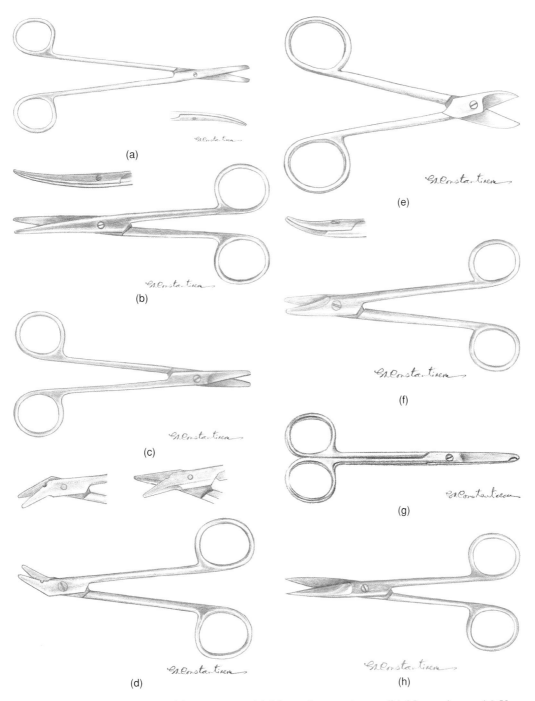

(a)

(b)

(c)

(d)

(e)

(f)

(g)

(h)

Figure 5.3   Common scissors used by surgeons: (a) Metzenbaum scissors, (b) Mayo scissors, (c) Vernon cartilage and wire scissors, (d) Roger wire cutting scissors, (e) Bantam wire cutting scissors, (f) Sistrunk scissors, (g) stitch scissors, and (h) sharp-sharp general operating scissors.

life of these expensive instruments. Scissors for cutting sutures should be used only for that purpose and for cutting fabric such as making a fenestration in a disposable sterile drape. Unlike tissue scissors, straight varieties of suture scissors are often preferred instead of curved scissors. The scissors used for cutting suture in the authors' didactic surgery laboratory and preferred by the author in clinical surgery are the Vernon cartilage and wire scissors (Figure 5.3c). These scissors have serrated edges on both blades, which help prevent suture slippage during the cut. Other wire scissors such as the Roger wire cutting scissors (Figure 5.3d), which have one serrated edge, and the Bantam wire cutting scissors (Figure 5.3e), which are available with or without one serrated edge, are also good for cutting suture. Some surgeons prefer to use the Sistrunk scissors (Figure 5.3f) for cutting suture, but these scissors are actually designed for cutting tissue and do not have the serrated edge advantage. Stitch scissors (Figure 5.3g) are used for cutting skin sutures to remove them; they are not intended for intraoperative use. In addition to the above types of scissors, some surgeons like to include in their surgical packs general operating scissors, such as the straight sharp-sharp operating scissors (Figure 5.3h), which are used for very precise dissection.

Instruments for manipulation of tissue are designed to allow the surgeon to precisely handle tissue without direct digital contact. The most commonly used tissue forceps are thumb forceps. Some examples are listed here from most to least traumatic: rat-toothed thumb forceps (Figures 5.4a and 5.4b), Brown-Adson thumb forceps (Figure 5.4c), and DeBakey tissue forceps (Figure 5.4d). Thumb forceps are held with the thumb and index finger in chopstick fashion (Figures 5.5a and 5.5b) to minimize tissue trauma. Thumb forceps are also used for handling needles during suturing. Needle grasping should be done delicately so as to preserve the tips of the thumb forceps. Damaged/dulled tips will add to tissue trauma when the forceps are used again to manipulate tissue. Ratcheted tissue forceps allow manipulation of tissues without repeated grasping. Examples of such forceps are the Allis tissue forceps (Figure 5.6a) and the Babcock tissue forceps (Figure 5.6b). For ideally minimizing tissue trauma, these forceps are avoided altogether. In fact, the Allis tissue forceps have been nicknamed the "Allis *trauma* forceps" to drive home this concept. If ratcheted tissue forceps are necessary, the Babcock tissue forceps are preferred because it is less traumatic than the Allis tissue forceps.

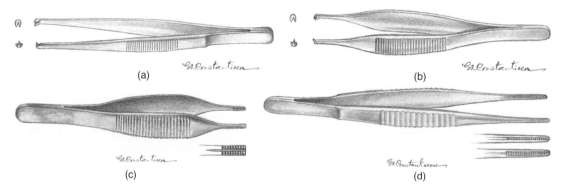

(a)

(b)

(c)

(d)

Figure 5.4   Common thumb forceps: (a) rat-toothed thumb forceps with narrow thumb and finger blades, (b) rat-toothed thumb forceps with wide thumb and finger blades, (c) Brown-Adson thumb forceps, and (d) DeBakey tissue forceps.

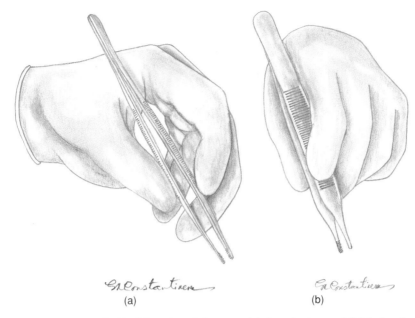

(a)   (b)

Figure 5.5   Proper method of holding thumb forceps: (a) thumb view and (b) index finger view.

Retraction of tissues is necessary for visualization of the targeted area of the surgery. Various retractors are available to achieve this objective. Retractors are classified into two major categories: handheld retractors and self-retaining retractors. Common handheld retractors include the Senn retractor (Figure 5.7a), Volkmann retractor (Figure 5.7b), Army-Navy retractor (Figure 5.7c), Meyerding retractor (Figure 5.7d), and Hohmann retractor

(Figure 5.7e). The rake portions of the Senn and Volkman retractors are available in sharp and blunt varieties. The Meyerding's tiny teeth help keep the retracted tissue confined behind the retractor and less likely to slip out compared to the smooth blades of the Army-Navy retractor. The Hohmann retractor is available in standard size and a small variety referred to as baby Hohmann retractors. Hohmann retractors are used most commonly in orthopedic

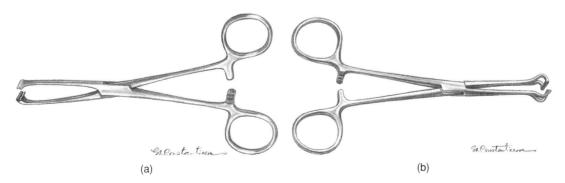

(a)   (b)

Figure 5.6   Ratcheted tissue forceps: (a) Allis tissue forceps and (b) Babcock tissue forceps.

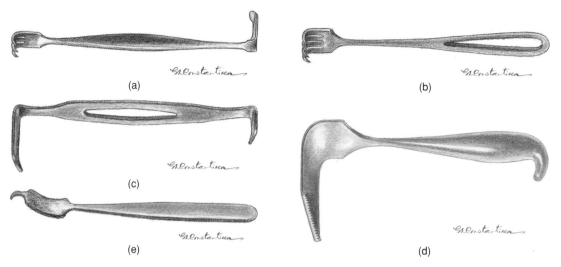

Figure 5.7 Common handheld retractors: (a) Senn retractor, (b) Volkmann retractor, (c) Army-Navy retractor, (d) Meyerding retractor, and (e) Hohmann retractor.

procedures by hooking and levering tissue over a bony area. Self-retaining retractors are handy when there is not enough intraoperative assistance or room for handheld retraction. Common self-retaining retractors include the Gelpi perineal retractor (Figure 5.8a), Weitlaner retractor (Figure 5.8b), Balfour retractor (Figure 5.8c), Finochietto rib retractor (Figure 5.8d), and Frazier laminectomy retractor (Figure 5.8e). The Gelpi and Weitlaner retractors are used to retract skin and superficial tissues. They can be used for deeper tissues as long as vital structures are not put at risk by the sharp points. The Weitlaner retractor is available with sharp or blunt tips. Balfour and Finochietto retractors are designed to hold body cavities open. The Balfour retractor is meant for keeping open celiotomy incisions, but can be used as a rib retractor. The Finochietto rib retractor is a specific rib spreader to keep open a thoracotomy incision. The Frazier laminectomy retractor may be used for thoracotomy incision

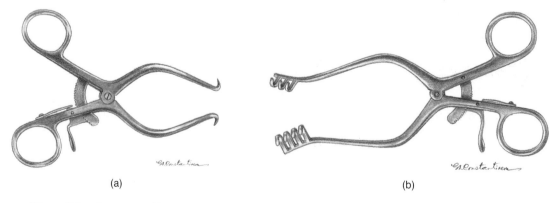

Figure 5.8 Common self-retaining retractors: (a) Gelpi perineal retractor, (b) Weitlaner retractor.

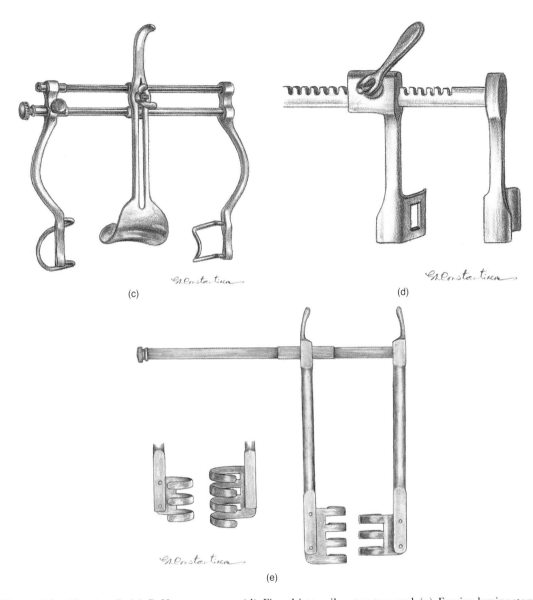

Figure 5.8   (*Continued*) (c) Balfour retractor, (d) Finochietto rib retractor, and (e) Frazier laminectomy retractor.

retraction if an appropriately sized Finiochietto rib spreader or Balfour retractor is not available. The Frazier laminectomy retractor is also helpful for retracting the sternohyoideus muscles during neck surgery.

Maintenance of good visualization requires proper hemostasis and clearing the surgical field of blood and effusions. Four common hemostatic forceps are the mosquito hemostatic forceps (Figure 5.9a), the Kelly hemostatic forceps (Figure 5.9b), the Rochester-Péan hemostatic forceps (Figure 5.9c), and the Rochester-Carmalt forceps (Figure 5.9d). The curved varieties of these forceps are more

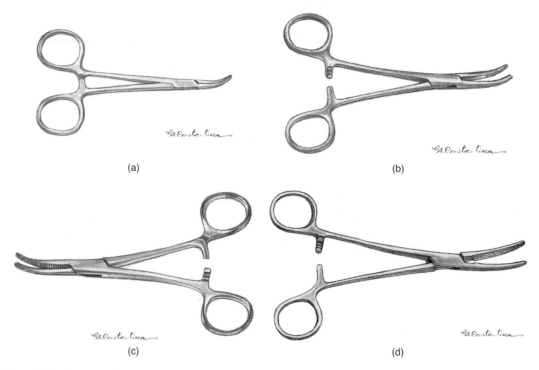

(a)

(b)

(c)

(d)

Figure 5.9 Common hemostatic forceps: (a) mosquito hemostatic forceps, (b) Kelly hemostatic forceps, (c) Rochester-Péan hemostatic forceps, and (d) Rochester-Carmalt forceps.

useful than the straight versions. Mosquito forceps are used to clamp small (approximately 1 mm diameter) vessels to prevent bleeding or to stop bleeding if the vessel is cut before forceps application. Kelly and Rochester-Péan forceps are designed for similar hemostasis of larger vessels. Mosquito, Kelly, and Rochester-Péan hemostatic forceps have serrations that are perpendicular to the jaws so that the vessel is less likely to slip when the hemostat is properly applied, that is, with the forceps' tip on the end of the vessel and the jaws oriented parallel to the vessel (see Chapter 12). Rochester-Carmalt forceps have serrations on the jaws that are parallel to the jaws. At the tip of the Rochester-Carmalt forceps, there are also perpendicular serrations. As such, this instrument is designed for maximal security of clamped tissue. The most common use for the Rochester-Carmalt forceps is for clamping vascular pedicles (i.e., ovarian pedi-

cle during ovariohysterectomy). The Rochester-Carmalt forceps are applied with the jaws perpendicular to the pedicle to take advantage of the serrations that are parallel to the jaws (see Chapters 12 and 18). Because of the crossed serrations at the tip, Rochester-Carmalt forceps could be used on vessels in a manner similar to mosquito and Kelly forceps, but are typically too large for that purpose.

Three common suction tips that are attached to suction tubing and vacuum source for aspirating blood and fluid from surgical fields are the Poole suction tip (Figure 5.10a), Yankauer suction tip (Figure 5.10b), and Frazier suction tip (Figure 5.10c). The Poole suction tip usually has a detachable guard with many tiny fenestrations to allow suction of the abdominal cavity without plugging by tissues such as omentum. The guard can be removed when more precise suctioning is desired in areas where

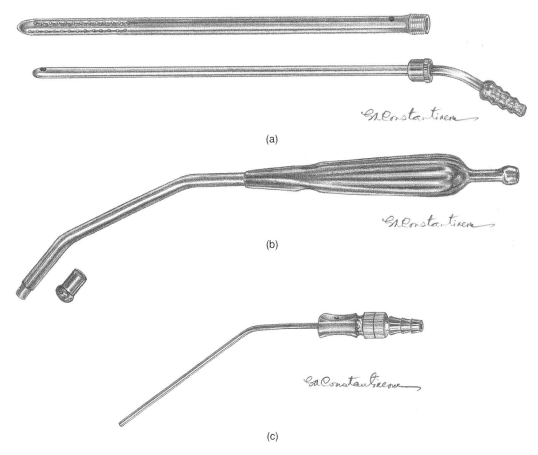

(a)

(b)

(c)

Figure 5.10 Common suction tips: (a) Poole suction tip, (b) Yankauer suction tip, and (c) Frazier suction tip.

tissues are less likely to plug the suction tip. The Yankauer suction tip is used commonly in the thoracic cavity where plugging with tissues is not likely. The Frazier suction tip is smaller than Poole and Yankauer tips and is used in small areas of fluid accumulation such as orthopedic and neurologic surgical approaches. The Frazier suction tip has a hole where the surgeon's thumb holds the instrument. Covering this hole provides high-pressure suction; leaving the hole uncovered provides low-pressure suction, which is less likely to suck tissues into the tip, thereby preventing unnecessary tissue trauma.

Closure of the surgical wound with suture requires needle holders (also referred to as needle drivers), thumb forceps, and suture scissors. A variety of sizes and styles of needle holders are available. The size and type chosen depend on the surgical procedure and sizes of suture and suture needle. A very commonly used needle holder is the Mayo-Hegar needle holder (Figure 5.11a). Another popular needle holder that incorporates suture scissors in the jaws is the Olsen-Hegar needle holder (Figure 5.11b). Caution must be exercised when using the latter needle holder to prevent premature cutting of suture.

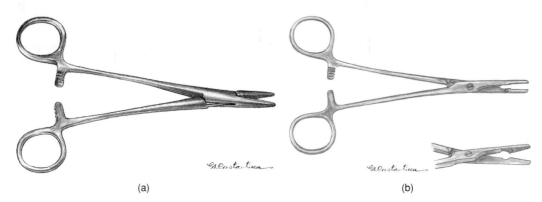

(a)   (b)

Figure 5.11 Common needle holders: (a) Mayo-Hegar needle holder and (b) Olsen-Hegar needle holder.

ADDITIONAL RESOURCES

Additional information about instrumentation in small animal surgery can be found in the following textbooks:

1. Fossum TW, ed. *Small Animal Surgery*, 3rd ed. St. Louis, Missouri: Mosby Elsevier, 2007.
2. Busch SJ, ed. *Small Animal Surgical Nursing Skills and Concepts.* St. Louis, Missouri: Mosby Elsevier, 2006.
3. Slatter D, ed. *Textbook of Small Animal Surgery*, 3rd ed. Philadelphia, Pennsylvania: Saunders, 2003.

Chapter 6

PACK PREPARATION FOR STERILIZATION

Fred Anthony Mann

The most common form of sterilization for gown and instrument packs is steam under pressure. Gas sterilization with ethylene oxide and plasma sterilization with hydrogen peroxide gas are used for materials other than stainless steel, linen, and nonwoven fabric ("paper") that would be damaged by steam sterilization. Because of health hazards associated with ethylene oxide gas, gas plasma sterilization is replacing ethylene oxide for materials that cannot be steam sterilized. However, gas plasma sterilization does have some limitations, one being that it cannot penetrate the walls of devices with lumens. As such, one cannot depend on the lumen of tubes to be sterile when gas plasma sterilization is used.

Surgical instruments should be adequately cleaned and lubricated before packing for sterilization. Immediately after usage in surgery, instruments should be presoaked in distilled water or in water mixed with a detergent solution designed for this specific purpose. Then, precleaning is performed by rinsing the instru-

Fundamentals of Small Animal Surgery, 1st edition.
By Fred Anthony Mann, Gheorghe M. Constantinescu and Hun-Young Yoon.
© 2011 Blackwell Publishing Ltd.

ments, preferably with distilled water to avoid mineral deposits that limit instrument life. The next step is to place the instruments (box locks open) in a basin containing warm water and a surgical instrument detergent. A soft brush is used to clean each instrument, paying attention to box locks and crevices. Each instrument is rinsed in distilled water and allowed to dry. At this point, one may use an ultrasonic cleaner with an enzymatic solution to assist in breaking down soils. After a final rinse with distilled water an instrument lubricant (commonly called "instrument milk") is applied by spraying or dipping, and the instruments are allowed to air dry prior to wrapping.

Instruments may be sterilized in individual wrappers (Figure 6.1) or grouped into packs for general or specified types of surgeries. When instruments are grouped into packs, surgical trays (Figure 6.2) are helpful in keeping instruments organized. A linen towel placed in the bottom of a stainless steel tray will help prevent sliding of instruments and pooling of moisture from the steam sterilization process. Double wrapping should be routine for surgical packs. Linen wrappers are less likely to tear than paper wrappers, but are more likely to absorb moisture and provide an avenue for microbial entry. Linen

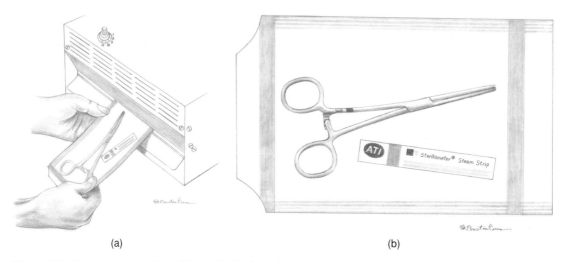

(a)   (b)

Figure 6.1 Instrument packaged in an individual disposable wrapper for sterilization: (a) heat sealing a plastic/paper wrapper and (b) completed individual instrument package ready for sterilization.

wrappers may be laundered and used many times, but they should be inspected for wear and tear before each use. Unsoiled paper wrappers may be reused once or twice, but the integrity of the material must be closely inspected.

Surgical gowns must be properly folded before wrapping. Slight variations in folding may be dictated by the style of gown, but the basic goal is to fold the gown inside out such that when the sterile pack is opened only the inside of the gown is touched as the gown is lifted out of the pack. Furthermore, folding must make sure that sleeves and other outer surfaces are not at risk for contamination as the gown is unfolded for donning. After the gown is folded inside out, accordion-pleated folding is done to reduce the gown to a size and shape suitable for wrapping (Figure 6.3).

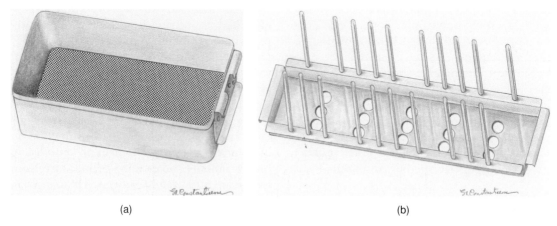

(a)   (b)

Figure 6.2 Surgical instrument trays for containing surgical instruments so that they can be wrapped for sterilization: (a) pan style and (b) rack style.

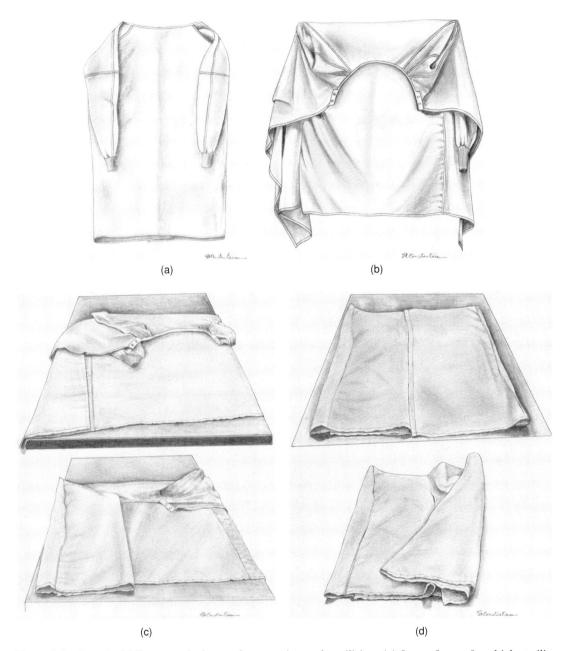

(a)

(b)

(c)

(d)

Figure 6.3   Steps in folding a surgical gown for wrapping and sterilizing: (a) front of gown for which sterility must be maintained, (b) folding neck down to expose the sleeve entry points, (c) folding right side inward to cover the right sleeve, (d) folding left side inward to cover the left sleeve and folding the gown in half lengthwise to result in a rectangular shape,

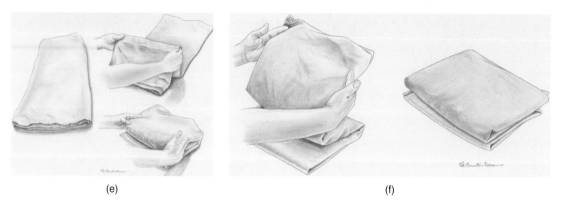

(e) (f)

Figure 6.3 (*Continued*) (e) folding the rectangular gown in an accordion pleat, and (f) finishing the accordion pleat with the sleeve hole in an upward corner (area of left hand).

Surgical drapes are typically prepared for wrapping by folding in accordion-pleated fashion so that the drape may be aseptically unfolded and applied while preserving one fold (Figure 6.4). Huck towels (towels for hand drying) are also folded in accordion-pleated fashion.

There are two basic methods of wrapping instrument, gown, and drape packs: (1) square method and (2) angled method. With the square method, the pack contents are oriented on the wrappers with the edges parallel to the edges of the wrappers (Figure 6.5). With the angled method, the pack contents are oriented on the wrapper with the edges in line with the corners of the wrappers (Figure 6.6).

Gowns, hand towels, drapes, and other linens to be sterilized in packs should be inspected for flaws, laundered, dried, and properly folded. Paper gowns and drapes are designed for one-time use and should not be sterilized after they have been soiled.

All packs should contain internal sterilization indicators (Figures 6.1 and 6.6a). Additionally, sterilization indicator tape should be applied externally to all wrapped packs (Figures 6.5f and 6.6g).

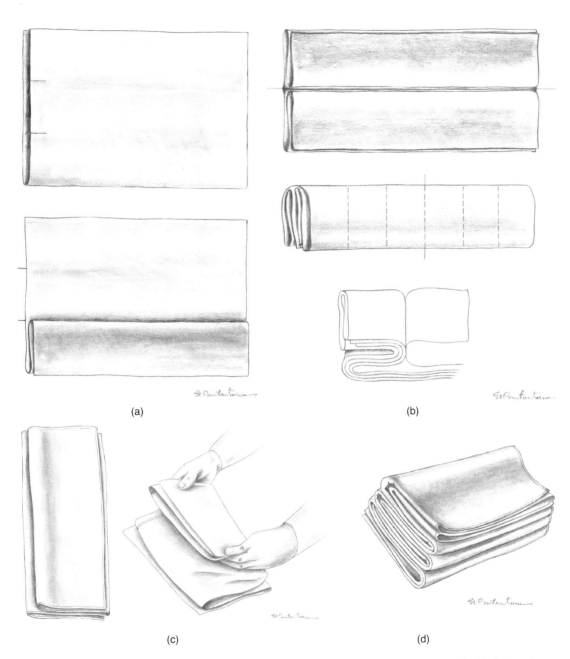

(a)

(b)

(c)

(d)

Figure 6.4   Steps in folding a surgical drape for wrapping and sterilization: (a) drape folded in half and one side accordion pleated, (b) both sides accordion pleated and the pleats folded toward each other to create a long rectangle, (c) accordion pleating of the rectangle, (d) finished accordion fold, and (e) (see page 40)

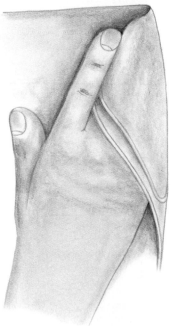

(e)

Figure 6.4 (*Continued*) (e) demonstration of how the drape would be unfolded, preserving one fold, and held for application to the surgical field.

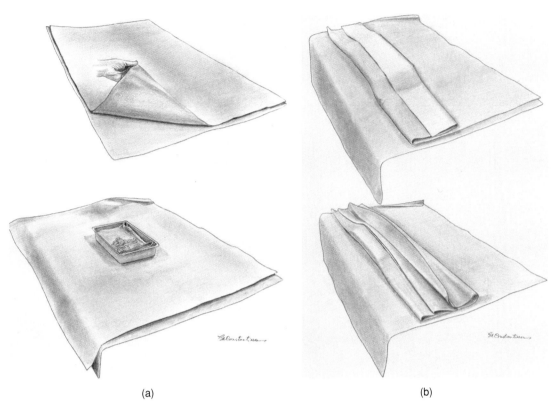

(a)   (b)

Figure 6.5   Square method of wrapping surgical packs: (a) instruments in an instrument tray placed on two wrappers with edges of the tray parallel to edges of the wrappers, (b) left edge accordion pleated with flap for grasping during pack opening (top drawing), and right edge pleated in like fashion and lapped over the left flap (bottom drawing),

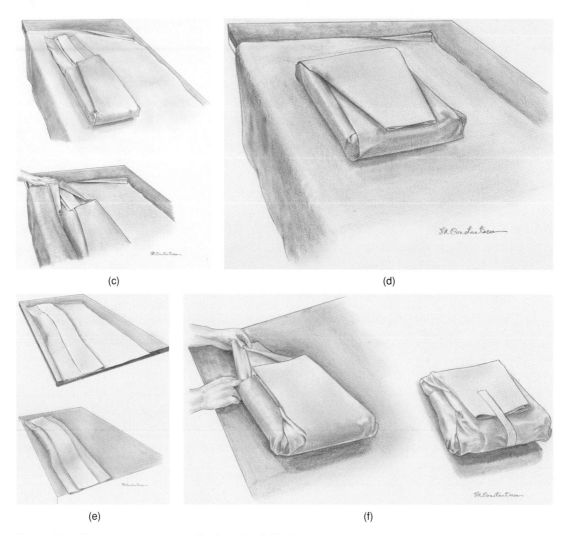

(c) (d)

(e) (f)

Figure 6.5 (*Continued*) (c) perpendicular sides folded over the right and left pleated folds, (d) completed inner wrap, (e) outer wrap left and right flaps folded in pleats identical to inner wrap, and (f) completed outer wrap secured with autoclave tape.

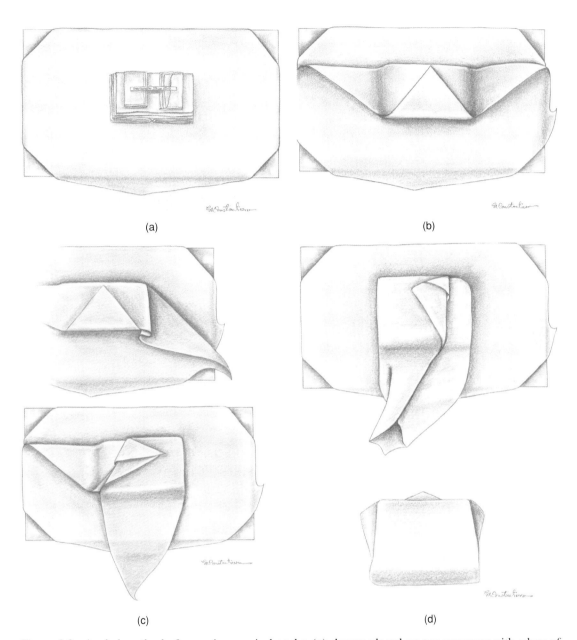

(a)   (b)

(c)   (d)

Figure 6.6   Angled method of wrapping surgical packs: (a) drapes placed on two wrappers with edges of drapes in line with the corners of the wrappers, (b) first edge folded so that the pleat creates a triangular tab for grasping during pack opening, (c) one side pleated to cover the triangular tab, (d) next side pleated to overlap the opposite side, and final side advanced to cover previous sides and tucked under the previous folds leaving a tab for pulling to open,

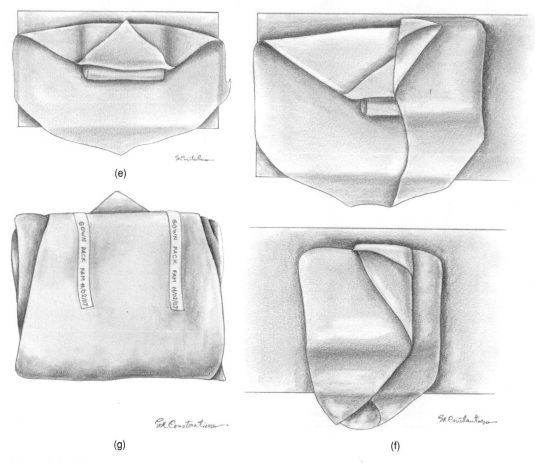

(e)

(g)   (f)

Figure 6.6 (*Continued*) (e) beginning of outer wrap identical to inner wrap, (f) folding of sides of wrap prior to tucking, and (g) completed outer wrap secured with autoclave tape.

ADDITIONAL RESOURCES

Additional information about surgical pack preparation and sterilization in small animal surgery can be found in the following textbooks:

1. Fossum TW, ed. *Small Animal Surgery*, 3rd ed. St. Louis, Missouri: Mosby Elsevier, 2007.

2. Busch SJ, ed. *Small Animal Surgical Nursing Skills and Concepts*. St. Louis, Missouri: Mosby Elsevier, 2006.

3. Slatter D, ed. *Textbook of Small Animal Surgery*, 3rd ed. Philadelphia, Pennsylvania: Saunders, 2003.

Chapter 7

OPERATING ROOM PROTOCOL

Fred Anthony Mann

Individuals that may be present during a surgical procedure include the surgeon, assistant surgeon, circulating nurse, and anesthetist. Certainly, in academic institutions, residents, interns, veterinary students, other trainees, and observers may also be present. Responsibilities of people inside the operating room revolve around maintaining an aseptic environment, contributing to the efficiency of the procedure, and ensuring safety for both the patient and the associated personnel. The purpose of this chapter is to discuss these responsibilities with the hope of allowing the reader to develop a fundamental understanding of proper operating room protocol.

Prior to entering the surgical suite, all personnel need to be properly attired. The specifics of surgical attire are illustrated in Chapter 8; however, a brief introduction follows. All personnel, regardless of their role, should have a surgical cap (+/− beard cover), a surgical mask covering their nose and mouth, and a clean pair of surgical scrubs. These scrubs should only be worn within the surgical suite and are not considered appropriate "street clothes." Ideally, footwear should be dedicated for use in the surgical suite, or protective shoe covers ("booties") should be donned over the individual's shoes; however, there is no established evidence that wearing shoe covering decreases surgical wound infection rate. A laboratory coat should never be worn into the surgical suite. Laboratory coats are worn over surgical scrubs while outside the surgical suite where the patients are prepared for surgery and in all parts of the building other than the operative theater.

The keys to efficiency in the surgical suite are preparedness and the ability to anticipate the next step of the procedure. Pertinent diagnostic imaging studies should be available in the surgical suite. These include radiographic images, computed tomography images, relevant ultrasound images, and/or magnetic resonance images. Hard copies of these images should be placed on the available light boxes, or if the facility is equipped with digital imaging capabilities, the images should be made available on a computer screen in the operating room. Having these images available, prior to entering the surgical suite, will aid the surgery team in localizing and visualizing the surgical site which, in effect,

Fundamentals of Small Animal Surgery, 1st edition.
By Fred Anthony Mann, Gheorghe M. Constantinescu
and Hun-Young Yoon.
© 2011 Blackwell Publishing Ltd.

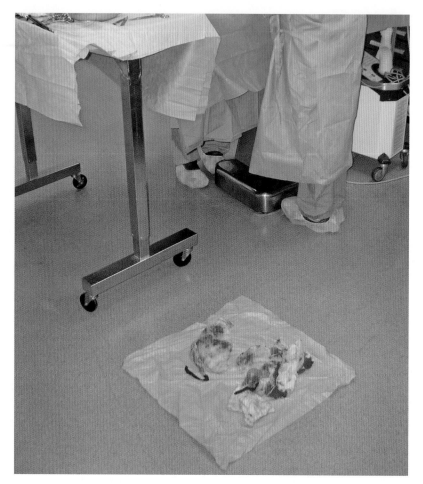

Figure 7.1   Floor target for discarding used gauze sponges and laparotomy pads.

will allow the surgeon to plan surgical margins (lumpectomies and mass removals) and avoid adjacent anatomical structures during the dissection. Other diagnostic reports should also be available and include complete blood counts, serum chemistries, ancillary blood tests (coagulation profiles, bile acid profiles, etc.), culture and susceptibility results, cytology reports, and histology reports. Having these results available will aid in decision-making and will hasten any paper work should additional samples need to be submitted.

Physical movements made during a surgery by scrubbed personnel should be aimed at improving the overall efficiency of the procedure. An assistant surgeon's responsibility is to maintain a clean and tidy instrument table. Used gauze sponges should be discarded onto a water-impermeable drape on the floor in order to easily account for them (Figure 7.1). Discarding sponges directly into a waste receptacle or allowing them to be removed from the room for whatever reason makes it difficult to verify that no sponges are left in the patient at the end of the procedure. Bloody instruments should be wiped free of debris and placed back on the instrument table in an orderly manner. Any organ or biologic material removed from the patient should be passed off to nonsterile personnel for appropriate processing. It is the assistant surgeon's responsibility to anticipate the surgeon's next move. Always think about the next step of the procedure and have the proposed implement ready to hand to the surgeon. Anticipation may be as simple as having a dry gauze sponge ready to blot away extraneous blood or fluid, or as complex as assembling a saw to create an osteotomy. When passing a ringed instrument, hold the instrument with the rings pointing downward (Figure 7.2). The surgeon will ask for the instrument by name and will extend his/her palm to receive the instrument (Figure 7.3). With a quick flick of the wrist, the assistant surgeon should forcefully place the ringed part of the instrument into the waiting palm of the surgeon (Figure 7.4). Forceful placement into the surgeon's hand permits the surgeon to confirm that the instrument is there without taking his/her eyes off the surgical field. A scalpel should be gently passed handle first into the waiting grasp of the surgeon (Figures 7.5–7.7). Scalpels are not forcefully passed. Sometimes, the surgeon will use hand signals to request specific instruments (Figures 7.8–7.12). Hand signals contribute to efficient use of intraoperative time as long as both the surgeon and assistant know the hand signals. Proper passage and receipt of surgical instruments will reduce the risk of dropping instruments either into the operative site or onto the floor. Consider that the instrument may be the only sterile one of its kind in the hospital, and an unlucky meeting with a nonsterile surface may delay the surgery while the contaminated instrument is being resterilized, or may force the surgical plan to be altered so that a less desirable instrument can act a replacement.

During the surgical procedure, it is imperative that all personnel focus on practicing and maintaining aseptic principles. Guidelines for aseptic technique are outlined in Chapter 3, and while all of these guidelines are considered appropriate operating room protocol, there are a few that are repeated in this chapter for emphasis. Talking and movement should be kept to a minimum to decrease exposure of the patient to airborne particles and to maintain focus on the surgical procedure and the patient. Scrubbed personnel should face the sterile field at all times. Gowns are considered sterile from just below the shoulder to the waist and from gloved finger tips to two inches above the elbow. Therefore, scrubbed personnel should not compromise the integrity of the sterile field with unnecessary movement. Only use properly sterilized instruments during a sterile surgical procedure. There should be a sterility indicator on the outside and inside of the surgical packs. Be sure to pay attention to these sterility indicators so that unsterilized instruments are not accidentally used. Some instruments will not be included in the surgery pack and instead will be sterilized in separate pouches. Do not use an instrument that is enclosed in a wet sterilization pouch. Instruments in pouches that have encountered moisture are no longer considered sterile. If a sterile instrument, contained in a sterile pouch, touches the open edge of that pouch while being opened, it is considered contaminated and a new instrument must be opened.

A sponge count (4 inch × 4 inch radiopaque gauze squares as well as laparotomy sponges) must be performed prior to the initial skin incision. The number of sponges is told to the anesthetist who records the number on the anesthesia log which will ultimately become part of the patient's permanent record. If additional sponges are added to the surgery table, these too should be counted and added to the sponge count on the anesthesia log. Prior to closing the surgical incision (specifically, prior to closing the linea alba for celiotomies and prior to intercostal space apposition for thoracotomies), both used and unused sponges must be counted to verify that the number of sponges remaining at the end of the procedure match the number of sponges opened throughout the procedure. A sterile assistant counts the sponges and laparotomy pads on the sterile field while a

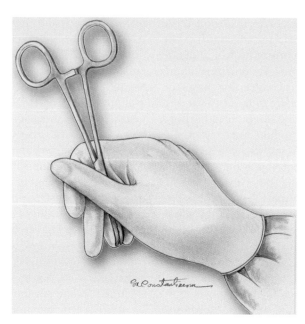

Figure 7.2   Passing a ringed instrument. The instrument should be handed to the surgeon closed (but not locked if it is a ratcheted instrument) with the rings at a downward angle, so the surgeon can grasp the instrument and immediately utilize it without adjusting his/her grip. Curved instruments should be passed with the tips curving upward.

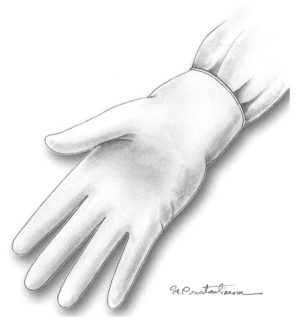

Figure 7.3   Preparing to receive a ringed instrument. The surgeon extends his/her palm after requesting a specific instrument.

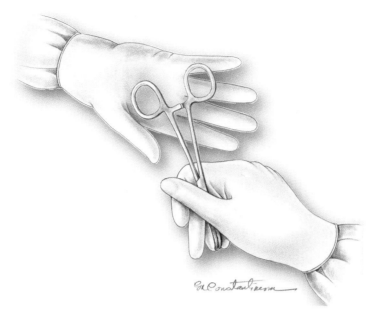

Figure 7.4   Receiving a ringed instrument. The instrument is snapped into the surgeon's palm with a definitive flick of the wrist.

nonsterile assistant counts the sponges that have been discarded from the sterile field (Figure 7.13). A statement confirming that the preincision and preclosure sponge counts match is written on the anesthesia log. The act of counting sponges will ensure that no sponges are inadvertently left behind inside a body cavity as a foreign body (referred to as a textiloma or gossypiboma). Should the sponge counts not match, a recount must be performed. If the count still does not match, the animal is routinely closed and two orthogonal radiographic views of the abdomen must be performed to visualize the rogue sponge or confirm that no sponge has been left behind. Obviously, radiopaque sponges must be used to radiographically confirm presence or absence of a retained sponge.

It is always advisable to minimize the number of people in the surgical suite. This will decrease the amount of talking and moving within the room and will directly decrease the probability that the patient will be exposed to po-

tential pathogens. Adhering to the principle of low noise and restricted movement is difficult in teaching institutions, but is nonetheless an important goal to target. The door of the operating room is to remain closed at all times and should only be opened for the passage of surgical supplies, appropriate personnel, and the patient. The storage of certain commonly used surgical supplies in the surgical suite is acceptable. These may include, but are not limited to, sterile gloves, suture material, skin staplers, gauze squares, and laparotomy sponges. Having commonly used supplies in the operating room decreases traffic by minimizing the need for personnel to move in and out of the room to retrieve the additional supplies.

Oversights and omissions are mistakes all human beings can make, including surgeons and other operating room personnel. To minimize such potentially devastating errors, some surgical teams use surgery safety checklists (Table 7.1). Use of such checklists is encouraged and can be customized for the surgical facility.

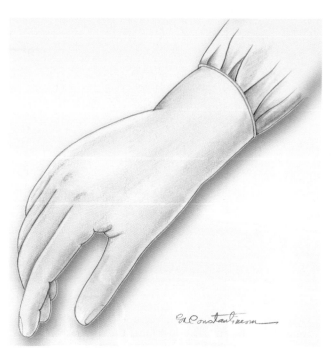

Figure 7.5   Preparing to receive a scalpel. The surgeon's dominant hand assumes the position of holding a scalpel, but without the thumb touching the fingers.

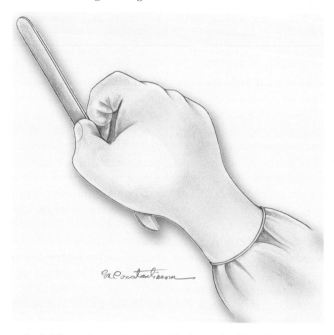

Figure 7.6   Passing a scalpel. The assistant should hold the scalpel handle with the blade pointed toward him/herself and the sharp edge down with the hand over the top of the handle.

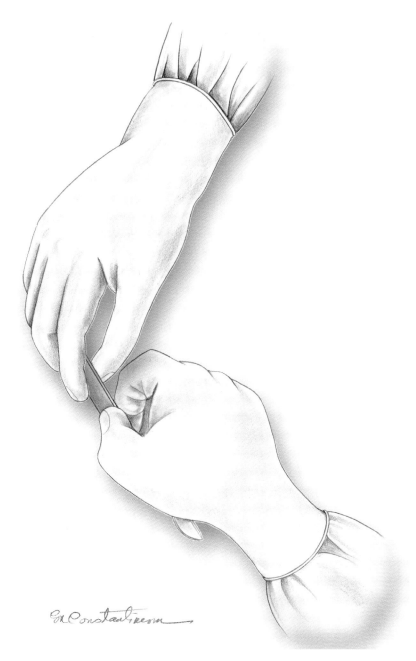

Figure 7.7   Receiving a scalpel. The surgeon will receive the scalpel handle in an over-the-top grip ready for cutting.

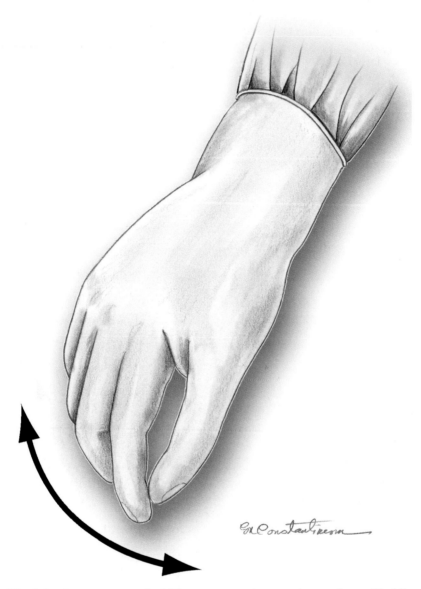

Figure 7.8   Hand signal to request a scalpel. The surgeon makes a cutting motion as if holding a scalpel and then opens the fingers to accept the handle.

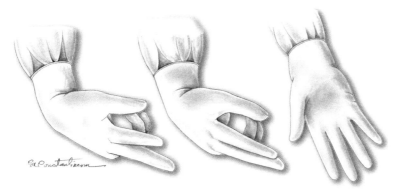

Figure 7.9   Hand signal to request scissors. The surgeon opens and closes the second and third fingers (pointer and middle fingers) as if scissors were opening and closing and then extends an open palm.

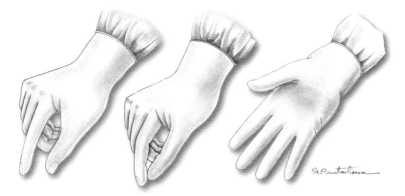

Figure 7.10   Hand signal to request thumb forceps. The surgeon taps the thumb and first (pointer) finger together like pinchers and then extends the open palm. If the dominant hand is already occupied by needle holders, the surgeon will signal for and receive the thumb forceps with the nondominant hand.

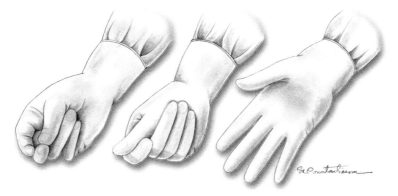

Figure 7.11   Hand signal to request hemostatic forceps. The surgeon snaps his/her fingers and extends an open palm.

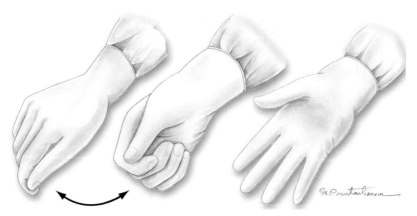

Figure 7.12 Hand signal to request a needle holder. The surgeon pantomimes a suturing motion and then extends the open palm.

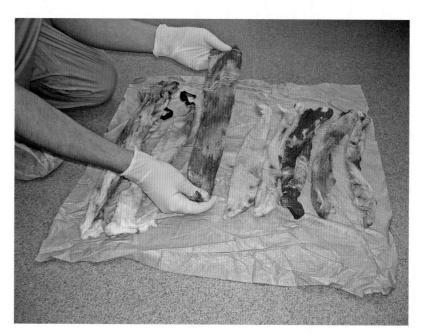

Figure 7.13 Performing a sponge count on a water-impermeable drape placed on the floor near the surgeon or assistant surgeon. A circulating assistant dons nonsterile examination gloves to count the sponges and laparotomy pads on the floor target, while the gowned assistant counts the sponges and laparotomy pads that remain on the sterile field. Gauze sponges and laparotomy pads should be separated from each other and opened fully to make certain more than one are not bunched together and inadvertently missed in the count.

Table 7.1   **Example of a surgery safety checklist**

DATE OF SURGERY: _____   CASE #: _____

PATIENT NAME: _____
PATIENT LABEL

SOFT TISSUE SURGERY INTRAOPERATIVE CHECKLIST

- ○ POSITIONING (per surgeon preference plus check the following)
    - ○ Leg ties – proper looseness
    - ○ Electrosurgery ground plate – proper contact and sufficient gel
    - ○ Acceptable warming devices – proper contact; away from eyes
- ○ PULL SPECIAL INSTRUMENTS
- ○ RADIOGRAPHS/ULTRASOUND/COMPUTED TOMOGRAPHY/OTHER DIAGNOSTICS
- ○
- ○ MISCELLANEOUS SURGICAL SUPPLIES FEE SHEET
- ○ VERIFY PATIENT
- ○ INTRODUCTION OF PARTICIPANTS
- ○ VERIFY SURGERY/PROCEDURES TO BE PERFORMED
- ○ REVIEW ANTICIPATED CRITICAL EVENTS/STEPS OF PROCEDURE
- ○ SPONGE/LAPAROTOMY PAD COUNT – PREOPERATIVE
- ○ ANTIBIOTICS GIVEN
- ○ BIOPSIES
- ○ CULTURE/SUSCEPTIBILITY
- ○ SPECIAL ONCOLOGY SAMPLES
- ○ SPONGE/LAPAROTOMY PAD COUNT – POSTOPERATIVE
- ○
- ○ URINARY CATHETER
- ○ FEEDING TUBE (TYPE: _____)
- ○ NASAL OXYGEN TUBE
- ○ ARTERIAL CATHETER MONITORING
- ○ CENTRAL VENOUS CATHETER
- ○ POSTOPERATIVE PAIN MANAGEMENT PLAN

> Check the circle when each checklist item is done.
>
> Check and write N/A if that item is not needed or otherwise not applicable.

ADDITIONAL RESOURCES

Additional information about operating room protocol in small animal surgery can be found in the following textbook and journal article:

1. Busch SJ, ed. *Small Animal Surgical Nursing Skills and Concepts.* St. Louis, Missouri: Mosby Elsevier, 2006.

2. Haynes AB, Weiser TG, Berry WR, et al. A surgical safety checklist to reduce morbidity and mortality in a global population. *N Engl J Med* 2009;360:491–499.

Chapter 8

SURGICAL ATTIRE

Fred Anthony Mann

The proper surgical attire depends on the location of the surgery personnel. In the sterile operating theater, a scrub suit (Figure 8.1) should be worn along with a surgical cap and mask (Figures 8.2–8.4). The surgical scrub suit should be worn with the shirt tail tucked. Undergarments should not be visible. For instance, no sleeves should extend past the scrub shirt sleeves and no collars should be visible above the "V" of the scrub shirt neck. A cap and mask should be donned immediately prior to entering the operating theater. The cap is put on first. Once the cap is in place, there should be no hair showing. That is, no hair should be extending from the borders of the cap. After the cap is in place, the mask is positioned such that the bottom tie is tied behind the neck and the top tie is tied behind the head. Both ties should be snug and the mask conformed to the face so that air filters through the mask during breathing. Breaths should not cause air flow out the top, sides, or bottom of the mask. Coughing can force air out the sides of a properly donned mask. As such, a person scrubbed for surgery should not turn his/her head to cough or else

droplets could be directed toward the sterile field. An alternative mask is a somewhat rigid mask (Figure 8.3) that conforms to the nose and mouth and is secured with a single elastic band that is positioned on the back of the head. This mask may be preferred by those who wear eyeglasses to help prevent fogging of glasses. However, traditional masks that tie behind the neck and head often have a moldable band at the bridge of the nose that conforms the mask to the face and minimizes the possibility of fogging eyeglasses. People with long hair, beards, and side burns require head gear that keeps hair from escaping. Special caps called hoods (Figure 8.4) are designed for this purpose.

Disposable surgical shoe covers ("booties") are required in many hospitals (Figure 8.5). Regardless of whether shoe covers are used, shoes should be clean and should be worn only at work, preferably only in the operating theater (Figure 8.6). Shoe covers should not be worn outside of the operating theater, because they can drag hospital debris into the operating rooms, thus defeating the purpose of wearing them. Likewise, it is best to wear shoes other

Fundamentals of Small Animal Surgery, 1st edition.
By Fred Anthony Mann, Gheorghe M. Constantinescu and Hun-Young Yoon.
© 2011 Blackwell Publishing Ltd.

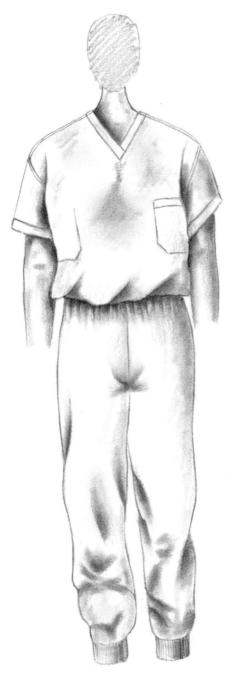

Figure 8.1 Surgical scrub suit. The shirt should be tucked into the pants.

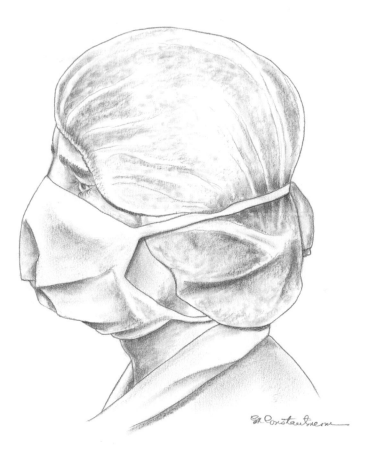

Figure 8.2 Bouffant surgical cap and standard surgical mask. Ears should be covered by this type of surgical cap. Both mask ties are tied behind the head. The method of crossing the mask ties and tying the bottom tie on the top of the head is inappropriate.

than those worn in the operating theater when traveling about the hospital.

Attire other than a scrub suit should be worn outside the operating theater. When a scrub suit is worn outside of the operating theater (such as in the animal preparatory area) it should be covered by a laboratory coat (Figure 8.7). Long laboratory coats are preferred because the intention is to protect as much of the scrubs as possible. The purpose of the laboratory coat is to protect the scrubs from hospital debris, such as dirt, dust, and hair. It is especially important that the laboratory coat be worn during clipping and rough preparation of the animal pa-

tient. The laboratory coat must not be worn in the operating theater.

Those in the operating theater who are not scrubbing for the surgical procedure should dress similarly to the surgeons. Alternately, there are other styles of operating room apparel that can be worn by those not performing surgery; however, it is important that this apparel is not worn outside the operating theater without appropriate covering. For brief visits into the operating theater, one may wear cap, mask, and shoe covers, and cover "street clothes" with a nonsterile surgical gown.

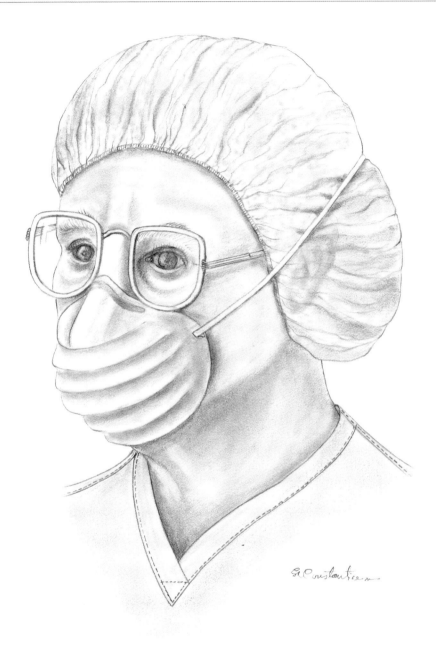

Figure 8.3   Rigid surgical mask.

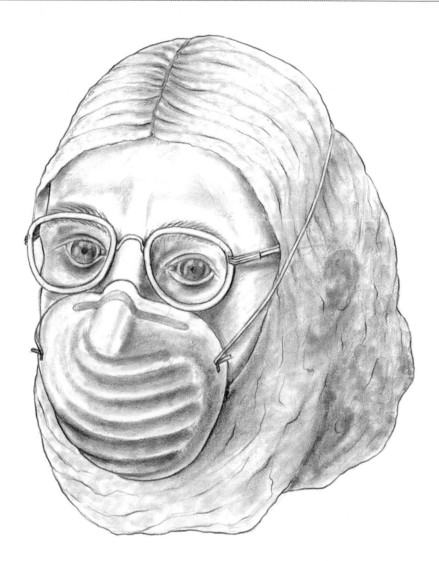

Figure 8.4 Surgical hood. Hoods are also called beard covers.

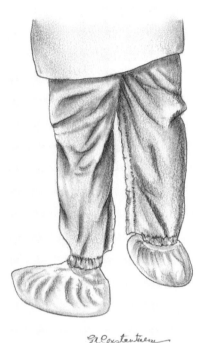

Figure 8.5   Shoe covers. If used, shoe covers should be donned immediately before entering the operating theater. They should not be worn outside of the operating theater. The laboratory coat illustrated in this figure would be removed immediately before entering the operating theater.

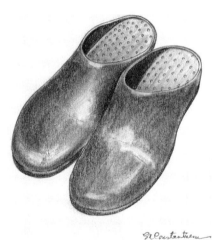

Figure 8.6   Surgical shoes. Commercially available surgical shoes are designed to facilitate comfort for surgeons who must stand in one position for long periods of time. These shoes are not necessarily designed for comfort in walking about the hospital. It is not necessary to have these specifically designed shoes, but the shoes chosen should be dedicated to the operating theater and not worn outside of the hospital, and preferably not worn outside of the operating theater.

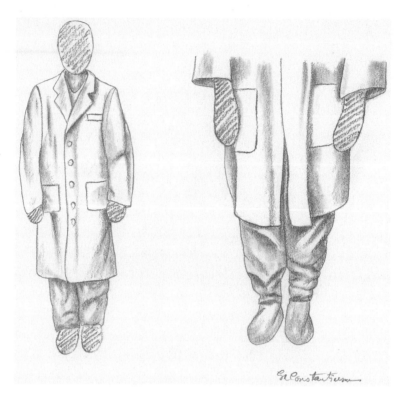

Figure 8.7   Laboratory coat. The laboratory coat should always cover the scrub suit outside of the operating rooms and should never be worn in the operating theater.

ADDITIONAL RESOURCES

Additional information about surgical attire in small animal surgery can be found in the following textbooks:

1. Fossum TW, ed. *Small Animal Surgery,* 3rd ed. St. Louis, Missouri: Mosby Elsevier, 2007.

2. Busch SJ, ed. *Small Animal Surgical Nursing Skills and Concepts.* St. Louis, Missouri: Mosby Elsevier, 2006.

3. Slatter D, ed. *Textbook of Small Animal Surgery,* 3rd ed. Philadelphia, Pennsylvania: Saunders, 2003.

Chapter 9

SCRUBBING, GOWNING, AND GLOVING

Hun-Young Yoon and Fred Anthony Mann

Surgical scrubbing is performed to remove as many microorganisms as possible from finger nails, hands, and forearms by mechanical washing and chemical antisepsis before participating in a surgical procedure. Commonly available scrub antiseptics include chlorhexidine gluconate, chlorhexidine diacetate, iodophors, triclosan, and chloroxylenol. Also, brushless rubs containing chlorhexidine gluconate, ethyl alcohol, or chloroxylenol are available. Whatever scrub agent is chosen, it is important to follow the manufacturer's written directions for scrub time and whether the use of a brush is recommended. Scrubbing is typically performed for five minutes. Scrub time is shorter for brushless rubs compared with traditional agents. Gowning is performed to build a barrier between the skin and the clothes of the surgical team member and the sterile surgical field. Likewise, gloving is performed to build a barrier between the hands of the surgical team member and the patient because hands cannot be sterilized. Proper scrubbing, gowning, and gloving tech-

niques are required to prevent microbial contamination during surgery.

Before surgical scrubbing, rings, watches, and jewelry should be removed, and gown and gloves need to be aseptically opened in the surgery area. For traditional surgical scrubbing, a nail pick and a brush (Figure 9.1) are needed as well as scrub agent. Surgical scrubbing should begin with a brief, general hand and forearm wash to remove surface debris. Then, the subungual areas of both hands are cleaned under running water using a nail pick (Figure 9.2). The next step is to apply the antimicrobial agent to wet fingers, hands, and forearms, using a brush and soft sponge. A brush is applied to the fingernails (Figure 9.3). A soft sponge is applied to the fingers, hands, and forearms. Each finger is divided into four sides (Figure 9.4) and a soft sponge is applied as ten up and down strokes to each of the four surfaces from the tip of the finger to the palm (Figure 9.5). Then, the palm, back, and sides of the hand are scrubbed as ten up and down strokes (Figure 9.6). The forearm is divided into four planes and a soft sponge is applied to the four planes from the wrist to the elbow (Figure 9.7). This process is repeated for the opposite fingers, hand, and forearm, and the used brush with sponge is discarded

Fundamentals of Small Animal Surgery, 1st edition.
By Fred Anthony Mann, Gheorghe M. Constantinescu and Hun-Young Yoon.
© 2011 Blackwell Publishing Ltd.

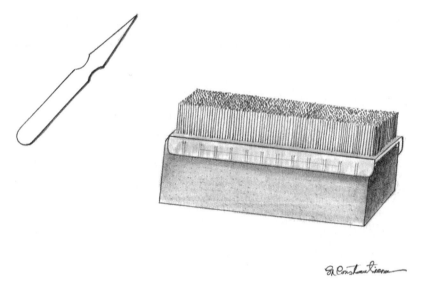

Figure 9.1   A nail pick (left) and a brush with a soft sponge (right) are used for scrubbing of the surgical team members.

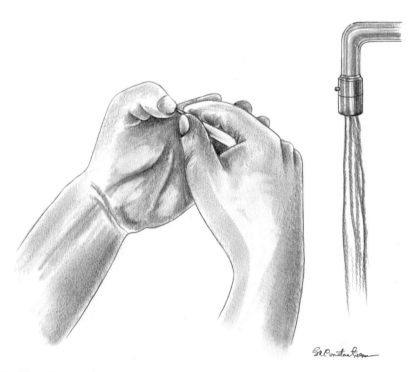

Figure 9.2   The subungual areas of both hands are cleaned under running water using a nail pick.

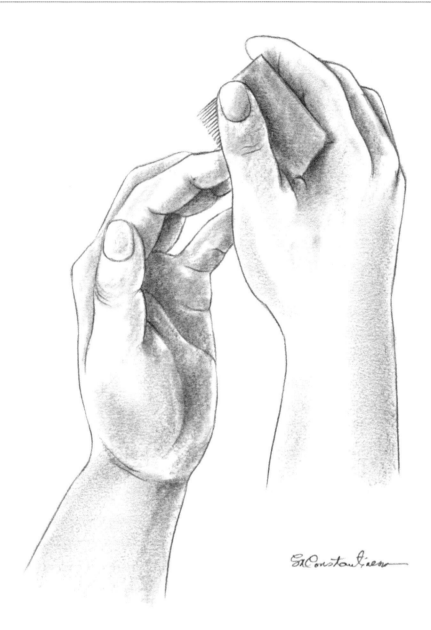

Figure 9.3 A brush with antiseptic scrub is applied to the fingernails.

in appropriate containers without contaminating the scrubbed skin. Then, water is allowed to run from the tips of the fingers to the elbows for rinsing (Figure 9.8). After rinsing, the remnant of water on fingers, hands, and forearms is allowed to drip off the elbows before drying in order to not contaminate a sterilized gown pack when grasping the sterile towel. The next step is to dry fingers, hands, and forearms with a sterile towel, which is typically located on the top of a sterilized gown in a sterile pack. One end of the towel is used to dry one hand and

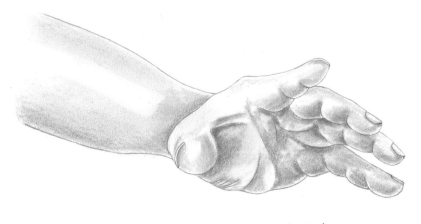

Figure 9.4   Each finger is divided into four sides for scrubbing.

forearm from fingers to the elbow, and then the opposite end on the opposite side of the towel is used to dry the other hand and forearm (Figure 9.9). Once the towel leaves the hand, it cannot go back up to the hand. During drying, the sterile towel should not touch any nonsterile surfaces other than the fingers, hands, and forearms. Bending forward and extending arms will prevent the sterile towel from touching the nonsterile scrub top.

For surgical scrubbing using brushless rubs, finger nails and hands must be clean. For the first scrubbing of each day, the subungual areas of both hands are cleaned under running water using a nail pick (Figure 9.2). Then, a brief, general hand and forearm wash and dry should be performed to remove surface debris. Hands and arms must be dry before applying scrubless rub solutions. Dispense one pump of the rub solution into the palm of one hand using a foot pedal (Figure 9.10) and dip the five fingertips of the opposite hand into the lotion to work it under the nails (Figure 9.11). The remaining lotion is spread over the hand (Figure 9.12)

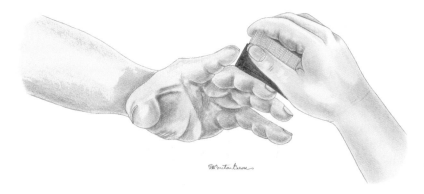

Figure 9.5   A soft sponge is applied to each of the four surfaces from the tip of the finger to the palm.

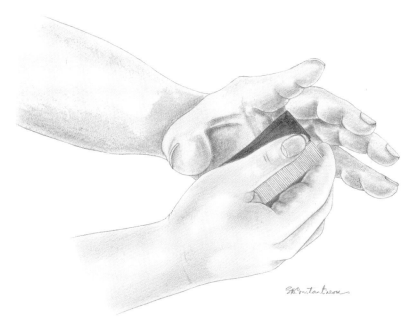

Figure 9.6   A soft sponge is applied to the palm, back, and sides of the hand.

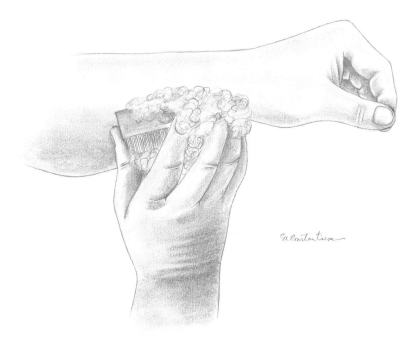

Figure 9.7   A forearm is divided into four sides and a soft sponge is applied to the four sides from the wrist to the elbow.

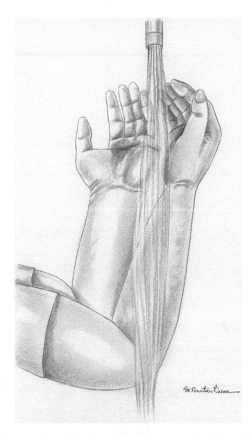

Figure 9.8 Water is allowed to run from the tips of the fingers to the elbows for rinsing.

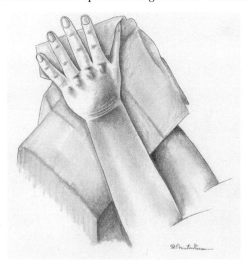

Figure 9.9 One end of a sterile towel is used to dry one hand and forearm from fingers to the elbow, and then the opposite end on the opposite side of the towel is used to dry the other hand and forearm.

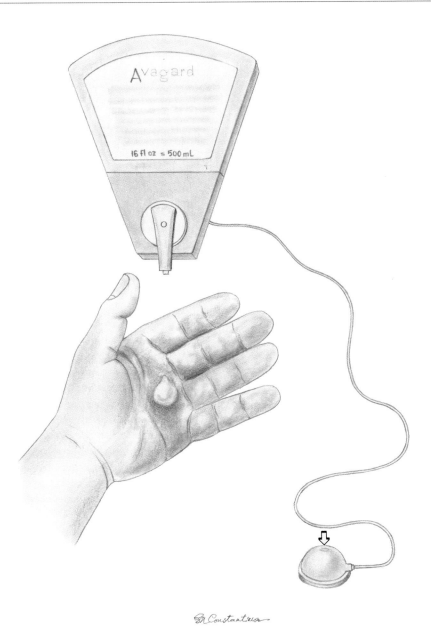

Figure 9.10 For surgical scrubbing using brushless rubs, one pump of solution is dispensed into the palm of one hand using a foot pedal.

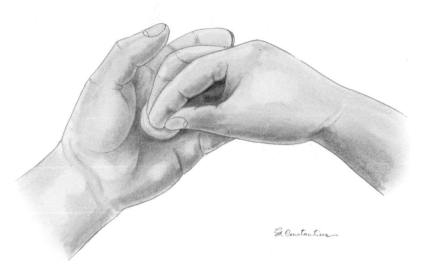

Figure 9.11 The five fingertips of the opposite hand are dipped into the brushless rub lotion to work it under the nails.

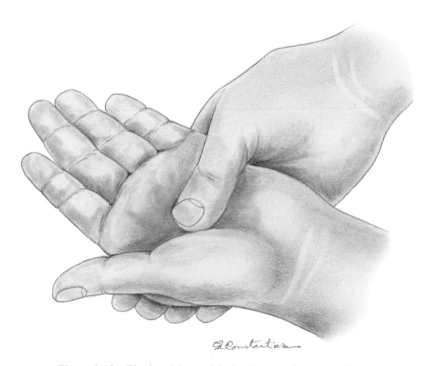

Figure 9.12 The brushless rub lotion is spread over the hand.

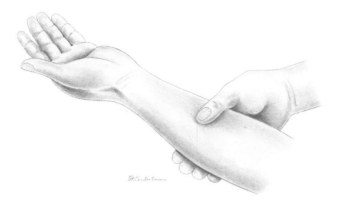

Figure 9.13   The remaining brushless rub lotion is spread over the forearm up to the elbow.

and up to the elbow (Figure 9.13). This process is repeated for the opposite fingers, hand, and forearm. A third pump of the scrub solution is dispensed into either hand to provide another rubbing of both hands and forearms (Figure 9.14). Both hands are allowed to dry before gowning and gloving.

Gowns are folded inside out in the packs. The folded gown is lifted out of the package and the surgeon steps away from the table. The next step is to identify the neckline and hold it while the armholes are found, and the gown is allowed to open (Figure 9.15). Both arms are advanced into the sleeves simultaneously, but the hands are not allowed to pass all the way through the cuffs in order to allow for closed gloving (Figure 9.16). An assistant secures the gown by closing the neck fasteners and tying the

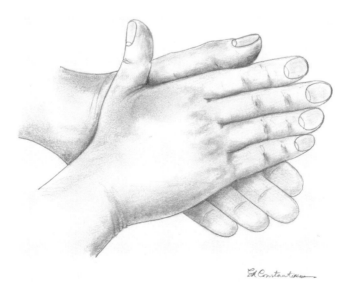

Figure 9.14   A third pump of the brushless rub solution is dispensed into either hand to provide another rubbing of both hands and forearms.

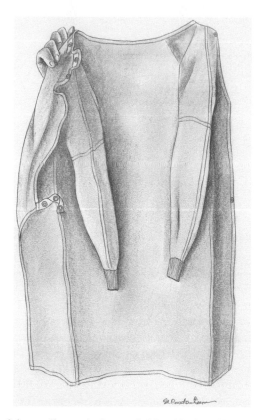

Figure 9.15 The neckline of the sterile surgical gown is identified and held while the armholes are found.

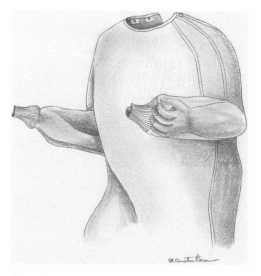

Figure 9.16 Both arms are advanced into the gown sleeves simultaneously, but the hands are not allowed to pass all the way through the cuffs in order to allow for closed gloving.

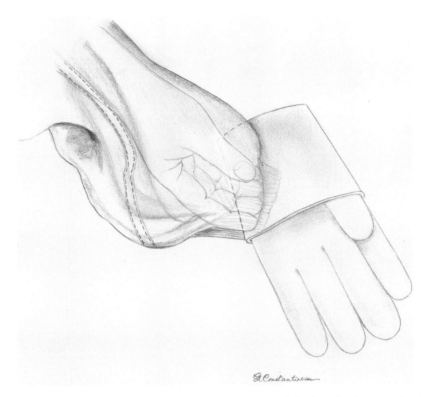

Figure 9.17 Closed gloving technique. One glove (left glove) is picked up by the opposite (right) hand, keeping fingers inside the cuff of the gown. The side of the glove is grasped.

inside waist tie. If a sterile-back gown is used, the appropriate tie is secured after gloving is done.

There are three methods of gloving: (1) closed gloving, (2) open gloving, and (3) assisted gloving. Both open and closed gloving enable the scrubbed personnel to glove themselves. Assisted gloving requires the assistance of another scrubbed-in team member. Closed gloving technique provides assurance against contamination because no bare skin is exposed in the process. For the closed gloving technique, one glove is picked up by the opposite hand, keeping fingers inside the cuff of the gown and grasping the side of the glove (Figure 9.17). The hands should remain within the cuffs of the gown until they are aseptically inserted into the gloves. The ventral rim of the glove is grasped with the hand that is to be gloved (Figure 9.18). The glove is laid on the palm with the fingers of the glove facing toward the elbow (Figure 9.19). Then, the dorsal rim of the glove is grasped with the opposite hand to open it wide (Figure 9.20). The rim of the glove is extended over the cuff of the gown with the index finger and thumb of the opposite hand (Figure 9.21). Then, the third, fourth, and fifth fingers are extended into the glove (Figure 9.22). The glove is advanced all the way over the gown cuff with the index finger and thumb of the opposite hand (Figure 9.23), thus completing one side of gloving (Figure 9.24). This process is repeated for opposite hand, but is easier because of the freedom of the gloved hand.

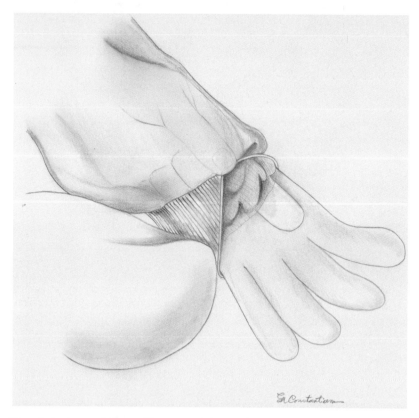

Figure 9.18 Closed gloving technique. The ventral rim of the (left) glove is grasped with the (left) hand that is to be gloved.

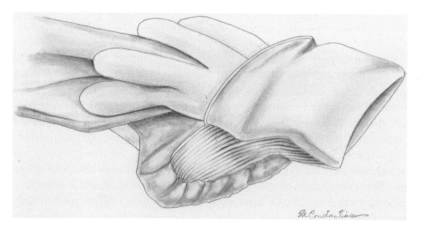

Figure 9.19 Closed gloving technique. The (left) glove is laid on the (left) palm with the fingers of the glove facing toward the elbow. The ventral rim of the glove is still grasped with the fingers of the (left) hand that is to be gloved.

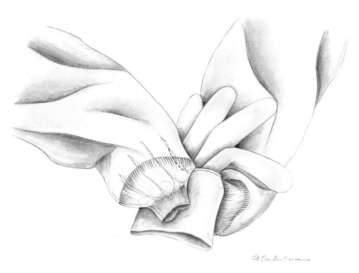

Figure 9.20 Closed gloving technique. The dorsal rim of the (left) glove is grasped with the opposite (right) hand to open it wide as the left fingers are extended into the glove. The right hand must stay entirely within the gown sleeve during gloving of the left hand.

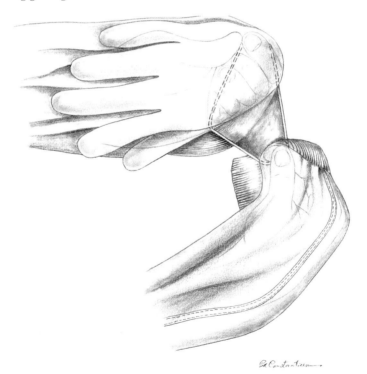

Figure 9.21 Closed gloving technique. The rim of the (left) glove is extended over the cuff of the gown with the index finger and thumb of the opposite (right) hand.

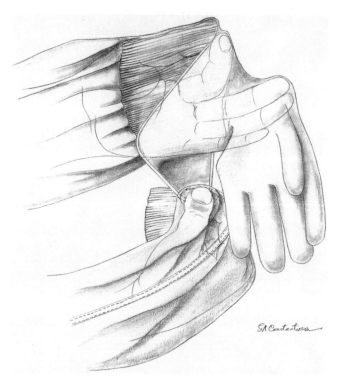

Figure 9.22   Closed gloving technique. The third, fourth and fifth fingers of the left hand are extended into the glove.

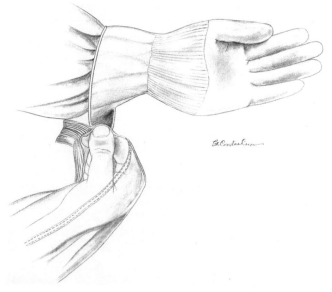

Figure 9.23   Closed gloving technique. The (left) glove is advanced all the way over the gown cuff with the index finger and thumb of the opposite (right) hand.

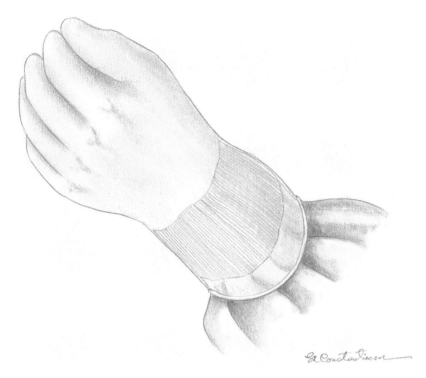

Figure 9.24   Closed gloving technique. One side of gloving (left hand) is completed.

Open gloving technique is used if one glove becomes contaminated during surgery and an assistant is not available to perform assisted gloving, or when only the hands need to be sterile and no gown is needed, such as for sterile surgical scrubs, minor surgical procedures, bone marrow biopsies, or catheterizations. For the open gloving technique, the skin surface (the folded cuff) of the first glove is grabbed between the thumb and the index finger of the opposite hand, and the hand is extended into the glove (Figure 9.25) without unfolding the cuff. Then, the gloved hand reaches under the folded cuff on the ventral surface of the second glove to pick it up (Figure 9.26). The cuff of the second glove is pulled to cover the entire cuff of the gown (Figure 9.27). Once the second glove is all the way on, the cuff of the first glove is unfolded using the gloved hand (Figure 9.28). Care is taken to avoid contamination of the gloved thumb during this process.

Assisted gloving is used when a sterile team member is available to assist in gloving another scrubbed-in team member. Assisted gloving may be performed as the initial gloving technique, or it can be performed to change contaminated gloves. Once a surgical glove is contaminated, a nonsterile assistant helps remove the glove (Figure 9.29). The entire hand (but none of the wrist) should be outside of the gown's cuff (Figure 9.30). A gowned and gloved assistant holds the palm of the glove toward the person needing the glove. The cuff of the glove is stretched wide by fingers placed on the outer surface of the glove (Figure 9.31). The thumbs of the assistant are not used to hold the glove, thereby preventing the assistant from accidentally touching the exposed hand of the person needing the glove (Figure 9.31). When there is a sterile glove on one hand, the sterile gloved hand can help introduce the other hand into a glove (Figure 9.32). The

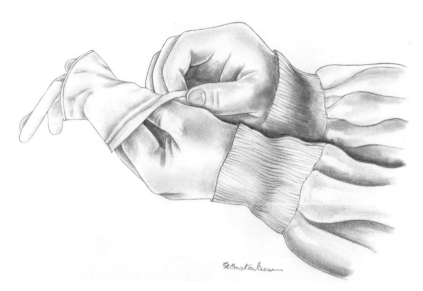

Figure 9.25   Open gloving technique. The skin surface (the folded cuff) of the first (left) glove is grasped between the thumb and the index finger of the opposite (right) hand, and the left hand is extended into the glove.

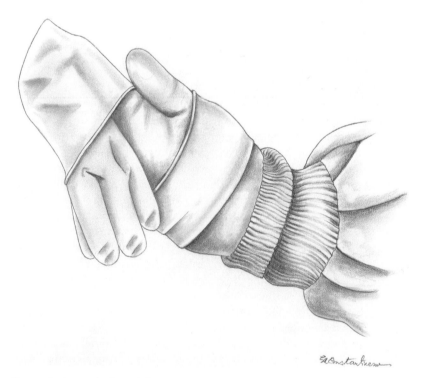

Figure 9.26   Open gloving technique. The gloved (left) hand reaches under the folded cuff on the ventral surface of the second (right) glove to pick it up.

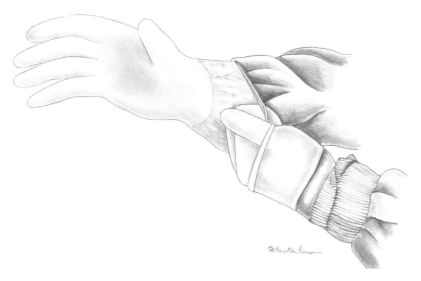

Figure 9.27   Open gloving technique. The cuff of the second (right) glove is pulled over the gown sleeve to cover the entire cuff of the gown.

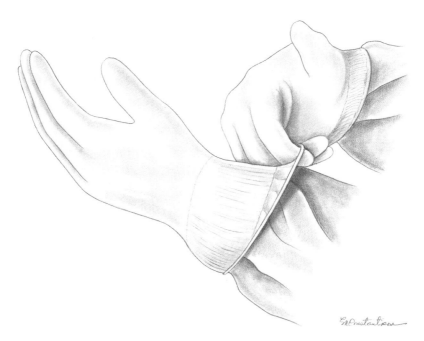

Figure 9.28   Open gloving technique. Once the second (right) glove is all the way on, the cuff of the first (left) glove is unfolded using the (right) gloved hand, making sure that no glove surface touches any exposed skin in the process.

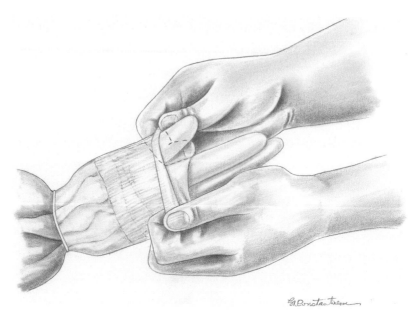

Figure 9.29   Degloving. When a glove is contaminated, a nonsterile assistant helps remove the glove by grasping the palm and the back of the glove.

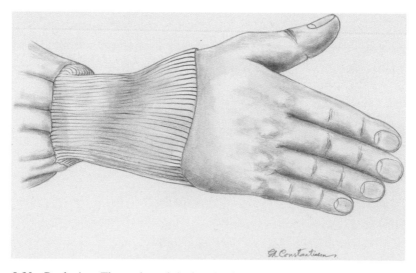

Figure 9.30   Degloving. The end result is that the fingers are located out of the gown's cuff.

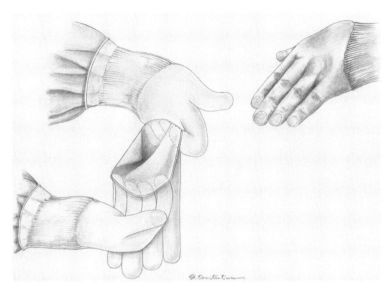

Figure 9.31 Assisted gloving technique. A gowned and gloved assistant has the cuff of the glove stretched wide by fingers placed on the outer surface of the glove. Then, the surgeon introduces the hand into the glove.

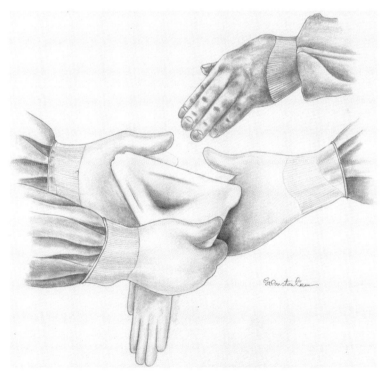

Figure 9.32 Assisted gloving technique. When there is a sterile glove on one (right) hand, that hand can help introduce the other (left) hand into a glove.

assistant pulls the cuff of the glove over the cuff of the gown as the hand is pushed into the glove.

If surgical gloves are contaminated at the beginning of the procedure before the surgeon's hands and wrists have had a chance to perspire, degloving can be performed in such a manner that the surgeon's hands stay entirely under the gown sleeves and cuffs. In this case, the surgeon has the option of putting on new sterile gloves using the closed gloving technique.

ADDITIONAL RESOURCES

Additional information about scrubbing, gowning, and gloving in small animal surgery can be found in the following textbooks:

1. Fossum TW, ed. *Small Animal Surgery*, 3rd ed. St. Louis, Missouri: Mosby Elsevier, 2007.
2. Busch SJ, ed. *Small Animal Surgical Nursing Skills and Concepts*. St. Louis, Missouri: Mosby Elsevier, 2006.
3. Slatter D, ed. *Textbook of Small Animal Surgery*, 3rd ed. Philadelphia, Pennsylvania: Saunders, 2003.

Chapter 10

SURGICAL PREPARATION AND ANIMAL POSITIONING

Hun-Young Yoon and Fred Anthony Mann

Surgical preparation is subdivided into initial preparation (nonsterile) and final preparation (sterile). Initial preparation includes hair clipping, urinary bladder expression, prepuce flushing, limb gloving and taping (for limb procedures), and rough scrubbing. Before initial preparation, ophthalmic antibiotic ointments or lubricants are placed on the cornea and conjunctiva. Once an animal has been stabilized under anesthesia, clipping begins. It is ideal to have an animal positioned for preparation in the same way as for the surgical procedure, but this is not always necessary. When clipping, one hand holds a clipper while the opposite hand tenses the skin to encourage easy movement of the clipper. The clipper should be held using a standard "pencil grip" (Figure 10.1) and initial clipping may be done along the hair growth pattern. Subsequent clipping should be against the pattern of hair growth to obtain a closer clip. Hair should be liberally clipped around the proposed incision site so that the incision can be extended within the sterile field as the

surgical procedure requires. A general guideline is to clip at least 4 cm on each side of the incision; however, clipping area depends on the size of the animal and the procedures [abdominal (Figure 10.2), orchiectomy (Figures 10.3 and 10.4), thoracic (Figure 10.5), neurologic (Figures 10.6–10.8), orthopedic (Figure 10.9), perineal (Figure 10.10), ocular (Figure 10.11), auricular (Figure 10.12), mandibular (Figure 10.13), nasal (Figure 10.14), and cranial (Figure 10.15) procedures] to be performed. After hair removal is completed, loose hair is removed with a vacuum. For limb procedures, the hair is removed from the surgical site and well beyond it. If exposure of the paw is unnecessary, the hair can be left on the paw (Figure 10.9). The animal's urinary bladder should be expressed to avoid inadvertent cystotomy when entering the abdominal cavity and to avoid urine soiling from urination during any surgical procedure. Expression of the urinary bladder may be contraindicated, or care should be taken to express the urinary bladder, if the abdomen has been traumatized. The urinary bladder can be expressed with the animal in either dorsal or lateral recumbence, but is more easily achieved with lateral recumbence. When expressing the urinary bladder, care should be taken to use

Fundamentals of Small Animal Surgery, 1st edition.
By Fred Anthony Mann, Gheorghe M. Constantinescu and Hun-Young Yoon.
© 2011 Blackwell Publishing Ltd.

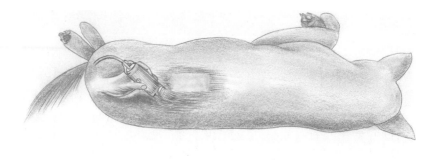

Figure 10.1   Clipping of hair. The clipper should be held using a standard "pencil grip", initially clipping along the hair growth pattern. Subsequent clipping should be against the pattern of hair growth to obtain a closer clip.

gentle, constant pressure rather than a pulsating action. In male dogs undergoing abdominal procedures, or any procedure involving the caudal half of the body, the prepuce is flushed with antiseptic solution before preparing the surgical site.

If not yet done, the animal is placed in its surgical position after clipping and vacuuming. Positioning depends on the proposed surgical site. The animal is positioned in dorsal recumbence [thoracoabdominal positioner (Figure 10.16) can be used] for abdominal procedures, ventral

cervical procedures, and median sternotomies. Lateral recumbence positioning is used for lateral thoracic approaches, auricular procedures, some oral procedures, and most ophthalmic procedures. Ventral recumbence positioning is used for dorsal spinal procedures and some ophthalmic procedures. The paw can be excluded from the surgical area by placing an examination glove over the distal extremity and covering the glove with tape (Figure 10.17). To avoid a tourniquet effect, the tape should not be applied too tightly. Then, the limb is carefully

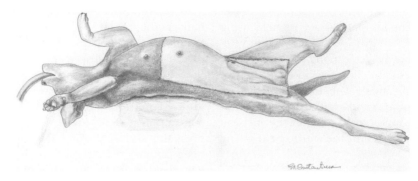

Figure 10.2   Clipping for an abdominal procedure. The clip extends cranially to the middle part of the ventral thorax, caudally to the base of the scrotum or vulva, and bilaterally to a line parallel with the fold of the flank.

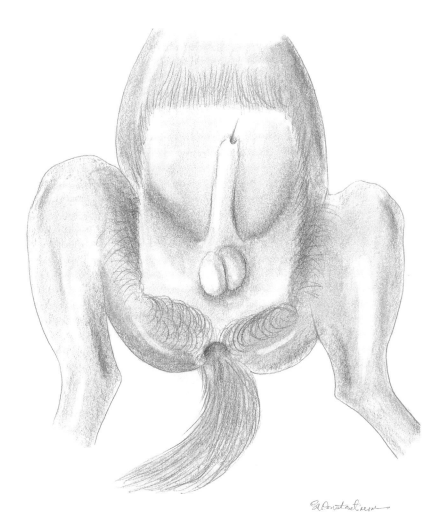

Figure 10.3 Clipping for canine orchiectomy. Clip the entire inguinal area, the entire prepuce, the scrotum, and a few centimeters caudal to the scrotum. The scrotum should be gently clipped first, while the clippers are still cool, to avoid scrotal skin irritation. Long hair in the periphery of the clipped region should be trimmed to prevent it from creeping under the drapes into the sterile field.

suspended with tape from an intravenous fluid stand for final prepping and draping (Figure 10.17). Two scrubs are performed: (1) a rough scrub outside the operating room and (2) a sterile scrub in the operating room.

The skin is scrubbed with germicidal solutions to remove debris and reduce bacterial populations. Depending on the area of the body

that is having surgery, one of three patterns of action is used to scrub the site: target, orthopedic, or perineal. The target pattern is primarily used to scrub surgical sites for abdominal, thoracic, and neurologic procedures. The first step is to take one of the rinsing sponges and wipe around the periphery of the clipped margin. This moistens the hair and flattens it down,

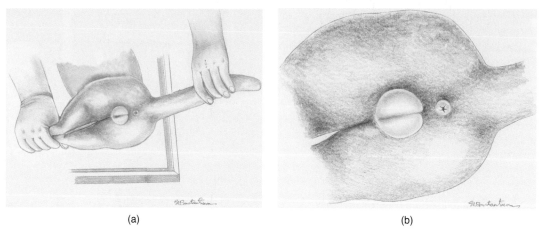

(a)   (b)

Figure 10.4   Preparation for feline orchiectomy. (a) With the cat in lateral recumbence, the thoracic limbs are pulled toward the head and the tail pulled dorsally. (b) Scrotal hair is plucked. Clipping is not routinely done for feline castration.

which helps prevent the hair from flying onto the clipped area. The second step is to scrub the surgical site with one scrub sponge using an antiseptic soap (typically, chlorhexidine or povidone iodine). Start at the proposed incision site and then move the sponge back and forth for enough strokes (approximately 30 strokes) to achieve gross cleansing. After scrubbing the intended incision site, move the sponge in a progressively outward circle until the hair is reached (Figure 10.18). Once the hair or any other contaminated area has been touched with

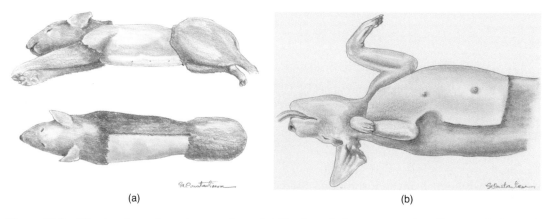

(a)   (b)

Figure 10.5   Clipping for a thoracic procedure. (a) For lateral thoracotomy, the clip extends from the cranial aspect of the scapula and the proximal part of the brachium, caudally to the middle part of the abdomen, ventrally to the sternum, and dorsally to the vertebral dorsal spinous processes. (b) For median sternotomy, the clip extends from cranial to the manubrium, caudally past the xiphoid to the mid-abdomen, and bilaterally to a line parallel with the fold of the flank, allowing plenty of space for aseptic intercostal thoracic tube placement.

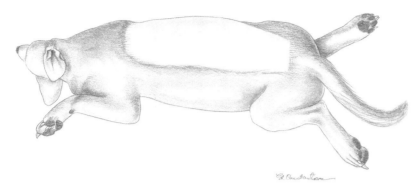

Figure 10.6   Clipping for thoracolumbar spinal surgery. The clip extends from the caudal cervical vertebrae and scapulae, caudally to the sacrum, and at least 4 cm lateral to midline bilaterally.

the sponge, the sponge must never return to the proposed incision site. The scrub should be repeated at least two more times. Dry or wet gauze can be used for rinsing off the chemical with same pattern as the scrub. The gauze does not need to be sterile for the rough scrub. The

second scrub pattern is that used with orthopedic surgeries. Once the limb is suspended, the rough scrub can begin. Begin at the tape edge of the suspended limb from distal to proximal, moving circumferentially around the limb. The scrub is repeated a minimum of three times

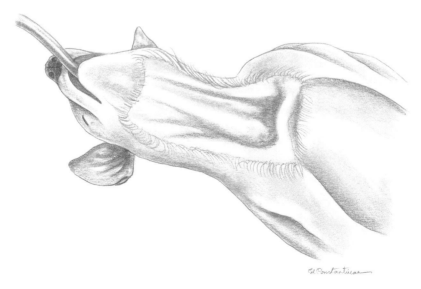

Figure 10.7   Clipping for a ventral approach to the cervical region. The clip extends from the middle part of the mandible, caudally to the manubrium, and bilaterally to the side of the neck at least 4 cm from the proposed incision, depending on the size of the animal.

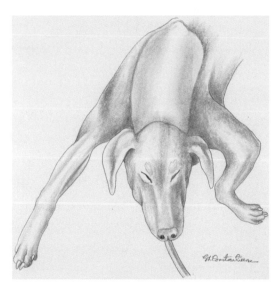

Figure 10.8 Clipping for a dorsal approach to the cervical region. The clip extends from the occipital protuberance, caudally to the cranial thoracic vertebrae, and bilaterally to the side of the neck at least 4 cm lateral to the proposed incision, depending on the size of the animal.

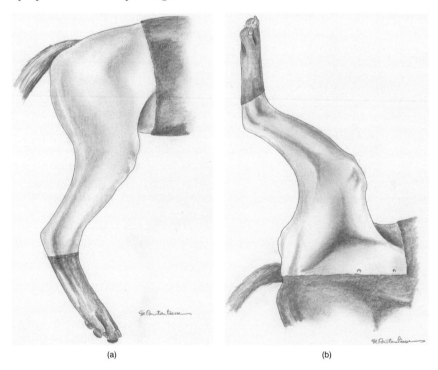

(a) (b)

Figure 10.9 Clipping for a pelvic limb procedure where exposure of the paw is not required. The entire limb should be clipped except for the paw such that the clip extends (a) dorsally past dorsal midline and (b) ventrally past ventral midline.

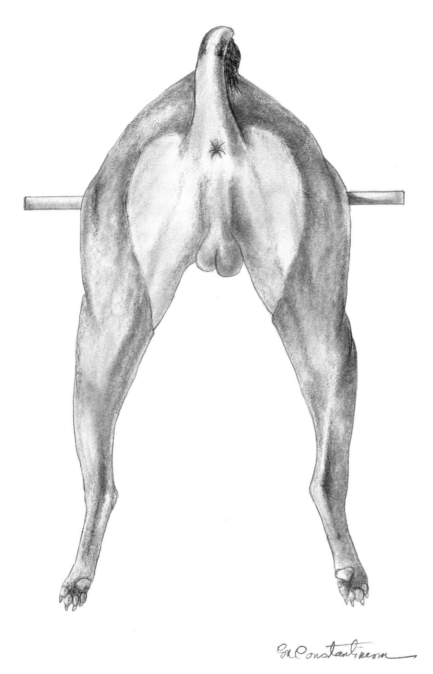

Figure 10.10   Clipping for perineal and perianal procedures. The animal will eventually be placed in ventral recumbence with pelvic limbs hanging over the padded edge of the surgical table. Therefore, the entire perineal and perianal areas are clipped, as well as the caudomedial aspects of the thighs.

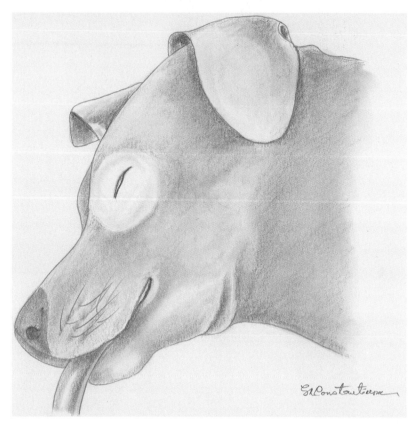

Figure 10.11 Clipping for an ophthalmic procedure. The periocular area is carefully clipped. The cilia on the upper lid are removed for intraocular procedures, such as a cataract procedure.

before rinsing. Rinsing is performed in the same pattern as the scrub. The third scrub pattern is that used with perineal surgeries. In most perineal surgeries, a purse-string suture should be placed around the anus before scrubbing (Figure 10.19). Then, perform a target pattern on the clipped area to the right and left of the anus. As with other patterns, the scrub is followed by a rinse. For deep area scrubbing, such as oral procedures, a cotton tip applicator soaked with antiseptic solution can be used to swab the oral mucosa.

After rough scrub prepping is complete, the animal is moved to the surgical suite and positioned so that the operative site is accessible to the surgeon. The animal is typically placed on a circulating warm water heating pad. If monopolar electrosurgery is used, the ground plate should be positioned under the animal and an appropriate quantity of contact gel should be applied. Adhesive ground plates require clipping of hair and contain conductive gel with the adhesive so that no additional contact gel should be applied. The body is braced in position with a thoracoabdominal positioner (Figure 10.16), sandbags, a vacuum-activated positioning device, or other stabilizing aid. Tape, a foam rubber tube, or rolled towels may be used to secure and elevate the head, neck, or body. The animal's limbs are tied to the table

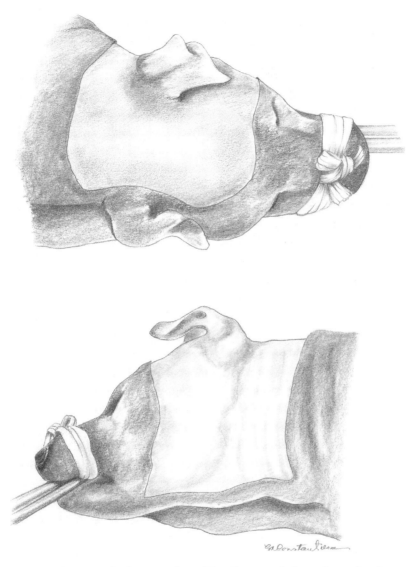

Figure 10.12   Clipping for an auricular procedure. The clip extends from the periocular area, caudally to the center of the neck, dorsally to the contralateral ear, and ventrally to the midline of the neck. Both sides of the pinna should be clipped.

using two loose loops, the distal loop being a half hitch (Figure 10.20). Care must be taken to apply these loops loosely to avoid ischemic injury to the distal limbs. For limb procedures, the limb should be carefully suspended with tape from an intravenous fluid stand (Figure 10.17).

It is very important for successful surgery to place and secure the animal in proper position on the operating table. The specific positioning depends on the procedure to be performed. For abdominal procedures, the animal is placed in dorsal recumbence with all four legs loosely

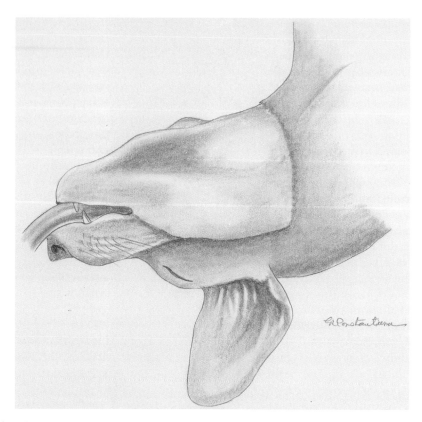

Figure 10.13   Clipping for a ventral approach to the mandible. The entire lower jaw is clipped. The clip extends caudally to the center of the neck.

secured to the operating table (Figure 10.21). Deep-chested dogs may require a thoracoabdominal positioner (Figure 10.21), bracing with sandbags, or some other stabilizing aid. Some operating tables are designed with adjustability to form a V-trough. For canine castration, the dog is placed and tied in the same position as for an abdominal procedure (Figure 10.22). For feline castration, the cat is placed in lateral recumbence with the pelvic limbs pulled toward the head (Figure 10.4). Some surgeons prefer dorsal recumbence for feline castration, which requires some sort of positioning aid. For thoracic surgery, the patient is placed in lateral (Figure 10.23) or dorsal (Figure 10.24) recumbence depending on the intended approach. The thoracic limbs are extended cranially as much as

possible and secured to the table, taking care to avoid ischemic injury that could occur if leg ties are too tight. For thoracolumbar spinal surgery (Figure 10.25), sandbags or rolled padding can be used to brace an animal and prevent leaning to one side. Tape applied across the scapulae and iliac wings helps provide stability. Thoracic limbs are extended cranially and the pelvic limbs are bent in a natural lying position. For a ventral approach to the cervical region (Figure 10.26), the thoracic limbs are secured caudally with ropes, and rolled padding is placed under the neck. The maxilla is secured to the table with tape to maintain symmetry. Lateral positioning aids along the thorax are usually also required to maintain straight positioning. For a dorsal approach to the neck (Figure 10.27),

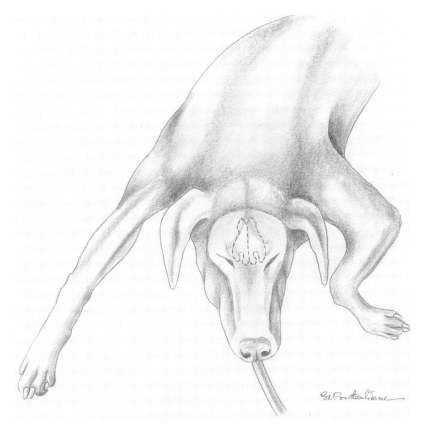

Figure 10.14   Clipping for a dorsal approach to the nasal cavity and/or frontal sinuses. The entire frontal sinus area and the nasal cavity region including the ocular area are clipped.

rolled padding is placed under the neck and the head is secured with tape over the occipital protuberance. For most orthopedic procedures, the animal is placed in lateral recumbence (Figure 10.28). If the right limb is the surgical site, the animal is placed in left lateral recumbence. If the left limb is the focus, the animal is positioned in right lateral recumbence. For a limb procedure where exposure of the paw is required (Figure 10.29), the entire limb, including the paw, should be clipped, and a towel clamp may be applied to the claw for manipulating the limb. For perineal procedures (Figure 10.30), the animal is typically placed in ventral recumbence. The thoracic limbs are secured to

the table and the pelvic limbs are tied so that they hang over the edge at the end of the table. Rolled towels are placed between the table and limbs for padding. The tail is fixed over the back with tape. For feline perineal urethrostomy, the cat may be placed in dorsal recumbence with pelvic limbs forward to facilitate access to abdomen if prepubic urethrostomy becomes necessary. For auricular procedures (Figure 10.31), the animal is placed in lateral recumbence. Vacuum-activated positioning devices or towels are used to brace the animal's head. The ear is manipulated with a towel forceps clamped on the end of the pinna and secured to an intravenous fluid stand with tape. For periocular

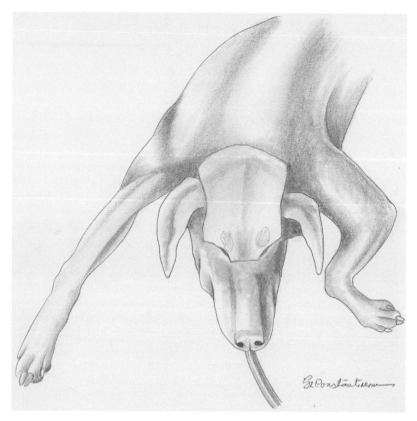

Figure 10.15 Clipping for a dorsal approach to the cranium. The entire dorsal skull including the upper ocular area and the bilateral skull is clipped. The periocular area is clipped when the rostral cranium must be approached.

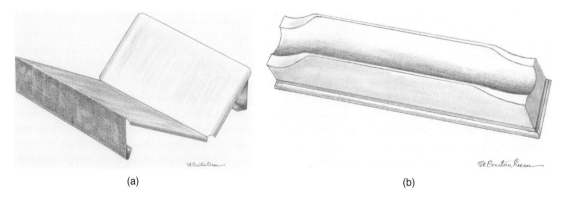

(a)   (b)

Figure 10.16 Thoracoabdominal positioner (a) for most dogs and (b) for small dogs and cats.

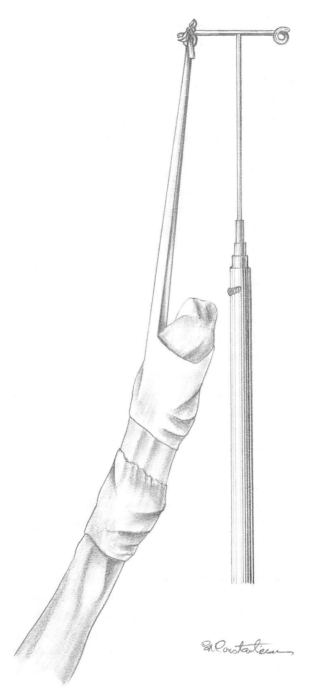

Figure 10.17   Positioning for a thoracic limb procedure where exposure of the paw is not required. The clipped paw is excluded from the surgical area by placing a latex glove over the distal extremity and securing the glove to the limb with tape. The glove should be covered with tape and the limb suspended with tape from an intravenous fluid stand.

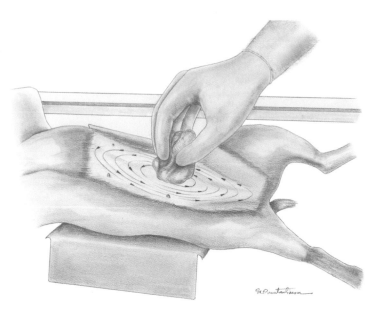

Figure 10.18 Abdominal preparation. With the animal secured in proper position, scrubbing is performed at the proposed incision site using circular motion, moving from the center to the periphery. Referred to as the rough scrub, this first scrub does not require the use of sterile gloves. A nonsterile examination glove is implied in this illustration.

procedures (Figure 10.32), the animal's head is placed on a folded towel or an elevated conforming rest (vacuum-activated positioning device) so that the eye can be positioned exactly as required. Intraocular procedures require the animal to be placed in dorsal recumbence. For extraocular procedures, the animal is placed in ventral or lateral recumbence. For oral procedures, the animal is placed in dorsal, ventral, or lateral recumbence. If an endotracheal tube

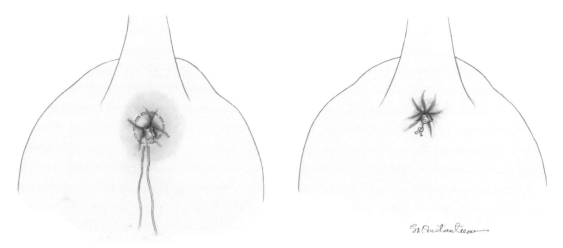

Figure 10.19 Anal purse-string suture. In order to prevent fecal contamination during perineal surgery, a purse-string suture is placed around the anus (left) and tied to occlude the anus (right). Prior to tightening the purse-string suture, a lubricated gauze tampon is placed in the rectum to contain feces.

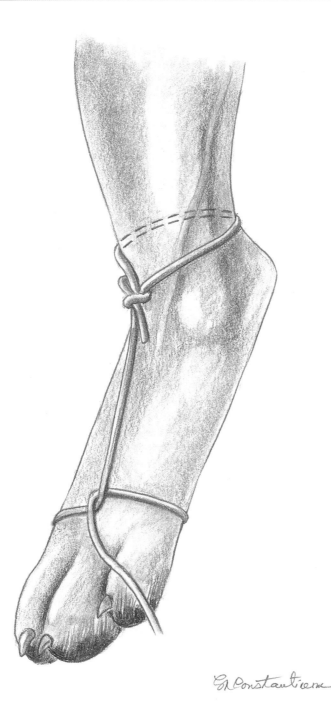

Figure 10.20 Securing limbs to the operating table. The limb is tied to the operating table using two loose loops, the distal loop being a half-hitch. Care is taken to make sure the loops do not compromise blood supply.

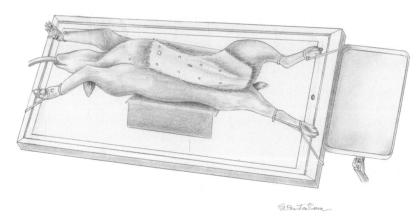

Figure 10.21   Positioning for an abdominal procedure. The animal is placed in dorsal recumbence with all four legs loosely secured to the operating table. Deep-chested animals must be placed in a thoracoabdominal positioner or braced by sandbags, towels, or other positioning aid to maintain straight positioning.

will interfere with the surgical field, it can be placed through the pharynx into the trachea via a lateral cervical incision (pharyngeal intubation). When positioning for a dorsal approach to the nasal cavity or the frontal sinuses, rolled padding is placed under the mandible and the mandible is secured to the table with tape (Figure 10.33).

The final sterile preparation is performed after the animal is positioned appropriately on the operating table. For the final sterile preparation, a sterile bowl and sterile gauze are used, and sterile gloves are worn. The germicidal scrub is poured into a sterile bowl. Sponges are handled with sterile sponge forceps or a gloved hand using aseptic technique.

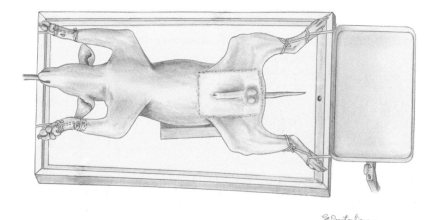

Figure 10.22   Positioning for canine castration. The animal is placed and tied in the same position as for an abdominal procedure (see also Figure 10.21).

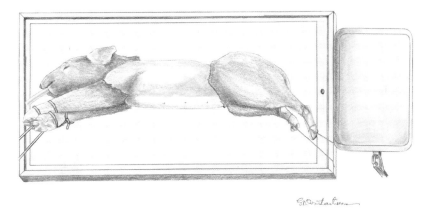

Figure 10.23   Positioning for lateral thoracotomy. The patient is placed in lateral recumbence. The thoracic limbs are extended cranially as much as possible and secured to the table.

Scrubbing is started at the incision site. A circular scrubbing motion is used, moving from the center to the periphery (Figure 10.34). Sponges should not be returned from the periphery to the center. Sponges are discarded after reaching the periphery. The final sterile preparation is performed in the same pattern as the initial nonsterile preparation. When using povidone-iodine and alcohol, the site is scrubbed alternatively with each solution three times to allow for five minutes of contact time. When the final povidone-iodine scrub is completed, a 10% povidone-iodine solution should be sprayed on the site. When chlorhexidine is used, the final chlorhexidine scrub is followed by spraying with chlorhexidine solution. Dry sterile gauze, instead of alcohol, is used to wipe away chlorhexidine scrub after each scrub application.

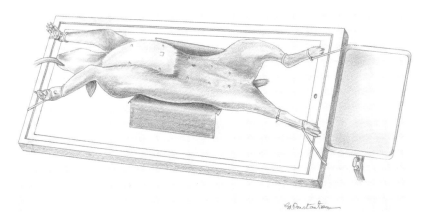

Figure 10.24   Positioning for median sternotomy. The animal is placed and tied in the same position as for an abdominal procedure. The thoracic limbs are extended cranially as much as possible and secured to the table, taking care to avoid vascular compromise by the leg ties. Deep-chested animals must be placed in a thoracoabdominal positioner, braced by sandbags, or stabilized with some other positioning aid to maintain straight positioning.

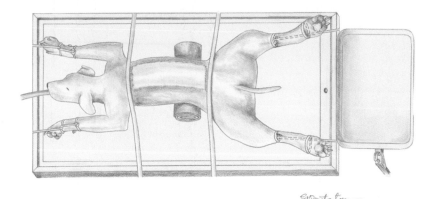

Figure 10.25 Positioning for thoracolumbar spinal surgery. The animal is symmetrically secured with ropes, and rolled padding is placed under the area where surgery will be performed. Tape can be used for additional stabilization across the shoulders and pelvic region. Lateral positioning aids (not shown) may also be helpful to maintain proper positioning.

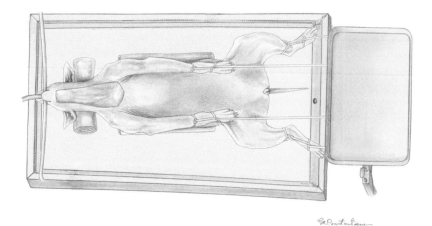

Figure 10.26 Positioning for a ventral approach to the cervical region. The thoracic limbs are secured caudally with ropes and rolled padding is placed under the neck. The maxilla is secured to the table with tape incorporating the canine teeth to maintain symmetry. Lateral positioning aids along the thorax may also be helpful to maintain proper positioning.

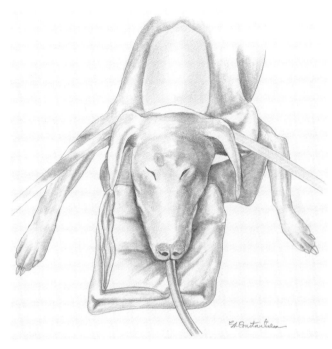

Figure 10.27 Positioning for a dorsal approach to the neck. Rolled padding is placed under the neck, and the head is secured to the table with tape on the occipital protuberance.

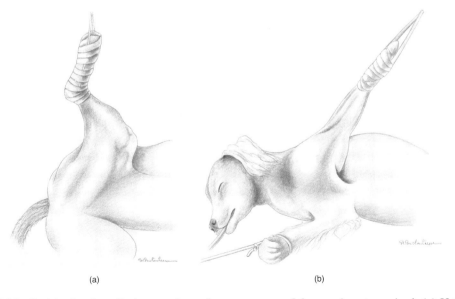

(a)   (b)

Figure 10.28 Positioning for a limb procedure where exposure of the paw is not required. (a) If the right limb is the surgical site, the animal is placed in left lateral recumbence. An examination glove is placed over unshaven paw and tape covers the examination glove. A tape stirrup is secured to the foot for handling the limb. (b) If the left limb is the focus, the animal is positioned in right lateral recumbence.

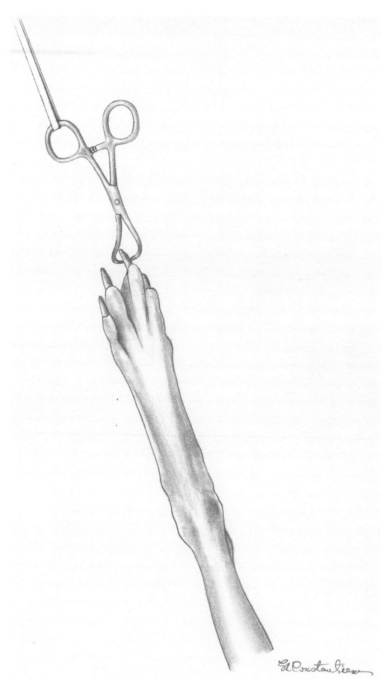

Figure 10.29   Positioning for a limb procedure where exposure of the paw is required. The entire limb including the paw should be clipped and the limb is secured with a towel clamp applied to the claw for manipulating the limb. Only the nail should be clamped so that there is no possibility of injuring the distal interphalangeal joint.

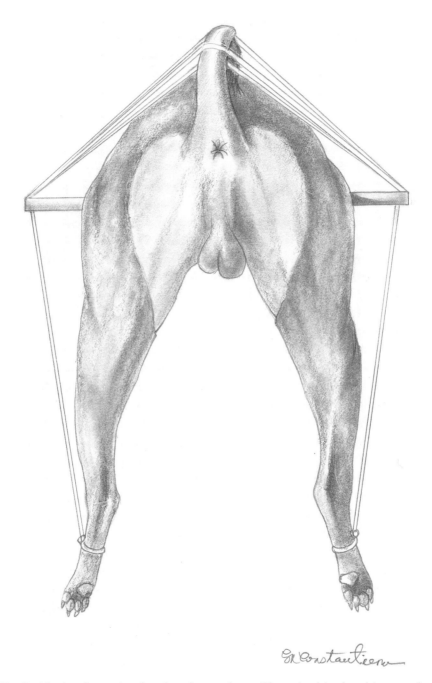

Figure 10.30 Positioning for perineal and anal procedures. The animal is placed in ventral recumbence with pelvic limbs hanging over the padded edge of the surgical table, and the tail is fixed over the back with tape. The pelvic limbs are secured over the edge at the end of the table. The table edge should be well padded to protect the limbs from pressure injury. Care must also be exercised to prevent distal limb ischemia caused by the leg ties. Using tape instead of rope may be preferred for securing the distal limbs.

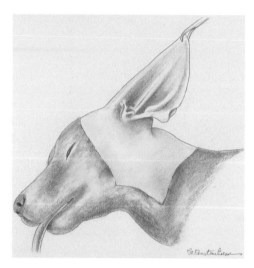

Figure 10.31   Positioning for auricular surgery. The ear is manipulated with a towel forceps clamped on the end of the pinna and attached to an intravenous fluid stand with tape.

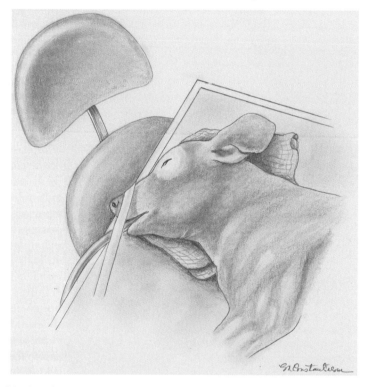

Figure 10.32   Positioning for periocular procedures. The animal is placed in lateral recumbence (for intraocular procedures, the animal is placed in dorsal recumbence). The animal's head is placed on towels (or vacuum-activated positioning devices) so that the eye can be positioned exactly as required. The nose is secured with tape.

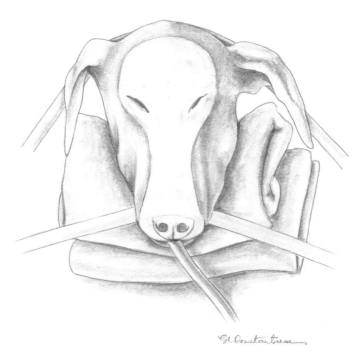

Figure 10.33 Positioning for a dorsal approach to the nasal cavity and/or frontal sinus. Rolled padding is placed under the mandible and the mandible is secured to the operating table with tape. Tape across the occipital protuberance further stabilizes the head.

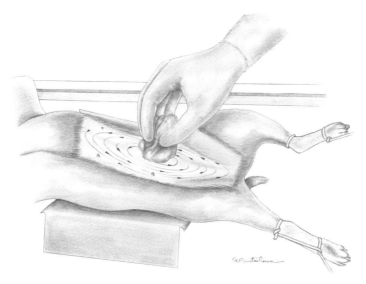

Figure 10.34 Abdominal preparation. After positioning the animal on the operating table, the final sterile preparation is performed in similar fashion as the rough scrub, except sterile gloves are worn and sterile supplies are used. Scrubbing is begun at the proposed incision site. A circular scrubbing motion is used, moving from the center to the periphery.

ADDITIONAL RESOURCES

Additional information about patient preparation in small animal surgery can be found in the following textbooks:

1. Fossum TW, ed. *Small Animal Surgery*, 3rd ed. St. Louis, Missouri: Mosby Elsevier, 2007.

2. Busch SJ, ed. *Small Animal Surgical Nursing Skills and Concepts*. St. Louis, Missouri: Mosby Elsevier, 2006.

3. Slatter D, ed. *Textbook of Small Animal Surgery*, 3rd ed. Philadelphia, Pennsylvania: Saunders, 2003.

Chapter 11

SURGICAL DRAPING

Hun-Young Yoon and Fred Anthony Mann

Draping isolates the surgical site from contaminated areas and provides a sterile working area. Once the animal has been positioned and the skin aseptically prepared, the animal is draped by a gowned and gloved surgical team member. There are two layers of drapes for patient draping. The first layer consists of four quarter drapes. The second layer consists of one full drape.

For placement of the first layer of drapes, the upper corners of the folded drape are grasped with three fingers (thumb, index, and third fingers), and the part of drape that is located toward the surgeon is unfolded (Figure 11.1). The most upper fold is left folded to provide two layers of barrier in the area closest to the proposed incision. The upper corners of the folded drape are inserted between the index and third fingers in scissor-like fashion with the flap of the retained fold away from the person placing the drape (Figure 11.2). Then, the hands are rotated so that the palms face away from the person placing the drape, allowing the drape corners to serve as barriers of protection as the drape is placed (Figure 11.2). Portions of the drapes that drop below table

level should be considered nonsterile because they are not within the surgeon's visual field and their sterility cannot be verified. Four quarter drapes are placed at the periphery of the prepared area according to the surgical procedures [abdominal (Figure 11.3), orchiectomy (Figure 11.4), thoracic (Figure 11.5), neurologic (Figure 11.6), orthopedic (Figure 11.7), perineal (Figure 11.8), ocular (Figure 11.9), auricular (Figure 11.10), oral (Figure 11.11), nasal (Figure 11.12), and cranial (Figure 11.13)] to be performed. The edge of each lateral drape should be approximately 2 cm from the proposed skin incision. If an abdominal incision extends to the pubis in male dogs, the prepuce should be clamped to one side with a sterile towel clamp before the placement of the first layer of drapes (Figure 11.14). The prepuce is clamped to the side opposite to the side where the surgeon stands. The prepuce is left unclamped and draped into the surgical field when intraoperative urethral catheterization is planned, such as with cystotomy for removal of urinary calculi. For canine orchiectomy, the first drape is placed over the preputial opening cranially (Figure 11.4a). Four quarter drapes are placed at the periphery of the prepared area and secured at the corners with sterile Backhaus towel clamps (Figure 11.4b). For lateral thoracotomy (Figure 11.5), the cranial and caudal

Fundamentals of Small Animal Surgery, 1st edition.
By Fred Anthony Mann, Gheorghe M. Constantinescu and Hun-Young Yoon.

Figure 11.1 A quarter drape as it is removed from the sterile pack. The upper corners of the folded drape are grasped with three fingers (thumb, index, and third fingers). The part of drape that is located toward the surgeon is unfolded, leaving folded the top portion of the drape held by the fingers. The remaining fold of the quarter drape faces the surgical area (side of drape shown in bottom picture) and the other side of the quarter drape faces the surgeon.

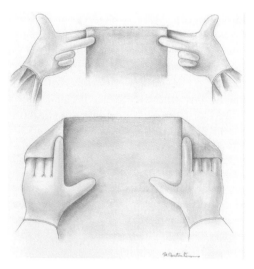

Figure 11.2 A quarter drape held for application to the patient. The upper corners of the folded drape are inserted between the index and third fingers in scissor-like fashion, and the hands are rotated with the palms away from the surgeon in order to protect the surgeon's gloves during drape application.

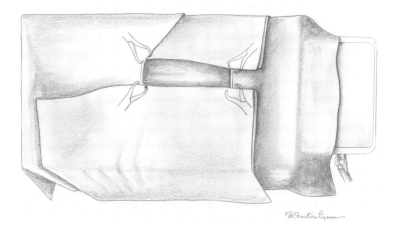

Figure 11.3   Draping for abdominal procedures. Placement of quarter drapes depends on proposed incision sites. The edge of each lateral drape should be approximately 2 cm from the proposed skin incision. The application of quarter drapes is followed by placement of a full drape that will be fenestrated. The order of quarter drape placement is somewhat dictated by surgeon preference, but progressing from caudal to right lateral to cranial to left lateral is recommended. Note: In this figure the progression is from caudal to left lateral to cranial to right lateral.

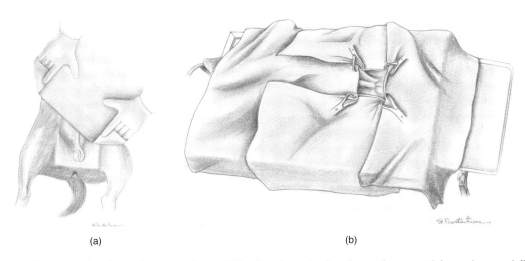

(a)   (b)

Figure 11.4   Draping for canine castration. (a) The first drape is placed over the preputial opening cranially. Note how the gloved fingers are protected from contamination. (b) Four quarter drapes are placed at the periphery of the prepared area and secured at the corners with sterile Backhaus towel clamps. The application of quarter drapes is followed by placement of a full drape that will be fenestrated.

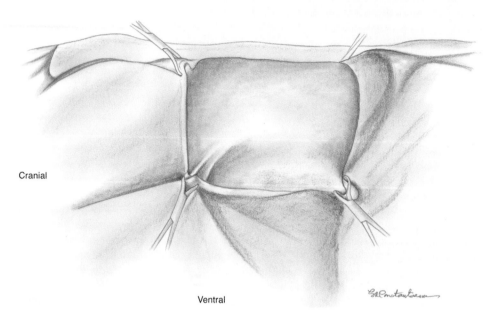

Cranial

Ventral

Figure 11.5 Draping for left lateral thoracotomy. The edges of the cranial and caudal drapes should be greater than 2 cm from the proposed skin incision, making sure that enough aseptically prepared skin is accessible for thoracostomy tube placement. The dorsal and ventral drapes should be placed on dorsal and ventral midlines. The application of quarter drapes is followed by placement of a full drape that will be fenestrated.

drapes should be placed first. The edges of the cranial and caudal drapes should be greater than 2 cm from the proposed skin incision. Caudally, there should be enough exposed aseptically prepared skin for thoracostomy tube placement. The dorsal and ventral drapes should be placed to allow incision from dorsal midline to ventral midline. For a dorsal approach to the cervical region (Figure 11.6), the cranial drape is placed caudal to the occipital protuberance, and the caudal drape is placed cranial to the thoracic vertebra. The lateral drapes are placed approximately 2 cm lateral to the proposed incision. For a pelvic limb procedure (Figure 11.7), the medial drape should cover the genitalia, and placement of the lateral drape depends on the proposed incision site. Four quarter drapes are placed and secured with sterile Backhaus towel clamps after the leg is hung. For a per-

ineal procedure (Figure 11.8), the first drape is placed dorsally. The second and third drapes are placed bilaterally. The three drapes are secured with two sterile Backhaus towel clamps. Another two towel clamps are used to secure drapes when the fourth drape is placed ventrally. Additional towel clamps can be used to secure the lateral parts of the bilateral drapes and ventral drape. For an ophthalmic procedure (Figure 11.9), three drapes are placed in triangulated fashion around the eye and secured with three Backhaus towel clamps. For an auricular procedure (Figure 11.10), four quarter drapes are placed around the ear with the entire pinna draped into the surgical field. If ear canal resection or ablation is performed, access to ear canals should be provided by drape placement. Drapes are used to isolate surgical fields involving the oral cavity (Figure 11.11)

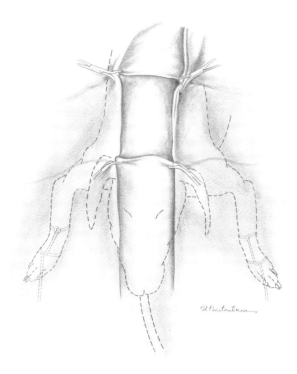

Figure 11.6   Draping for a dorsal approach to the cervical spine. The cranial drape is placed caudal to the occipital protuberance, the caudal drape is placed cranial to the thoracic vertebrae, and the lateral drapes are applied approximately 2 cm lateral to the proposed incision. The application of quarter drapes is followed by placement of a full drape that will be fenestrated.

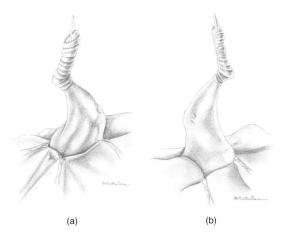

(a)   (b)

Figure 11.7   Draping for a left pelvic limb procedure. (a) Placement of the lateral drape depends on the proposed incision site. (b) The medial drape should cover the penis and scrotum in males, and the vulva in females. Four quarter drapes are placed and secured with sterile Backhaus towel clamps after the leg is hung. The application of quarter drapes is followed by sterile wrapping of the distal limb, which will be pulled through a fenestrated full drape.

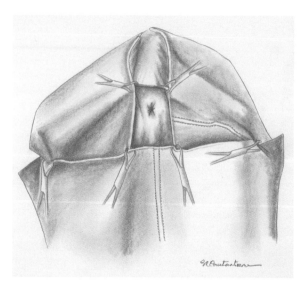

Figure 11.8 Draping for a perineal procedure. The first drape is placed dorsally. The second and third drapes are placed bilaterally. The three drapes are secured with two sterile Backhaus towel clamps. Another two towel clamps are used to secure drapes when the fourth drape is placed ventrally. Additional towel clamps can be used to secure the lateral parts of the bilateral drapes and ventral drape. The application of quarter drapes is followed by placement of a full drape that will be fenestrated.

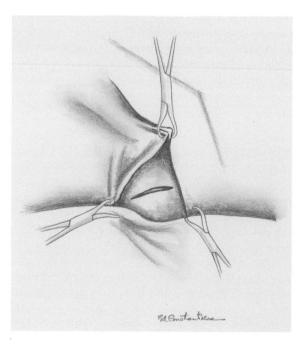

Figure 11.9 Draping for an ophthalmic procedure. Three drapes are placed around the eye and secured with three Backhaus towel clamps. The application of the triangulated drapes is followed by placement of a full drape that will be fenestrated.

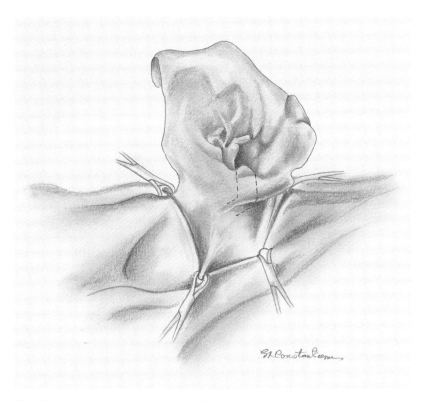

Figure 11.10   Draping for an auricular procedure. Four quarter drapes are placed around the ear with the entire pinna draped into the surgical site. If ear canal resection or ablation is performed, access to ear canals should be provided by drape placement. The application of quarter drapes is followed by placement of a full drape that will be fenestrated.

despite the inability to eliminate all oral bacteria. For bilateral mandibulectomy, the rostral drape is placed between the upper jaw and the lower jaw to the level of the lip commissure, and the caudal drape is placed caudal to the end of the mandibules (Figure 11.11a). For unilateral mandibulectomy, the mandible is isolated with four drapes and four Backhaus towel clamps (Figure 11.11b). One drape is placed over the endotracheal tube (Figure 11.11b). For intraoral or lateral approach to the maxilla, the maxilla is isolated with four drapes and four Backhaus towel clamps (Figure 11.11c). One drape is placed over the endotracheal tube (Figure 11.11c). The hair should be clipped for a lateral approach to the maxilla prior to prepping and

draping. For a dorsal approach to the nasal cavity or the frontal sinus (Figure 11.12), the caudal drape is placed immediately caudal to the frontal sinus and the rostral drape is placed near the nasal planum. Lateral drapes are placed approximately 1 cm lateral to the proposed incision. For a dorsal approach to the cranium (Figure 11.13), the rostral drape is placed at the caudal portion of the frontal sinus and the caudal drape is placed at the occipital protuberance. Placement of lateral drapes depends on the amount of access to the skull that is needed.

Once drapes are placed, they should not be readjusted toward the incision site because this carries bacteria onto the prepared skin. Drapes

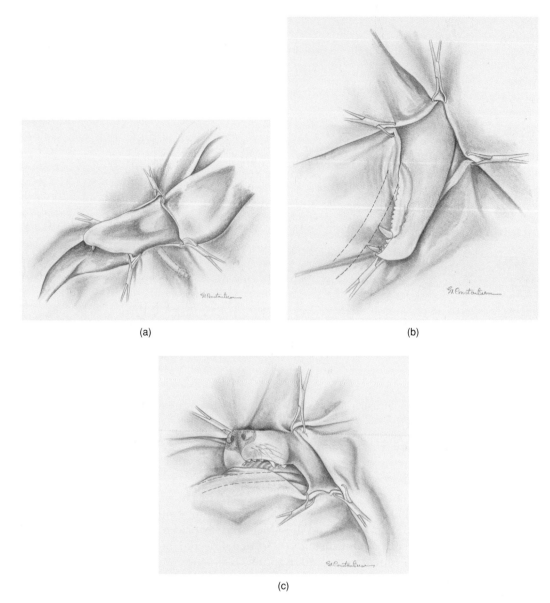

(a)

(b)

(c)

Figure 11.11 Draping for oral procedures. (a) For bilateral mandibulectomy, the rostral drape is placed between the upper jaw and the lower jaw to the level of the lip commissure, and the caudal drape is placed caudally to the end of the mandibules. (b) For unilateral mandibulectomy, the mandible is isolated with four drapes and four Backhaus towel clamps. One drape is placed over the endotracheal tube. (c) For intraoral or lateral approach to the maxilla, the maxilla is isolated with four drapes and four Backhaus towel clamps. One drape is placed over the endotracheal tube. The hair should be clipped for a lateral approach to the maxilla. The application of quarter drapes is followed by placement of a full drape that will be fenestrated.

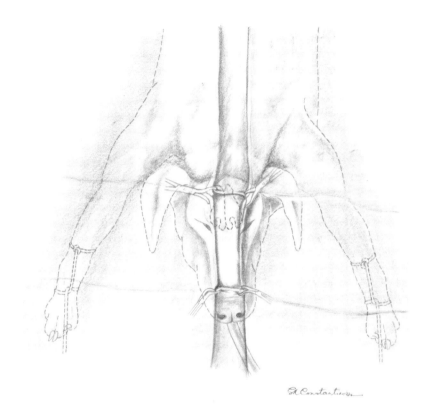

Figure 11.12   Draping for a dorsal approach to the nasal cavity or frontal sinuses. The caudal drape is placed at the caudal portion of the frontal sinuses and the rostral drape is placed on the rostral portion of the nasal cavity. Lateral drapes are placed approximately 1 cm lateral to the proposed incision. The application of quarter drapes is followed by placement of a full drape that will be fenestrated.

placed too close to the incision may be pulled away from the incision. The first layer of drapes is secured to the patient's skin by Backhaus towel clamps (Figure 11.15). The tips of the towel clamps are placed through the skin. Once the tip of the towel clamp penetrates the skin, it is considered nonsterile and should not be removed and repositioned. Typically, four towel clamps are used, one at each quarter drape junction. If the proposed incision site is long, additional Backhaus towel clamps can be added. For celiotomy and thoracotomy, these additional clamps are applied after fenestrating the full drape. The clamp is placed through both the

full drape and underlying quarter drape at the fenestration and quarter drape edges (Figure 11.16).

For the placement of the second layer of drape, a specially folded full drape is placed on the proposed incision site (Figure 11.17). It is bilaterally unfolded first (Figure 11.18a), then it is unfolded cranially and caudally (Figure 11.18b). The full drape is placed over the animal, the entire surgical table, and the instrument table to provide a continuous sterile field (Figure 11.19). Full drapes that are not folded specifically for this type of draping (i.e., folded in standard accordion fashion) may require an

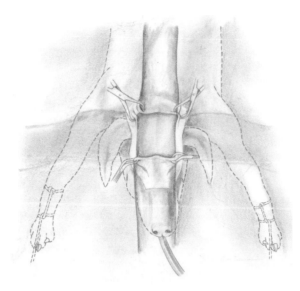

Figure 11.13 Draping for a dorsal approach to the cranium. The rostral drape is placed on the caudal portion of the frontal sinuses and the caudal drape is placed on the occipital protuberance. Placement of lateral drapes depends on the amount of access to the skull that is needed. The application of quarter drapes is followed by placement of a full drape that will be fenestrated.

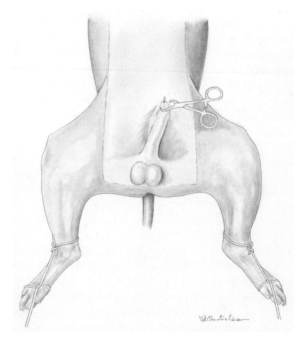

Figure 11.14 Prepuce placement for abdominal incisions. The prepuce should be aseptically clamped to one side with a sterile towel clamp before the placement of the first layer of drapes. Note: A right-handed surgeon typically clamps the prepuce to the dog's left side.

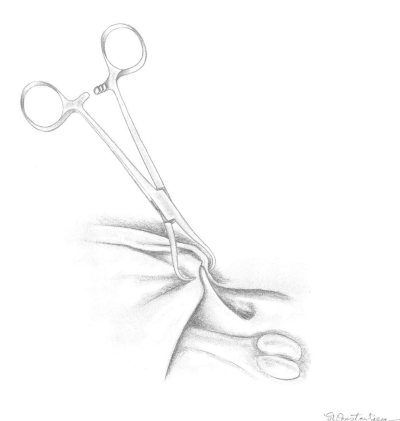

Figure 11.15   Placement of towel clamps. Two adjacent drapes and skin should be included between the tips of the towel clamps when drapes are secured with sterile Backhaus towel clamps.

assistant for placement, particularly when this drape is large. An appropriately sized hole is made in the full drape over the proposed incision site (Figure 11.20). Some full drapes are already fenestrated and care must be taken to place the fenestration in the correct spot. Additional towel clamps can be used to secure the full drape to the four quarter drapes to prevent shifting. These additional towel forceps should be strategically placed (Figure 11.16) and as few as possible should be used so that they do not interfere with surgery. It is common for suture to become tangled on these exposed clamps during closure of the incision.

After an appropriately sized hole is made in the full drape, the skin incision is performed. After incising the subcutaneous tissue so that the skin edges retract sufficiently, the technique referred to as "toweling in" may be performed.[1] A drape is placed along one edge of the incision parallel to the edge of the incision line and covering the other edge (Figure 11.21). One fold is left in the drape so that the folded edge will be secured to the skin edge, and when the secured drape is flipped, the flap fold will be against the full drape. The purpose of toweling in is to further isolate the surgical wound from the patient's skin. While no recent studies have

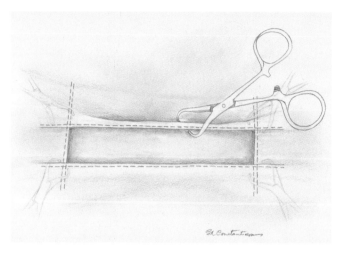

Figure 11.16 Placement of additional towel clamps. If the proposed incision site is long, additional Backhaus towel clamps can be added between the cranial and caudal clamps after fenestration of the full drape.

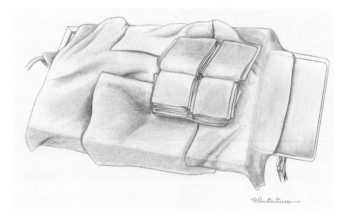

Figure 11.17 Application of the outer layer of drape (full drape). A folded full drape is placed on the proposed incision site.

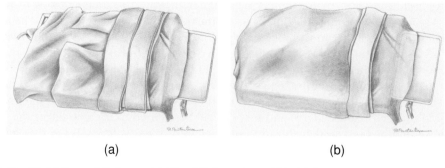

(a) (b)

Figure 11.18 Unfolding a full drape. (a) The full drape is unfolded bilaterally first and (b) then unfolded cranially and caudally.

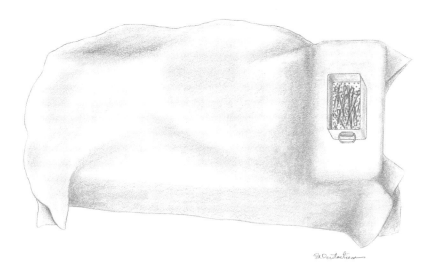

Figure 11.19   Completed application of a full drape. The full drape is placed over the animal, the entire surgical table, and the instrument table (Mayo stand) to provide a continuous sterile field.

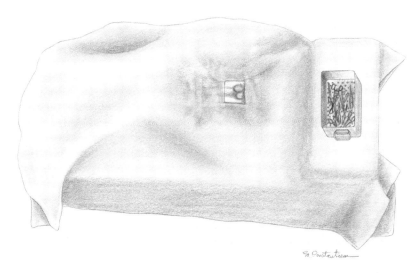

Figure 11.20   Making a hole in a full drape. An appropriately sized hole is made at the proposed incision site. Note: Some full drapes are already fenestrated and care must be taken to place the fenestration in the correct spot.

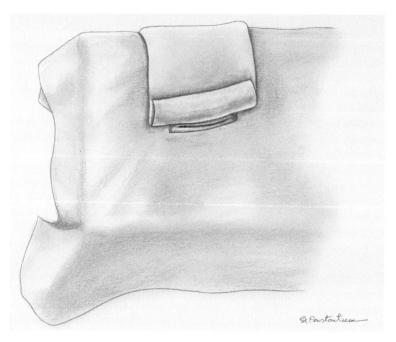

Figure 11.21 Toweling in. After the skin and subcutaneous tissue have been incised, a drape is placed along one edge of the incision line parallel to the edge of the incision line and covering the other edge. One fold is left in the drape so that the folded edge will be secured to the skin edge. When the secured drape is flipped, the flap fold will be against the full drape.

substantiated the claim of a 1962 study[2] that toweling in actually decreases infection rates compared to when it is not done, isolating the surgical wound in this manner offers some other advantages. For example, instruments are less likely to fall under the full drape and quarter drapes, and particulate matter from under the drapes is less likely to gain access to the exposed tissues. The latter is of particular concern when warm air flow devices are being used to prevent patient hypothermia. Toweling in also helps prevent tissue desiccation that occurs when warm air flow devices push air from under the quarter and full drapes, causing air to blow across the exposed tissues. The method of toweling in involves attaching drapes to the edges of the skin incision with clips (Figure 11.22), towel clamps (Figure 11.23), or a continuous suture pattern. After making a linea alba or intercostal incision, the edges of the incision are covered with laparotomy sponges and Balfour or Finochietto rib retractors (Figures 11.24 and 11.25). Surgeons who do not towel in, use these laparotomy sponges to provide additional barrier from exposed skin. Some surgeons will apply an adhesive drape (3M™ Ioban™ 2 Antimicrobial Incise Drape, 3M Health Care, St. Paul, MN) to the skin and full drape prior to making a skin incision, especially in very small patients, to serve the function of toweling in. It is debatable whether plastic adhesive draping significantly contributes to reduction of surgical infections,[3] but this technique affords other advantages of surgical field isolation similar to toweling in.

For orthopedic procedures involving long bones and joints, access to the entire limb is necessary. The limb is suspended above the

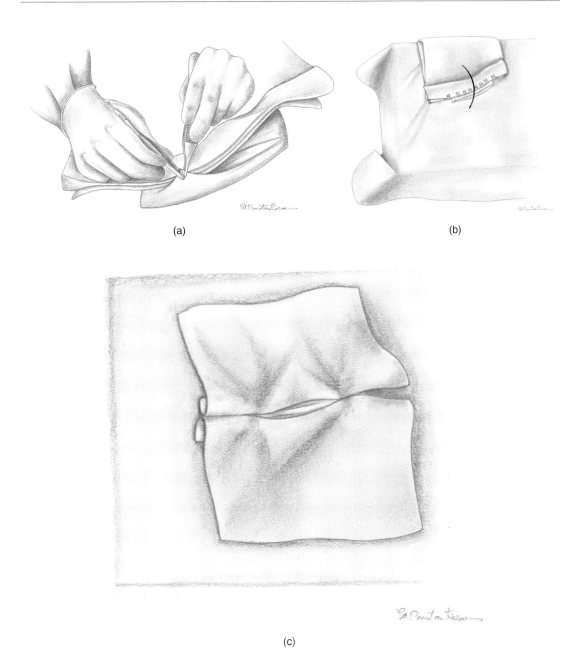

(a)

(b)

(c)

Figure 11.22   Toweling in using clips. (a) The drape is attached to the edge of the skin incision with clips. (b) After the second drape is applied, two additional clips are placed, one cranially and one caudally, to attach both drapes at the level of the beginning and end of the incision. Then, the second drape is turned over on the opposite side. (c) Both drapes are attached to the edges of the skin incision.

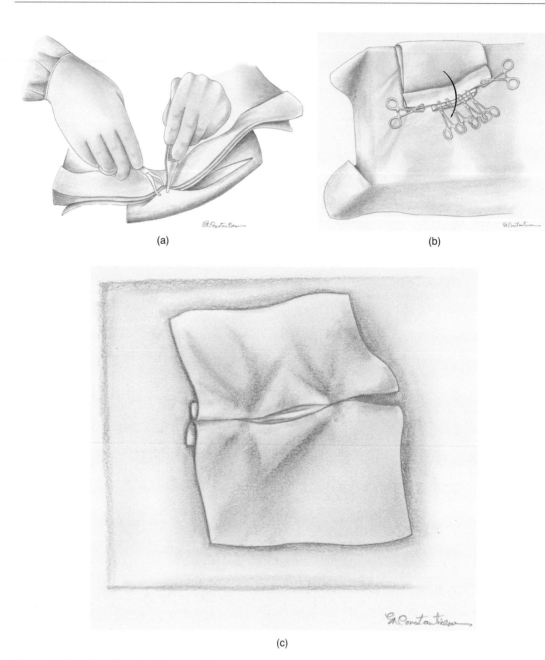

(a)

(b)

(c)

Figure 11.23   Toweling in using towel clamps. (a) The drape is attached to the edge of the skin incision with towel clamps. (b) After the second drape is applied, two additional towel clamps are placed, one cranially and one caudally, to attach both drapes at the level of the beginning and end of the incision. Then, the second drape is turned over on the opposite side. (c) Both drapes are attached to the edges of the skin incision.

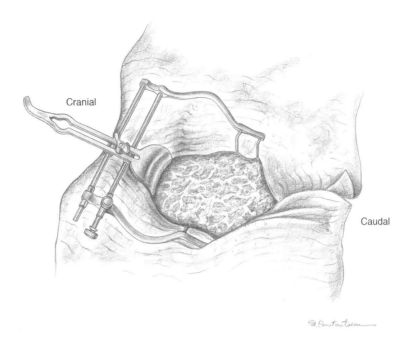

Figure 11.24 Placing laparotomy sponges and Balfour retractors in an abdominal procedure. After incising the linea alba, the incision edges are covered with laparotomy sponges. Balfour retractors are used to retract the abdominal wall.

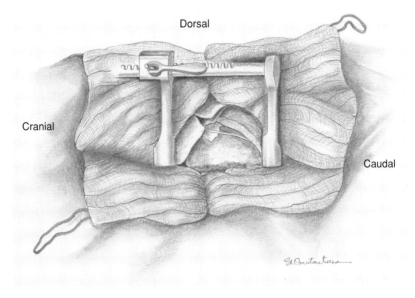

Figure 11.25 Placing laparotomy sponges and Finochietto retractors in left lateral thoracotomy. After making an incision between ribs, the incision edges are covered with laparotomy sponges. Finochietto retractors are used to retract the thoracic wall.

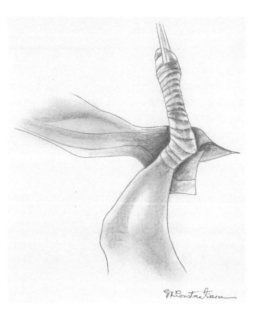

Figure 11.26 Small sterile drape used to wrap the distal limb. The drape should cover all of the taped area. The tape holding the elevated limb is cut by a nonsterile assistant while the sterile surgical member grasps the limb in the small sterile drape.

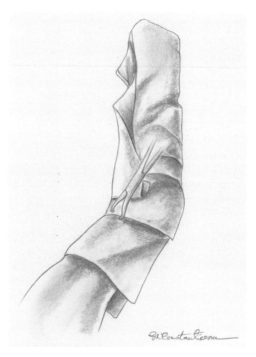

Figure 11.27 Attaching a small sterile drape that is wrapped around the distal limb. After it is wrapped, the drape is secured to the skin with sterile Backhaus towel clamps.

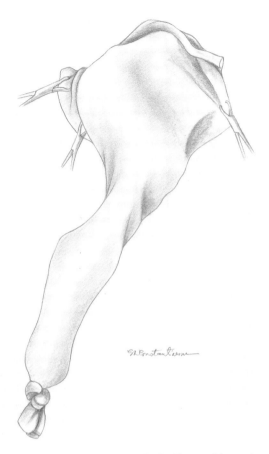

Figure 11.28   Sterile stockinette used to cover the entire limb. The stockinette is carefully unrolled down the limb and secured with sterile Backhaus towel clamps at the base of the limb on the body, clamping through the stockinette and underlying quarter drapes.

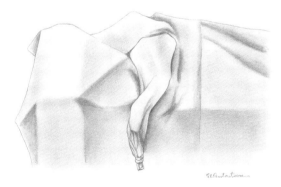

Figure 11.29   Full drape for limb procedure. The limb covered with a stockinette is placed through a fenestration in the full drape.

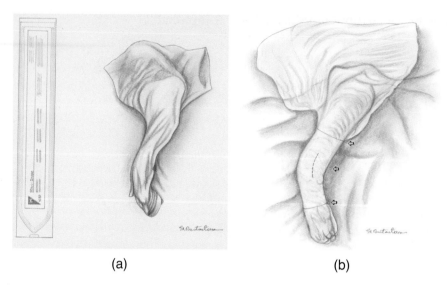

(a)   (b)

Figure 11.30   Combination of sterile plastic adhesive and stockinette for an orthopedic limb procedure. (a) Plastic adhesive drape (left) may be applied to the stockinette (right) over the proposed incision site. (b) Then, a fenestration (hashed line) is made in the plastic adhesive-stockinette combination (arrows) at the proposed incision site.

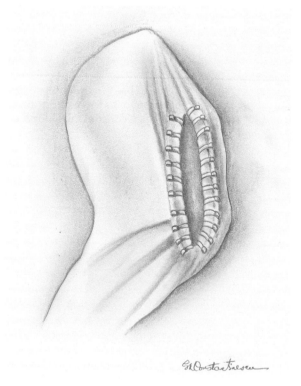

Figure 11.31   Toweling in for a limb procedure. The fenestration edges of the adhesive-stockinette combination are attached to the edges of the incised skin by clips after the skin incision is made.

surgery table or elevated by an assistant. The limb is isolated at its base by four quarter drapes and the drapes are secured with towel clamps (Figure 11.7). A small sterile drape is used to wrap the distal portion of the limb (Figure 11.26). The tape holding the elevated limb is cut while the sterile surgical member grasps the limb in the small sterile drape. The drape should cover all taped area and is secured with a towel clamp (Figure 11.27). Then, a stockinette is rolled up the limb to a point proximal to the proposed incision and secured with towel clamps at the base of the limb on the body (Figure 11.28). The limb is placed through a fenestration of a full drape (Figure 11.29). For toweling in of orthopedic procedures on long bones, a stockinette, plastic adhesive drape, or adhesive-stockinette combination can be used (Figure 11.30). When using an adhesive-stockinette combination, a fenestration is made over the proposed incision site, and the edges of this fenestration are sutured to the incised skin edges or secured to the incised skin edges using clips (Figure 11.31). The plastic adhesive drape at the surgical site is advantageous as a waterproof barrier.

REFERENCE

1. Knecht CD, Allen AR, Williams DJ, Johnson JH. *Fundamental Techniques in Veterinary Surgery*, 3rd ed. Philadelphia, Pennsylvania: Saunders Co, 1987:17–18.
2. Shepherd RC, Kinmonth JB. Skin preparation and towelling in prevention of wound infection. *Br Med J* 1962;2:151–153.
3. Webster J, Alghamdi A. Use of plastic adhesive drapes during surgery for preventing surgical site infection. *Cochrane Database Syst Rev* 2007(4):CD006353. DOI: 10.1002/14651858. CD006353.pub2.

ADDITIONAL RESOURCES

Additional information about draping in small animal surgery can be found in the following textbooks:

1. Fossum TW, ed. *Small Animal Surgery*, 3rd ed. St. Louis, Missouri: Mosby Elsevier, 2007.
2. Busch SJ, ed. *Small Animal Surgical Nursing Skills and Concepts*. St. Louis, Missouri: Mosby Elsevier, 2006.
3. Slatter D, ed. *Textbook of Small Animal Surgery*, 3rd ed. Philadelphia, Pennsylvania: Saunders, 2003.

Chapter 12

INSTRUMENT HANDLING

Hun-Young Yoon and Fred Anthony Mann

Successful accomplishment of small animal surgical procedures requires proper handling of surgical instruments. Proper instrument handling can minimize tissue trauma and avoid instrument damage.

Two general categories of instruments are ringed instruments and nonringed instruments. For ringed instruments, the thumb and fourth finger are usually placed in the upper and lower rings, respectively, and the index finger can be placed along the shank for added control and stability (Figure 12.1). For nonringed instruments, handling varies depending on the specific instrument.

The Backhaus towel forceps is placed using the ringed instrument handling technique. The tips of the Backhaus towel forceps are closed to secure surgical drapes to each other and to the patient's skin by clamping with the thumb and fourth finger (Figure 12.2).

There are three basic grips for holding a scalpel: fingertip grip (Figure 12.3), palm grip (Figure 12.4), and pencil grip (Figure 12.5). For the fingertip grip, the scalpel handle is held with the tips of fingers. The index finger can be placed either on the back of the scalpel blade

(Figure 12.3a) or on one side of the scalpel handle (Figure 12.3b). The fingertip grip is recommended for long incisions because arm movement is used instead of finger movement. For the palm grip, the scalpel handle is held with the palm while the thumb is placed on the back of the scalpel blade (Figure 12.4). This grip is recommended when great pressure must be applied to incise tissue. As with the fingertip grip, arm motion is used rather than finger motion. For the pencil grip, the scalpel handle is held like gripping a pencil in conventional pencil holding fashion (Figure 12.5). The pencil grip is best suited for short, precise incisions because finger movement is used instead of arm movement. With the scalpel blade inverted, the pencil grip is used to make the stab incision in the linea alba for celiotomy while thumb forceps hold the linea alba upward (Figure 12.6).

There are two basic grips for holding surgical scissors: the forehand grip and the backhand grip. For the forehand grip, the thumb and fourth finger (wide-based tripod grip) are placed in the upper and lower rings (Figure 12.7a), or the thenar eminence and fourth finger (thenar eminence-fourth finger grip) are placed out of the upper ring and in the lower ring, respectively (Figure 12.7b). For the backhand grip method, the thumb and index finger (thumb–index finger grip; Figure 12.8a) or the

Fundamentals of Small Animal Surgery, 1st edition.
By Fred Anthony Mann, Gheorghe M. Constantinescu and Hun-Young Yoon.
© 2011 Blackwell Publishing Ltd.

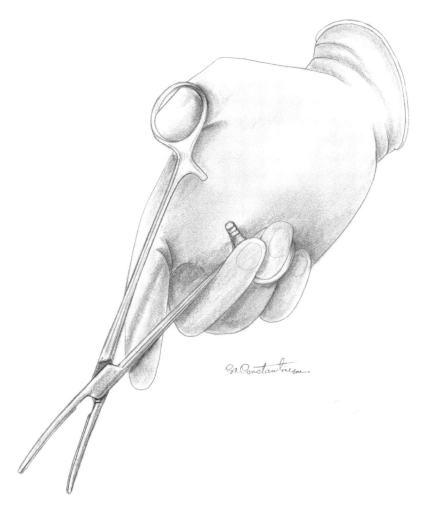

Figure 12.1   Ringed instrument (such as the Rochester-Carmalt shown in this picture) handling: The thumb and fourth fingers are placed in the rings, and the index finger is placed along the shank for added control and stability. [Note: There are other acceptable methods for holding needle holders and scissors, but other ringed instruments are held in this fashion.]

thumb and fourth finger (thumb–fourth finger grip; Figure 12.8b) are placed in the upper and lower rings. The scissor grip method that best utilizes the three scissor forces (closing, shearing, and torque) is the wide-based tripod grip. The thenar eminence–fourth finger grip provides adequate shearing force, reduced closing force, and practically no torque compared with the wide-based tripod grip. A backhand thumb–index finger grip (Figure 12.8a) is used when the surgeon must execute reverse cutting toward the surgeon's dominant side (from left to right for a right-handed surgeon). Alternately, the backhand thumb–fourth finger grip (Figure 12.8b) may be used for reversed cutting, but this method requires more body shifting than the backhand thumb–index finger grip.

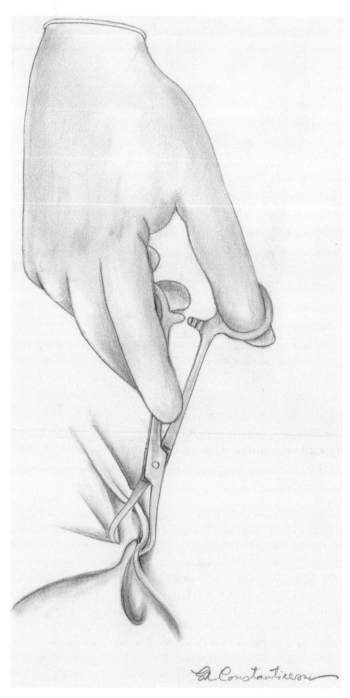

Figure 12.2   Backhaus towel forceps handling: The Backhaus towel forceps is clamped using the thumb and fourth fingers to secure surgical drapes to each other and to the patient's skin.

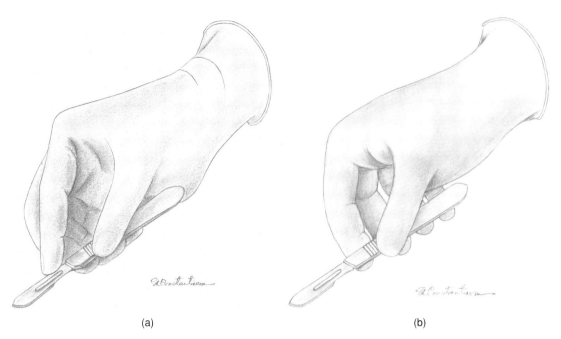

(a)   (b)

Figure 12.3   Scalpel handling (fingertip grip): For the fingertip grip, the scalpel handle is held with the tips of fingers. The index finger can be placed either (a) on the back of the scalpel blade or (b) on one side of the scalpel handle.

There are three basic methods of cutting tissues with scissors: scissor cutting (Figure 12.9a), push cutting (Figure 12.9b), and blunt dissection (Figure 12.9c). Scissor cutting and push cutting constitute sharp dissection (Figures 12.9a and 12.9b). Scissor cutting is most applicable for short incisions and heavy fascia. Long incision of delicate tissue is often initiated with a scissor cut and continued by push cutting (Figure 12.9b). Blunt dissection is used to separate anatomical structures, such as when developing skin flaps. Blunt dissection is typically avoided, because it is more traumatic than sharp dissection and tends to created excessive dead space.

There are two basic grips for holding instruments for manipulation of tissue. Thumb forceps are held with the thumb and index finger in chopstick fashion as mentioned in Chapter 5 (Figures 5.5a and 5.5b). Ringed instruments such as the Allis tissue forceps and the Babcock tissue forceps are handled using the ringed instrument handling technique (Figure 12.1). When tissue forceps are used, the minimum amount of tissue is grasped, and the minimum amount of pressure necessary to hold the tissue is applied to minimize tissue trauma. Thumb forceps are usually held in the surgeon's nondominant hand and used to assist cutting tissue (Figures 12.9a and 12.9c) and suturing (Figure 12.10). When in use, thumb forceps are grasped in chopstick fashion. When temporarily not in use, thumb forceps are carried in the palmed position, leaving the thumb, index finger, and middle finger free (Figure 12.11). While gentle holding of thumb forceps will minimize tissue trauma, it is also important to use the appropriate tissue forceps for the structure to be grasped. Rat-toothed thumb forceps or Brown-Adson thumb forceps are used to

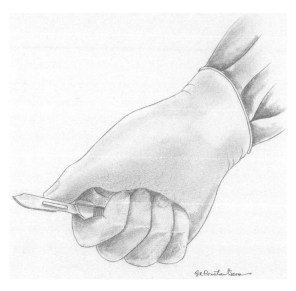

Figure 12.4   Scalpel handling (palm grip): For the palm grip, the scalpel handle is held with the palm, and the thumb is placed on the back of the scalpel blade.

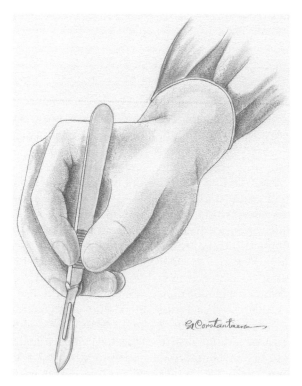

Figure 12.5   Scalpel handling (pencil grip): For the pencil grip, the scalpel handle is held in conventional pencil gripping fashion.

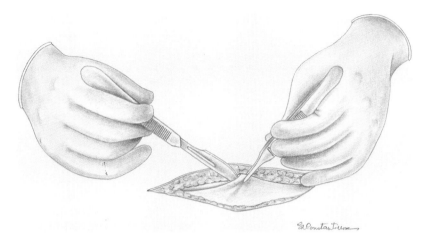

Figure 12.6   Scalpel handling (inverted pencil grip): Inverted blade press cutting (stab incision) is applied using the pencil grip to incise the linea alba while the adjacent linea alba is lifted with thumb forceps.

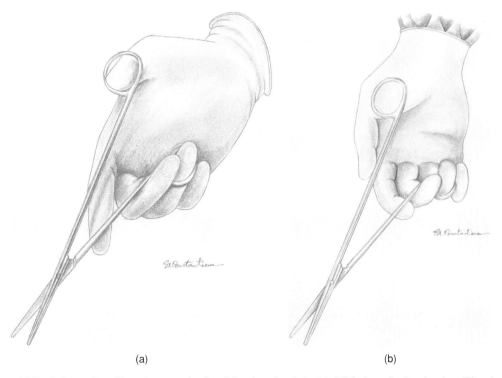

(a)   (b)

Figure 12.7   Scissors handling (two methods of forehand grip): (a) Wide-based tripod grip—The thumb and fourth finger are placed in the upper and lower rings of the scissors. (b) Thenar eminence–fourth finger grip—The thenar eminence stabilizes the upper ring, and the fourth finger occupies the lower ring.

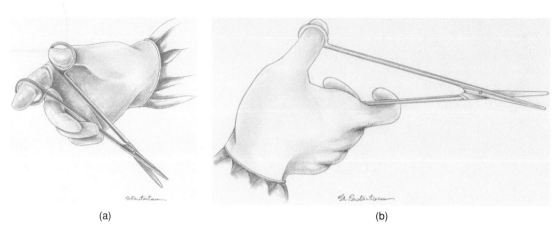

(a)   (b)

Figure 12.8   Scissors handling (two methods of backhand grip): (a) Thumb–index finger grip—The thumb and index finger are placed in the scissor rings with the scissors pointing backwards. (b) Thumb–fourth finger grip—The thumb and fourth finger are kept in the scissors' upper and lower rings while the hand is turned backwards.

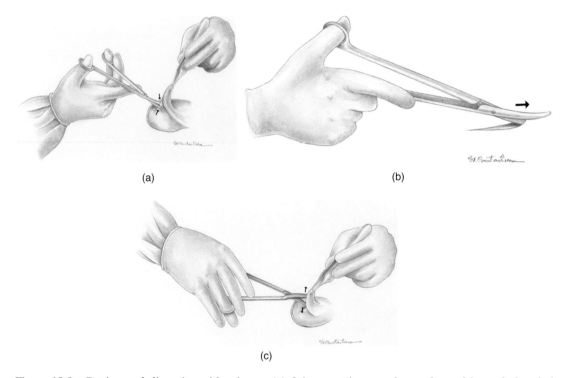

(a)   (b)

(c)

Figure 12.9   Cutting and dissecting with scissors: (a) Scissor cutting may be performed in underhanded fashion (as demonstrated here) or overhanded fashion (usually preferred). (b) Push cutting is likened to cutting wrapping paper and is properly executed using the midportion of the scissor blades with the blades partially open. (c) Blunt dissection is generally reserved for separating anatomical structures, such as when elevating skin and subcutaneous from underlying fascia to create a skin flap.

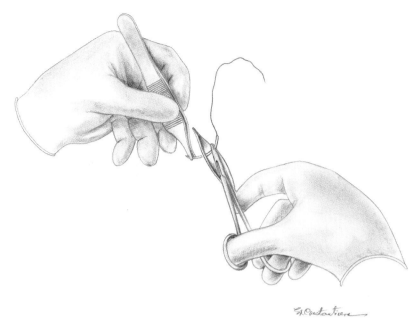

Figure 12.10 Thumb forceps for needle handling: The thumb forceps is used to pull the needle through the tissue after the needle holder is disengaged.

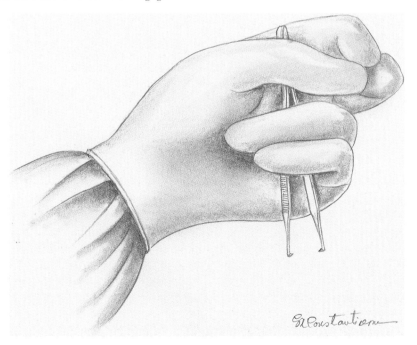

Figure 12.11 Thumb forceps when temporarily not in use: The thumb forceps is carried in the palmed position, leaving the thumb, index finger, and middle finger free.

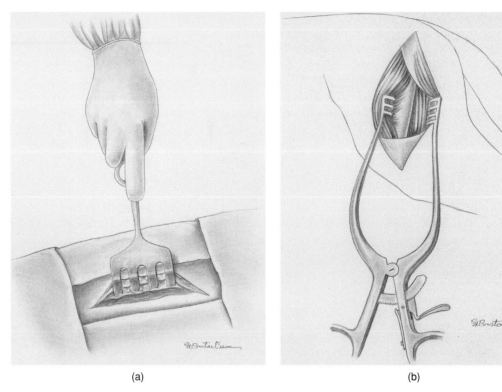

(a)   (b)

Figure 12.12   Retractors: (a) Hand held (Volkmann) retractor placed to visualize the targeted area of the surgery using an assistant's hand. (b) Self-retaining (Weitlaner) retractor placed to visualize the targeted area of the surgery without an assistant.

manipulate skin and other dense tissues, Brown-Adson thumb forceps can be used to grasp suture needles, and DeBakey tissue forceps are used for viscera and other delicate tissues. Ratcheted tissue forceps (such as Allis and Babcock tissue forceps) are used for manipulation of tissues without repeated grasping. Such application is usually more traumatic than thumb forceps and is, therefore, limited to grasping structures that will be excised, especially when Allis tissue forceps are used. Babcock tissue forceps are less traumatic than Allis tissue forceps; therefore, some surgeons will use Babcock tissue forceps to manipulated structures that they do not intend to excise.

Retractors are used to obtain proper visualization of the targeted area of the surgery. Healthy tissue withstands the pressure of retractors, but too much pressure may cause neurovascular compromise and tissue damage. If too little retraction is provided, however, the surgeon is not able to see clearly, and the procedure may be compromised. Finding a proper medium is very important to achieve successful accomplishment of retractor application. Both hand held retractors and self-retaining retractors (Figure 12.12) are available in sharp and blunt varieties. Care should be taken not to traumatize tissues or damage vessels and nerves during retractor application, especially when

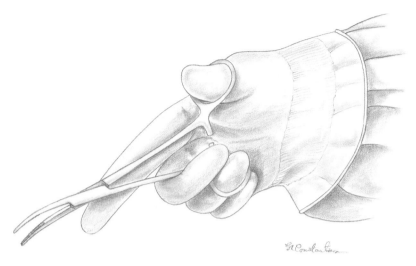

Figure 12.13   Hemostatic forceps handling: A single (Kelly) hemostat is held in the dominant hand using the wide-based tripod grip with the thumb and fourth finger in the instrument rings.

retractors with sharp blades are used. With blunt blades, pressure damage can occur if the retractor is applied too forcefully to the tissue. Self-retaining retractors are indispensable in working without an assistant (Figure 12.12b). The major hazard of self-retaining retractors is trauma or ischemia at the point of contact. During lengthy procedures, it is advisable to release self-retaining retractors periodically (every 15 minutes) to prevent prolonged ischemia of wound edges.

Correct application of hemostatic forceps aids visualization by affording proper hemostasis and minimizing the amount of blood in the surgical field. For placing hemostatic forceps, a single hemostat is grasped with the dominant hand in the wide-based tripod grip (Figure 12.13), and a thumb forceps is used in the opposite hand for manipulation of tissues surrounding the bleeding point. There are two methods for application of hemostatic forceps: tip-clamping method (Figure 12.14a) and jaw-clamping method (Figure 12.14b). For occluding small superficial bleeders, the tip-clamping method is used. The tip of the hemostat is pointed toward the vessel and the tip is used to grasp the smallest amount of tissue, preferably only the bleeding vessel itself (Figure 12.14a). After the hemostatic forceps is applied, the instrument is turned so that the tip is facing upward to facilitate ligature application. For occluding vessels within pedicles, the jaw-clamping method can be used. In this case, hemostatic forceps are applied perpendicular to the vessel with the tip facing upward (Figure 12.14b). The jaw is used to grasp the pedicle, taking care to avoid inadvertent grasping of adjacent structures. When a surgical assistant is not available and hemostats are applied in succession, multiple hemostats can be carried with the palm of dominant hand (Figure 12.15). Hemostasis can also be achieved by the use of electrosurgery. The assistant may electrocoagulate tissue or a vessel or may elevate the hemostat that is on the vessel so that the surgeon can activate electrocoagulation against the hemostatic forceps.

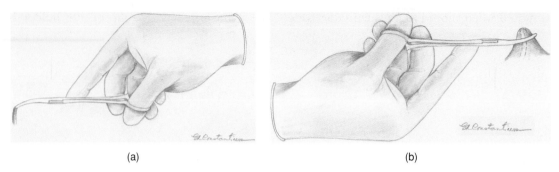

(a) (b)

Figure 12.14 Hemostatic forceps application: (a) Tip-clamping method for occluding small bleeders—The tip of the hemostat is pointed toward the vessel and the tip is used to grasp the smallest amount of tissue, preferably only the bleeding vessel itself. Then, the hemostat is turned so that the tip faces upward (not shown). (b) Jaw-clamping method for occluding vessels within tissue pedicles—Hemostatic forceps are applied perpendicular to the vessel with the tip facing upwards. The hemostatic forceps are left with the tip facing upward.

Clearance of blood from the surgical field is accomplished with surgical sponges and suction. Three common suction tips are the Poole, Yankauer, and Frazier (See Chapter 5; Figure 5.10). The Poole suction tip usually has a detachable guard with many tiny fenestrations to allow suction of the abdominal cavity without plugging by tissues, such as omentum. Unguarded suction tips can be used in the abdominal cavity, provided that a sponge is placed over the tip to prevent tissue from being sucked into the single opening. The Poole guard can be

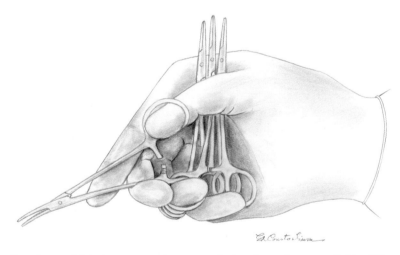

Figure 12.15 Carrying multiple hemostats when a surgical assistant is not available: When hemostats are applied in succession, multiple hemostats can be carried with the palm of the dominant hand.

removed when more precise suctioning is desired in areas where tissues are less likely to plug the suction tip. The Yankauer suction tip is used commonly in the thoracic cavity and deep pockets where plugging with tissues is not likely. The Frazier suction tip is smaller than Poole and Yankauer tips and is used in small areas of fluid accumulation, such as orthopedic and neurologic surgical approaches. The Frazier suction tip has a hole where the surgeon's thumb holds the instrument. Covering this hole provides high-pressure suction. Leaving the hole uncovered provides low-pressure suction which is less likely to suck tissues into the tip and, therefore, less likely to cause unnecessary tissue trauma.

There are four basic methods of grasping a needle holder: (1) thumb–fourth finger grip, (2) thenar eminence grip, (3) palm grip, and (4) pencil grip. In the thumb–fourth finger grip, the fingers are used to control opening and closing of the instrument (Figure 12.16a). This method provides excellent control and is recommended for novice surgeons. In the thenar eminence grip, the thenar eminence, thumb, and fourth finger are used to control opening and closing of the instrument. The thenar eminence is placed on the upper ring and the fourth finger is placed in the lower ring while the thumb placed along the shaft of the instrument (Figure 12.16b). This method provides good mobility, and, therefore, is recommended for continuous suture patterns. In

the palm grip method, the needle holder is gripped with the palm and the five fingers (Figure 12.16c). This method provides strong driving force for placing sutures in tough tissues but less precise control compared to the thumb–fourth finger grip. In the pencil grip method, a needle holder is grasped like gripping a pencil in conventional fashion (Figure 12.16d). Spring-opening needle holders with finger pressure, such as the Castroviejo needle holder, are usually held with a pencil grip. This method facilitates fine movements of the fingers; therefore, the pencil grip is appropriate for delicate work, such as vascular and ophthalmic surgery. Regardless of the method of grasping a needle holder, the needle is generally grasped perpendicular to the long axis of the needle holder and near the tip of the needle (Figure 12.17a) for greatest driving force, near the midpoint of the needle (Figure 12.17b) for general-purpose suturing, and near the suture attachment of the needle (Figure 12.17c) for suturing delicate tissues and spanning long distances. When driving or extracting the needle, a single rotating motion of the hand is most efficient. The thumb forceps is used to pull the needle through the tissue after the needle holder is disengaged (Figure 12.10). In addition to driving needles, the needle holder is used to load the scalpel blade onto the scalpel handle (Figure 12.18a) and to remove the scalpel blade from the scalpel handle (Figure 12.18b).

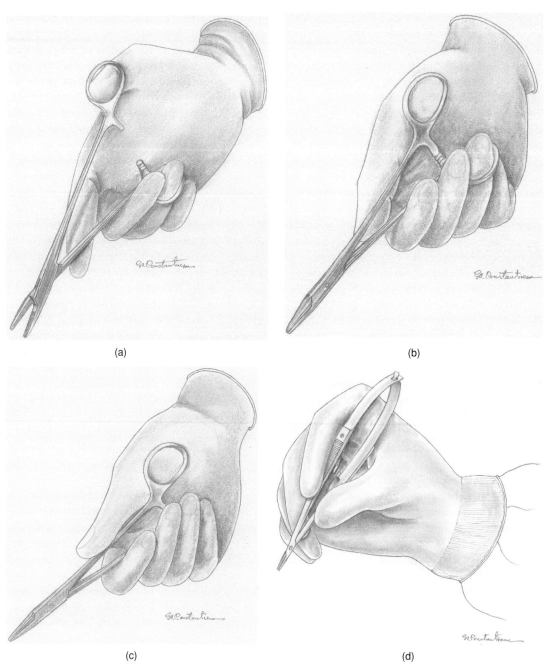

(a)

(b)

(c)

(d)

Figure 12.16 Handling needle holders: (a) The thumb–fourth finger grip—The thumb and fourth finger are used to control opening and closing of the instrument. (b) The thenar eminence grip—The thenar eminence, thumb, and fourth finger are used to control opening and closing of the instrument with the thenar eminence at one ring, the fourth finger in the other ring, and the thumb placed along the shaft of the instrument. (c) The palm grip—The needle holder is gripped with the palm and the five fingers. (d) Pencil grip—A Castroviejo needle holder is grasped like gripping a pencil in conventional pencil-holding fashion.

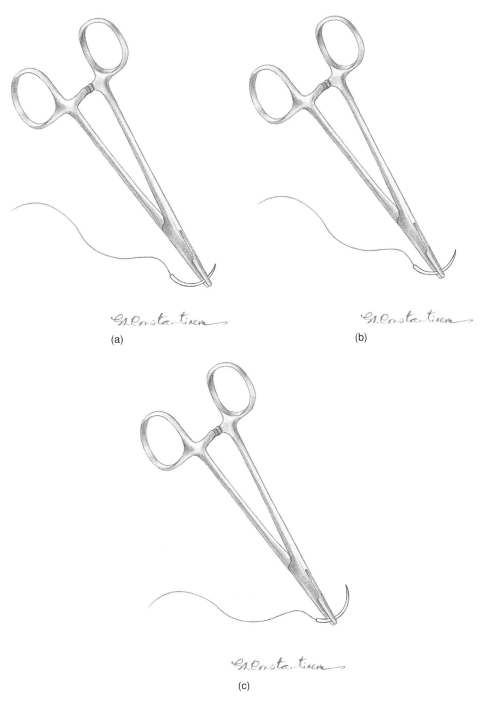

(a)

(b)

(c)

Figure 12.17   Holding a suture needle: A needle is generally grasped perpendicular to the long axis of the needle holder: (a) near the tip of the needle for greatest driving force; (b) near the midpoint of the needle for general-purpose suturing; or (c) near the suture end of the needle for suturing delicate tissues and for spanning the greatest distance.

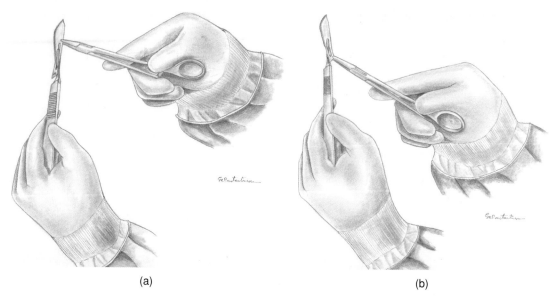

(a)   (b)

Figure 12.18   Loading and removing a scalpel blade: A needle holder is used (a) to grasp the back of the scalpel blade to load the blade onto the scalpel handle, and (b) to grasp the end of the scalpel blade closest to the handle to remove the scalpel blade from the scalpel handle.

ADDITIONAL RESOURCES

Additional information about instrument handling in small animal surgery can be found in the following textbooks:

1. Fossum TW, ed. *Small Animal Surgery*, 3rd ed. St. Louis, Missouri: Mosby Elsevier, 2007.

2. Busch SJ, ed. *Small Animal Surgical Nursing Skills and Concepts*. St. Louis, Missouri: Mosby Elsevier, 2006.

3. Slatter D, ed. *Textbook of Small Animal Surgery*, 3rd ed. Philadelphia, Pennsylvania: Saunders, 2003.

Chapter 13

SURGICAL KNOT TYING

Hun-Young Yoon and Fred Anthony Mann

Proper surgical knot tying is required for successful hemostasis and wound closure. Failure of a surgical knot can result in hemorrhage or wound dehiscence, both which can result in significant patient morbidity. There are three basic surgical knots: square knot, surgeon's knot, and slip knot. A granny knot is never considered to be an appropriate surgical knot. There are two general methods of tying knots: hand ties and instrument ties.

A knot consists of at least two throws laid on top of each other and tightened. Two consecutive simple throws result in a square knot, slip knot, or granny knot (Figure 13.1). A square knot is produced by reversing direction on each successive simple throw and maintaining even tension on both strands as each throw is tightened. Failure to maintain even tension on both strands or applying upward tension on strands often results in a slip knot. A granny knot results from failing to reverse direction on successive simple throws. The most reliable configuration for a knot is superimposition of a square knot. The granny knot and slip knot are not usually recommended because they are subject to slippage. However, a slip knot can be intentionally used when tying knots in deep cavities or where maneuvering space is limited. Then, the slip knot is covered with at least one square knot to prevent loosening. A surgeon's knot is similar to a square knot except that one strand is passed through the loop twice on the first throw. The surgeon's knot can be advantageous for ligation of thick vascular pedicles or during wound closures when tissue tension precludes adequate tightening of the first throw of a square knot.

Hand ties are particularly useful in confined or difficult to reach areas or when sutures have been preplaced, as in thoracotomy closure. Hand ties require that suture ends are left longer than is needed for an instrument tie. There are two-hand (Figure 13.2) and one-hand (Figure 13.3) techniques for hand tying, and both can be done in right-handed or left-handed fashion. In this chapter, only the ties most commonly used by the principal author are illustrated. Two-hand technique allows good control and accuracy, but it is awkward for tying

Fundamentals of Small Animal Surgery, 1st edition.
By Fred Anthony Mann, Gheorghe M. Constantinescu
and Hun-Young Yoon.
© 2011 Blackwell Publishing Ltd.

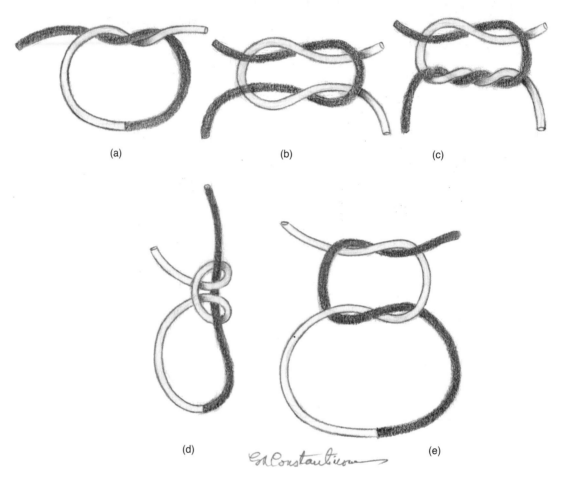

Figure 13.1 Types of knots: (a) single throw, (b) square knot, (c) surgeon's knot, (d) slip knot, and (e) granny knot.

in deep cavities and confined spaces. One-hand technique is more adaptable to deep cavities and confined spaces, but the first knot may need to be a slip knot. Instrument ties (Figure 13.4) are more commonly used than hand ties in veterinary practice because there is less waste of suture; however, the veterinarian should be accomplished in both hand and instrument tying to be prepared for any situation that will require one or the other.

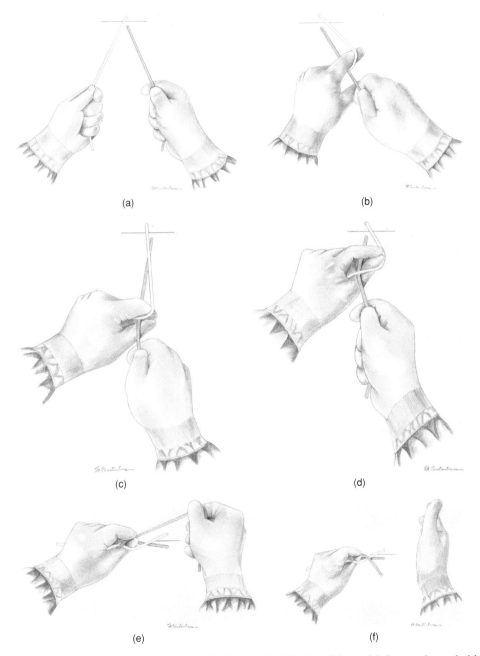

(a)

(b)

(c)

(d)

(e)

(f)

Figure 13.2   Two-hand knot tying technique (left-handed). (a) The right and left strands are held in the palm of the each hand and placed between the index finger and thumb of the each hand. (b) The left strand is hooked along the medial aspect of the left index finger, and the left thumb is passed below and around the right strand (the left thumb is placed to the right of the right strand). The shape of the strands resembles a backward "4". (c) The tips of the left index finger and thumb are put together. (d) The tips of the left index finger and thumb, still together, are placed upward through the loop formed by the strands. (e) The right strand is grasped between the left index finger and thumb. (f) The right strand is released from the right hand.

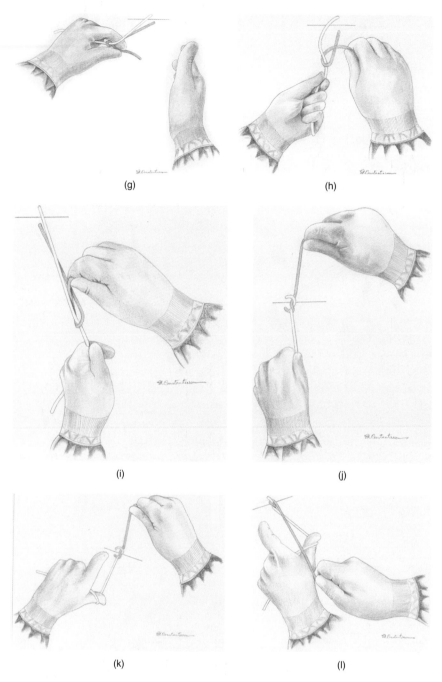

(g)   (h)

(i)   (j)

(k)   (l)

Figure 13.2   (*Continued*) (g) The right strand is pushed downward through the suture loop. (h) The right strand is returned to the right hand. (i) Even tension is applied to the suture ends as the throw is tightened. (j) Single throw is completed. (k) The left strand is hooked along the lateral aspect of the left thumb (the left thumb is placed to the left of the left strand). (l) The right strand is brought between the index finger and thumb of the left hand, forming another backward "4".

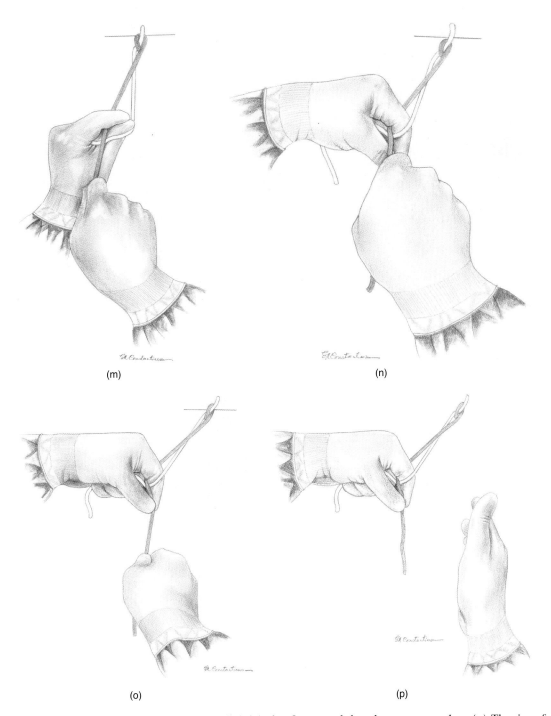

(m)

(n)

(o)

(p)

Figure 13.2   (*Continued*) (m) The tips of the left index finger and thumb are put together. (n) The tips of the left index finger and thumb, still together, are placed downward through the loop formed by the strands. (o) The right strand is grasped between the left index finger and thumb. (p) The right strand is released from the right hand.

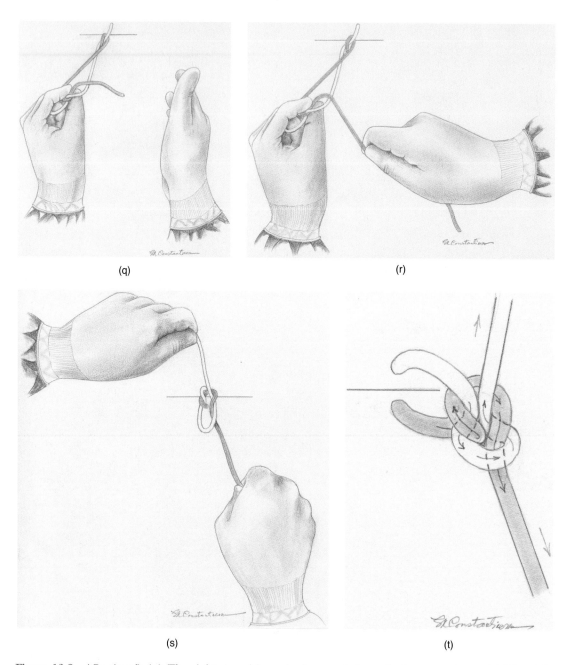

(q)

(r)

(s)

(t)

Figure 13.2 (*Continued*) (q) The right strand is pushed upward through the suture loop. (r) The right strand is returned to the right hand. (s) Even tension is applied to the suture ends to tighten the square knot. (t) The square knot is completed.

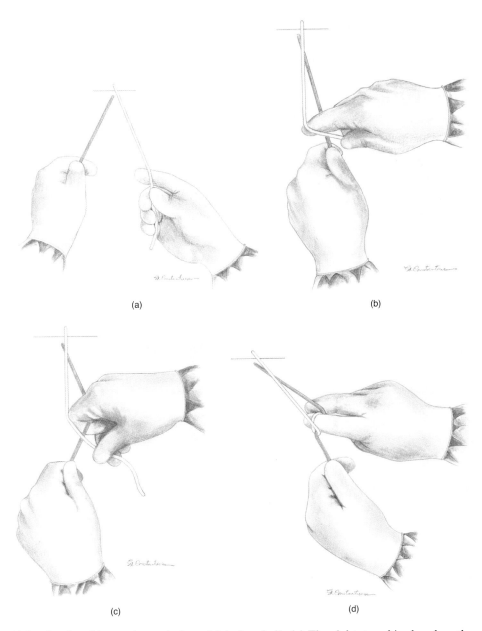

(a)

(b)

(c)

(d)

Figure 13.3   One-hand knot tying technique (right-handed). (a) The right strand is placed on the palm of the right hand and held between the third finger and thumb of the right hand. The left strand is held in the left hand in similar fashion, but is grasped by the left thumb and the index finger. (b) The right strand is brought to the left over the left strand (the index finger of the right hand is placed between the two strands) such that the strand resembles a "4". (c) The distal phalanx of the index finger of the right hand is flexed. (d) The right strand is drawn through the suture loop using the dorsal surface of the nail of the right index finger.

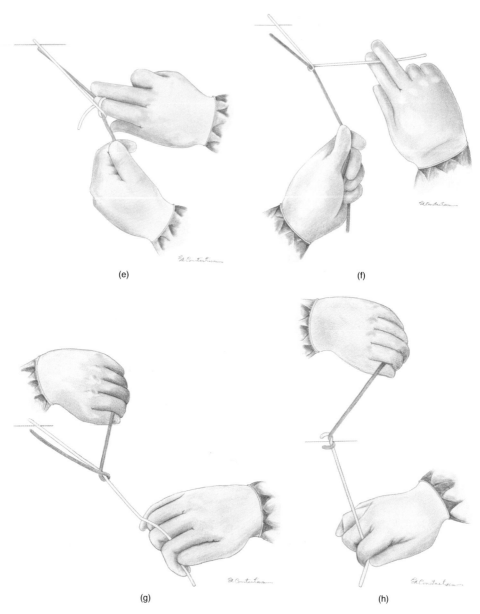

(e) (f)

(g) (h)

Figure 13.3 (*Continued*) (e) The right strand is pulled through the loop by the tips of the index and third fingers of the right hand. (f) The right strand is pulled all the way through the loop using the index and third fingers. (g) The right hand grip is shifted to the thumb and index finger, and even tension is applied to the two strands as the left hand moves away from and the right hand moves toward the surgeon. (h) Single throw is completed.

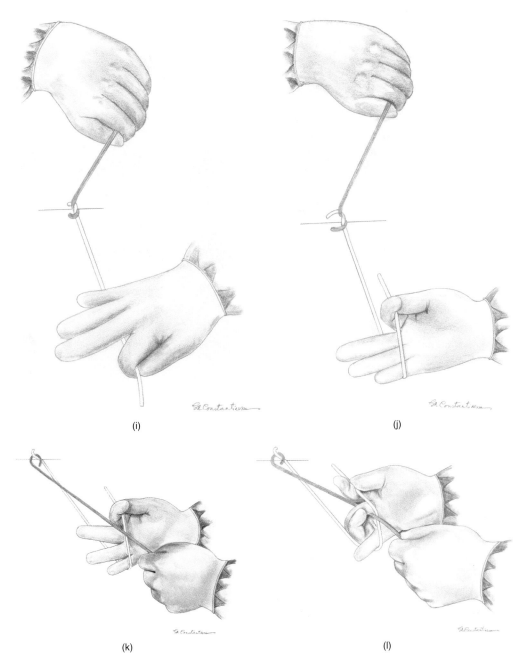

(i)

(j)

(k)

(l)

Figure 13.3 (*Continued*) (i) The third, fourth, and fifth fingers of the right hand are unfolded. (j) The right hand is flipped over (supinated). (k) The left strand is brought between the right index and third fingers, forming another "4". (l) The distal phalanx of the right third finger is flexed, and the right strand is drawn through the loop using the dorsal surface of the nail of the right third finger.

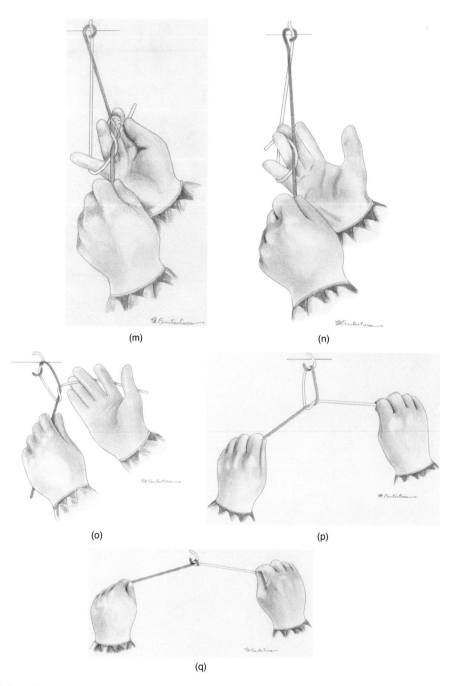

(m)

(n)

(o)

(p)

(q)

Figure 13.3 (*Continued*) (m) The right strand is grasped between the third and fourth fingers of the right hand. (n) The thumb–index finger grip is released, and the right strand is held entirely by the third and fourth fingers to pull it through the loop. (o) The right strand is pulled downward through the loop. (p) The right hand is pronated, and the right strand is regrasped between the right thumb and index finger. Then, even tension is applied to the two strands to tighten the square knot as the left hand moves toward and the right hand moves away from the surgeon. (q) The square knot is completed.

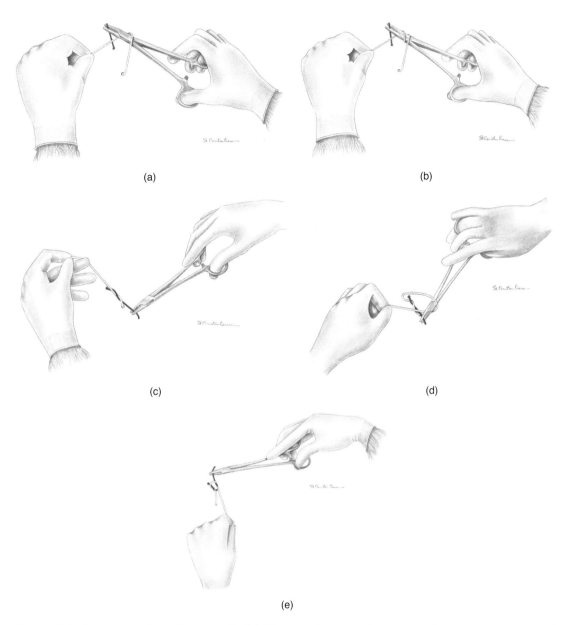

Figure 13.4   Instrument tie (right-handed). (a) The strand nearest the operator is wrapped once around the needle holder to form a loop, and the end of the far piece of suture is grasped with the needle holder. (b) The strand nearest the operator can be wrapped twice for a surgeon's throw. (c) The strand in the needle holder is brought toward the operator, and the strand in the opposite hand is moved away from the operator, as even tension is applied to the two strands. (d) The strand farthest from the operator is wrapped once over the needle holder to form a loop, and the end of the strand nearest the operator is grasped with the needle holder. (e) The strand is pulled through the loop away from the operator, and even tension is applied to the two strands to tighten the knot.

ADDITIONAL RESOURCES

Additional information about knot tying in small animal surgery can be found in the following textbook and manuals:

1. Fossum TW, ed. *Small Animal Surgery*, 3rd ed. St. Louis, Missouri: Mosby Elsevier, 2007.

2. Edlich RF, Long WB. *Surgical Knot Tying Manual*, 3rd ed. Norwalk, Connecticut: Covidien, 2008.

3. Ethicon, Inc. *Knot Tying Manual*. Somerville, New Jersey: Ethicon, Inc., 2005.

Chapter 14

SUTURE MATERIALS AND BASIC SUTURE PATTERNS

Carlos H. de M. Souza and Fred Anthony Mann

Suture materials are essential to veterinary surgery. They must provide stable wound closure and support until tissue healing has occurred. The ideal suture material should have excellent handling characteristics, knot security, and high tensile strength per diameter ratio. The suture material should be easily sterilized, nontoxic, nonallergenic, nonteratogenic, noncarcinogenic, and should not promote bacterial colonization. In addition, the ideal suture material should be absorbed without causing tissue reaction, and its absorption rate should not be influenced by the presence of inflammation or changes in body pH. Since there is no single suture material that fulfills all of the above criteria, the surgeon must choose the one that best applies to the particular animal and tissue being sutured.

Suture materials are classified as absorbable or nonabsorbable, natural or synthetic, and monofilament or multifilament, based on composition and structure. Materials that lose tensile strength within 60 days of implantation are classified as absorbable; whereas most suture materials will eventually be absorbed. The truly nonabsorbable sutures are polypropylene and stainless steel. Natural materials are absorbed through enzymatic degradation by macrophages. Synthetic materials are absorbed through nonenzymatic hydrolysis of ester bonds, with final byproducts being carbon dioxide and water. With hydrolytic absorption, the rate of suture degradation is not affected by inflammation or infection. Absorbable suture materials commonly used in veterinary practice include: surgical gut, polyglactin 910 (Coated Vicryl, Ethicon, Inc., Summerville, NJ), polyglycolic acid (Dexon II, Covidien Animal Health and Dental Division, Mansfield, MA), poliglecaprone 25 (Monocryl, Ethicon, Inc., Summerville, NJ), glycomer 631 (Biosyn, Covidien Animal Health and Dental Division, Mansfield, MA), glycolide/lactide copolymer (Polysorb, Covidien Animal Health and Dental Division, Mansfield, MA), polydioxanone (PDS II, Ethicon, Inc., Summerville, NJ), and polyglyconate (Maxon, Covidien Animal Health and Dental Division, Mansfield, MA). Table 14.1 summarizes properties of these commonly used absorbable suture materials.

Fundamentals of Small Animal Surgery, 1st edition.
By Fred Anthony Mann, Gheorghe M. Constantinescu and Hun-Young Yoon.
© 2011 Blackwell Publishing Ltd.

Table 14.1 **Properties of some common absorbable suture materials**

Name	Approximate loss of tensile strength at 14 days (%)	Complete absorption (days)	Strength[a]	Handling[a]	Reactivity (rank)[b]	Knot security
Chromic gut	50	90	+	++	6	+
Polyglactin 910	30	56–70	+++	+++	5	+++
Polyglycolic acid	35	90	+++	+++	3	+++
Poliglecaprone	60–80	90–110	+++	++++	4[c]	++++
Polydioxanone	20	180–240	++++	+++	2	++
Polyglyconate	25	180	++++	++++	1	++++
Glycomer 631	25	90–180	NA	NA	2	NA
Glycolide/lactide copolymer	20	56–70	NA	NA	NA	NA

[a]Worst = +; best = + + + +.

[b]Lowest reactivity = 1; highest reactivity = 6. [Note: While the tissue reactivity of gut is significant, the relative reactivity of the synthetic absorbable suture materials does not seem to be of noticeable clinical importance.]

[c]Studies in rats show poliglecaprone to be less reactive than polydioxanone.

Nonabsorbable suture materials include natural and synthetic fibers. Silk is the most commonly used nonabsorbable natural fiber. Synthetic nonabsorbable suture materials include polyester (Ethibond, Ethicon, Inc., Summerville, NJ; Mersilene, Ethicon, Inc., Summerville, NJ; and TiCron, Covidien Animal Health and Dental Division, Mansfield, MA), polybutester (Novafil, Covidien Animal Health and Dental Division, Mansfield, MA), nylon, polymerized caprolactam (Braunamid, Jorgensen Laboratories, Inc., Loveland, CO), polypropylene, and stainless steel. Natural fibers incite significant tissue reaction; thus, synthetic nonabsorbable materials are usually preferred. A number of discrepancies exist in the veterinary literature related to the characteristics of specific suture materials. The information below (including the tables) is derived from selected literature,[1–10] suture company catalogues, http://ecatalog.ethicon.com/sutures, http://www.covidien.com/syneture, and the personal experience of the authors.

ABSORBABLE SUTURE MATERIALS

Surgical gut (catgut) is a natural multifilament suture made from either intestinal submucosa (ovine) or serosa (bovine). It consists of 90% collagen. When cured with chromic salts, surgical gut has increased strength, less inflammatory reaction, and slower absorption. Surgical gut is absorbed by enzymatic digestion and phagocytosis by macrophages. Inflammation, infection, and catabolic states increase the rate of absorption. Chromic gut is difficult to handle, has poor knot security when wet, and has become less popular due to wide availability of greater quality synthetic absorbable sutures.

Polyglactin 910 is a braided multifilament synthetic suture material made of 90% glycolide and 10% L-lactide. Coating of polyglactin 910 with calcium stearate and a second copolymer (polyglactin 370) increases handling characteristics and decreases tissue drag, but also decreases knot security. Polyglactin 910 has greater initial strength than surgical gut and polyglycolic acid. It elicits minimal inflammatory reaction and is absorbed by hydrolysis. Polyglactin 910 is best used in tissues that heal with a rapid increase in tensile strength, such as the urinary bladder and the gastrointestinal tract. When compared to polydioxanone, polyglactin 910 has been shown to elicit less inflammatory reaction in the linea alba of cats. A rapidly absorbed type of polyglactin 910 (Vicryl-Rapide, Ethicon, Inc., Summerville, NJ) was developed for situations where the surgeon desires to minimize the time tissues are exposed to suture material. Vicryl-Rapide is polyglactin 910 that is irradiated to increase absorption rate. Vicryl-Rapide is reported by the manufacturer to be the fastest-absorbing synthetic suture, losing 50% of its tensile strength at 5 days and 100% at 10–14 days.

Polyglycolic acid is a multifilament braided synthetic suture material with greater initial strength than surgical gut. Also, in comparison to surgical gut, polyglycolic acid incites less inflammatory reaction. Polyglycolic acid is absorbed by hydrolysis and has a pattern of loss of strength similar to polyglactin 910. It has good handling characteristics, but tissue drag and relatively low knot security are drawbacks. Polyglycolic acid may be less desirable for use in the oral cavity and in infected urinary bladder due to the alkaline pH, which increases its absorption rate. Polyglycolic acid can be used in intestinal anastomosis and in circumstances where long-term tensile strength is not a requirement.

Poliglecaprone 25 is a monofilament synthetic suture material made from copolymers of glycolide and epsilon caprolactone. It has greater initial tensile strength than chromic gut and is designed to lose most of its tensile strength over 14 days. Poliglecaprone 25 is used in tissues that gain tensile strength rapidly, such as urinary bladder and subcutaneous tissue. Poliglecaprone 25 has excellent handling characteristics and knot security. Very few studies have investigated the tissue reaction caused by poliglecaprone 25 in comparison to other synthetic sutures. In rat studies, poliglecaprone 25

has caused less tissue reaction than polyglactin 910 and polydioxanone. Poliglecaprone 25 has been shown to cause mild inflammatory reaction when used to close the linea alba of cats.

Glycomer 631 is a synthetic monofilament suture made of a combination of glycolide, dioxanone, and trimethylene carbonate. It displays very little tissue drag. Glycomer 631 loses 25% of its tensile strength in 2 weeks. Effective wound support is maintained for 3 weeks and absorption is complete in 3–6 months.

Glycolide/lactide copolymer is a braided synthetic suture covered with a copolymer of caprolactone, glycolide, and calcium stearoyl lactylate. The manufacturer indicates that effective wound support is maintained for three weeks and absorption is complete in 56–70 days.

Polydioxanone is a monofilament synthetic suture made from a polymer of paradioxanone. It has greater tensile strength compared to surgical gut and lower tissue drag compared to braided absorbable sutures. Polydioxanone has notable memory, which decreases its handling quality, and has the lowest knot security of the synthetic absorbable sutures. Polydioxanone loses approximately 20% of its tensile strength in two weeks and is used in tissues where long-term strength is needed, such as the linea alba. Polydioxanone may cause more skin reaction than poliglecaprone 25 and glycomer 631, but tissue reactions can be expected to be minimal with all three of these suture materials.

Polyglyconate is a monofilament synthetic suture material with properties similar to polydioxanone. It maintains approximately 75% of its tensile strength in 14 days. Polyglyconate has less memory and suture kinking and better knot security than polydioxanone. Like polydioxanone, polyglyconate incites minimal tissue reaction.

Antimicrobial sutures have been promoted to decrease the chance of surgical wound infection. Polyglactin 910 (Coated Vicryl PLUS, Ethicon, Inc., Summerville, NJ), poliglecaprone 25 (Monocryl PLUS, Ethicon, Inc., Summerville, NJ), and polydioxanone (PDS II

PLUS, Ethicon, Inc., Summerville, NJ) are currently available with the impregnated antibacterial triclosan. In vitro studies show that triclosan can inhibit the growth of staphylococcal species, but clinical studies showing the effects of triclosan-impregnated sutures on infection rates are not currently available. Blinded studies have not shown differences in the handling characteristics of traditional versus triclosan-impregnated sutures.

NONABSORBABLE SUTURE MATERIALS

Silk is the only natural nonabsorbable suture material in common use today. Silk is a braided multifilament suture made from the cocoon of the silk worm. Silk elicits intense inflammatory reaction and has marked capillarity. It is inexpensive, has excellent handling characteristics, and has excellent knot security. Coating (wax or silicone) decreases suture capillarity and the tissue's inflammatory response at the expense of knot security. Silk must not be applied in infected tissues since it will decrease the number of bacteria necessary to cause a wound infection. Also, silk and can cause granulomas when used in hollow viscera. Silk loses most of its tensile strength in 6 months. Today, silk is still commonly used in vascular surgery (not as vascular grafts) and as inexpensive and dependable ligature material.

Polyester is a nonabsorbable multifilament material made from polyethylene terephthalate. Polyester is stronger than surgical gut and silk and does not lose significant strength over time. Polyester incites a severe inflammatory reaction and has marked tissue drag. Coating with polybutilate decreases tissue drag and increases handling characteristics at the expense of knot security. Polyester must not be used in infected wounds.

Polybutester is formed from a monofilament copolymer of polybutyline and polytetramethylene. It elicits minimal tissue reactivity and displays good handling characteristics and knot security. Polybutester has high elasticity (up to 30%) without losing tensile strength and can be used in tissues where prolonged wound healing is expected to occur, such as linea alba and tendons. In addition, because the suture allows significant compliance, polybutester has been used in venous and arterial anastomosis and skin.

Nylon is a polyamide nonabsorbable suture material derived from hexamethylenediamine and adipic acid. It is available as monofilament and multifilament, but monofilament is more widely used. Nylon has good handling characteristics and knot security, although memory and stiffness are negative factors. Nylon is commonly used as a skin suture due to its elastic capabilities, which are important since post surgical inflammation and edema are common, and nonelastic suture will cut the swelling tissue. Nylon is metabolized over 2–3 years by hydrolysis. In this process, adipic acid is released, which has antibacterial effects. Most suture companies distribute nylon suture. One company distributes a fluorescent monofilament nylon suture (Fluorescent Supramid, S. Jackson, Inc., Alexandria, VA) that makes the suture easy to find at the time of removal.

Polymerized caprolactam is another polyamide suture. It is a twisted multifilament suture that is coated with a polyethylene sheath to minimize capillarity. Polymerized caprolactam has superior tensile strength compared to nylon, catgut, and silk, and incites less tissue reaction when compared to catgut and silk. Excessive swelling with the possibility of sinus formation has been reported; therefore, polymerized caprolactam should be reserved for skin suturing only.

Polypropylene is a nonabsorbable synthetic suture material that displays minimal tissue drag and moderate strength and knot security. It tends to be stiff and have significant memory, which decreases its handling characteristics. Polypropylene is the one of the least thrombogenic sutures available and is commonly used in vascular surgery. Most suture

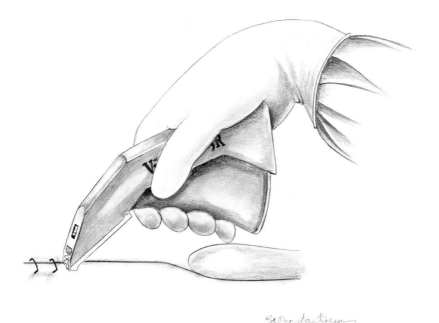

Figure 14.1   Skin closure using stainless steel staples.

companies distribute polypropylene suture. One company distributes a fluorescent monofilament polypropylene suture (Fluorofil, Intervet/Schering-Plough Animal Health, Millsboro, DE) that makes the suture easy to find at the time of removal.

Stainless steel is biologically inert and the strongest of the suture materials. It is commonly used in orthopedics in the form of stainless steel implants, but is uncommonly used as a suture material. Stainless steel suture has a tendency to cut through tissue and has poor handling characteristics. Although stainless steel sutures are not routinely used for closure of soft tissues, stainless steel skin staples (Figure 14.1) are becoming increasingly popular due to easy application and improved speed in closure, compared to conventional suturing.

BASIC SUTURE PATTERNS

A variety of suture patterns have been described for use in veterinary surgery. The use of a spe-
cific suture pattern may vary depending on the area being sutured, the length of the incision, the tension at the suture line, and the specific need for apposition, inversion, or eversion of the tissues.

Suture patterns can be broadly categorized as interrupted or continuous. Commonly employed interrupted suture patterns include the simple interrupted (Figure 14.2), cruciate (Figure 14.3), figure-of-eight (Figure 14.4), and interrupted intradermal (Figure 14.5). Commonly used continuous suture patterns include simple continuous (Figure 14.6), continuous intradermal (Figures 14.7 and 14.8), and Ford interlocking (Figure 14.9). Some suture patterns, like the Lembert (Figure 14.10) can be either interrupted or continuous. Typically, continuous patterns such as the Cushing (Figure 14.11), Connell (Figure 14.12), and continuous Lembert (Figures 14.10a and 14.10b) are used when inversion is desired, but an interrupted pattern such as the interrupted Lembert (Figure 14.10c) or Halsted (Figure 14.13) is

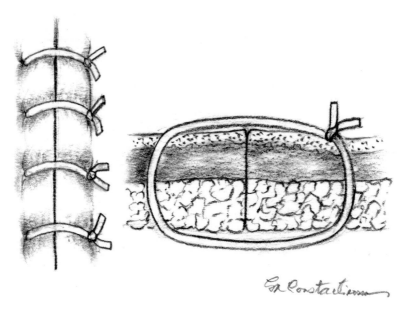

Figure 14.2   Simple interrupted sutures (skin closure demonstrated).

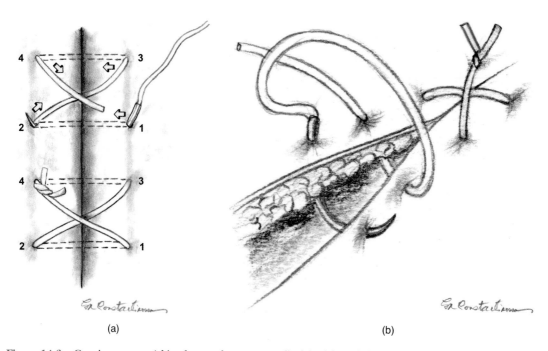

(a)   (b)

Figure 14.3   Cruciate suture (skin closure demonstrated): (a) with and (b) without suture passes numbered.

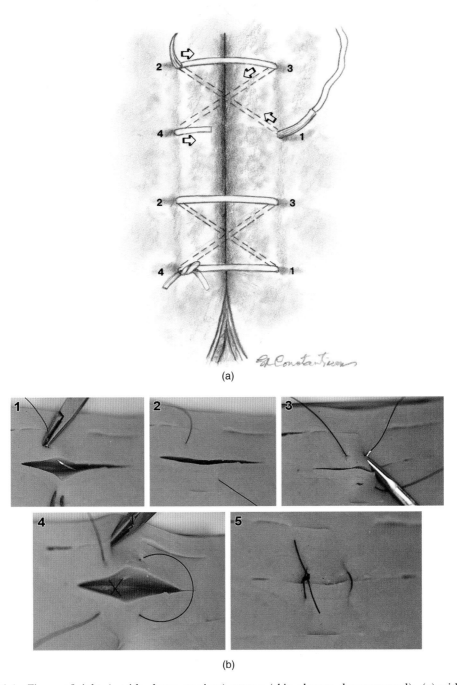

(a)

(b)

Figure 14.4   Figure-of-eight (upside down cruciate) suture (skin closure demonstrated): (a) with suture passes numbered and (b) with nylon suture on a model. [Note: It is difficult to illustrate proper suture tightness on this model; therefore, this figure-of-eight suture appears tighter than would be desired for ordinary small animal skin incision closure.]

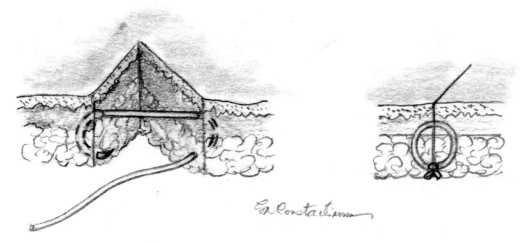

Figure 14.5   Interrupted intradermal (subcuticular) suture with buried knot.

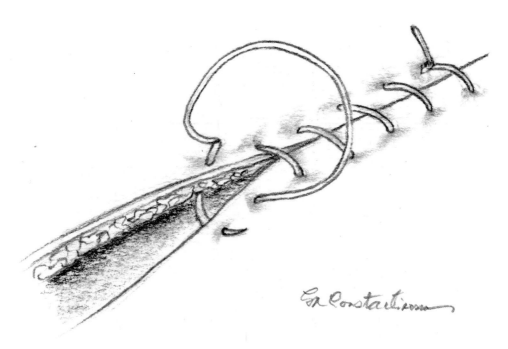

Figure 14.6   Simple continuous suture pattern. Skin closure is demonstrated; however, this pattern is more commonly used in subcutaneous tissues and for linea alba closure.

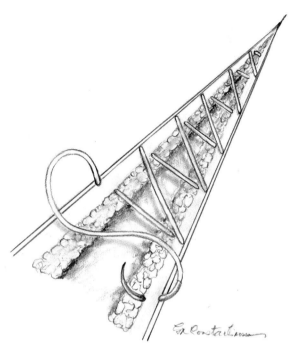

Figure 14.7   Continuous intradermal (subcuticular) suture pattern with vertical suture bites. The needle enters perpendicular to the skin edge.

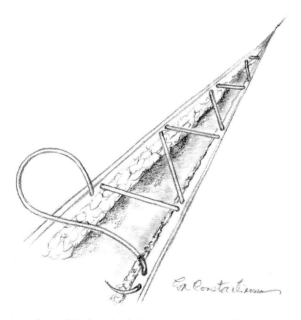

Figure 14.8   Continuous intradermal (subcuticular) suture pattern with horizontal suture bites. The needle enters parallel to the skin edge.

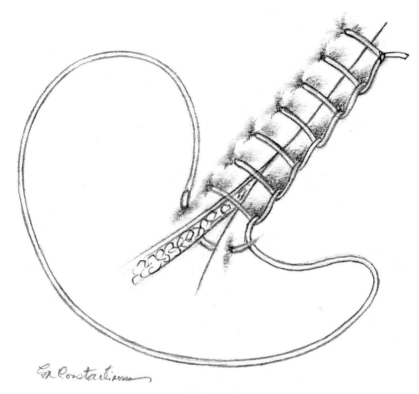

Figure 14.9 Ford interlocking suture pattern.

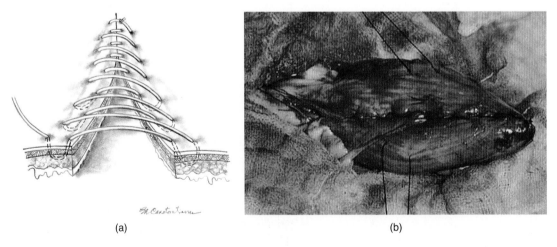

(a)   (b)

Figure 14.10 Lembert suture pattern: (a) continuous pattern, such as for gastric or urinary bladder closure, showing suture passage without the tightening that is usually done with each passage; (b) final appearance of continuous Lembert pattern in a urinary bladder demonstrating how this suture is not readily apparent on the serosal surface when properly tightened; and

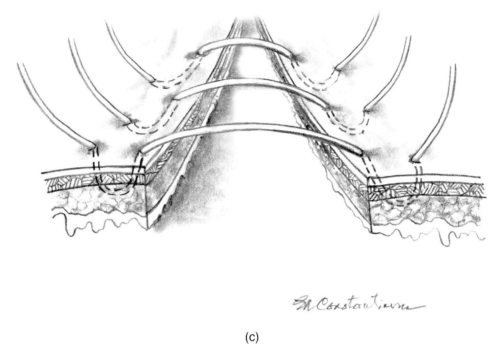

(c)

Figure 14.10 (*Continued*) (c) interrupted Lembert suture.

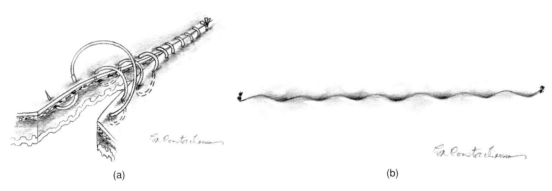

(a)

(b)

Figure 14.11 Cushing suture pattern: (a) demonstration of suture passage and (b) final appearance when properly tightened. Note the scalloped appearance of the finished product with no suture showing except for the knot at each end.

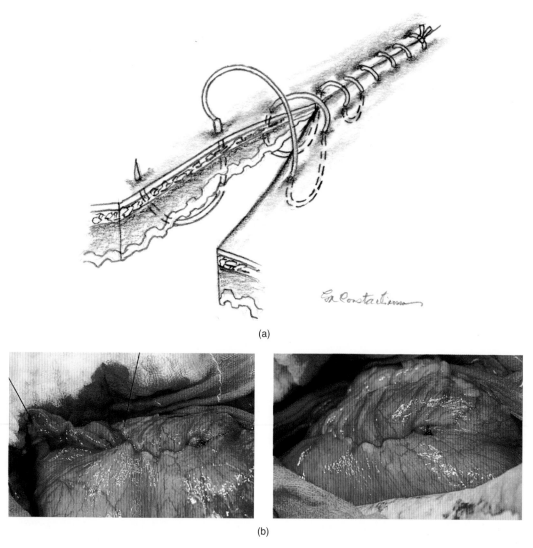

(a)

(b)

Figure 14.12 Connell suture pattern: (a) demonstration of suture passage and (b) final appearance when properly tightened (same as drawing in Figure 14.11b) in a gastrotomy closure. Note the scalloped appearance of the finished product with no suture showing except for the knot at each end (only one end visible, which is to the right in the photograph of the finished product).

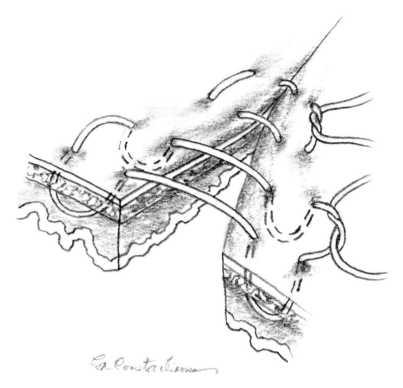

Figure 14.13   Halsted suture pattern.

occasionally used to invert tissue. Eversion of tissue can be accomplished with a vertical mattress (Figure 14.14) or horizontal mattress (Figure 14.15) suture pattern. A specialized mattress suture, the Mayo mattress (also called the vest over pants suture, Figure 14.16), results in overlapping of one tissue edge over the other. One situation where the Mayo mattress is used is in hernia repair. The Mayo mattress is especially useful for closing the linea alba in repair of a ventral abdominal hernia or dehiscence.

Suture patterns are also categorized in three different groups: appositional, inverting, and tension-relieving sutures. Appositional sutures (Table 14.2; Figures 14.2–14.9 and 14.17) are ideal when there is no excessive tension on the incision, and are commonly used for closure of skin, intestine, and urinary bladder. Wound healing will be optimal and scar forma-

tion minimized with good apposition of wound edges. Inverting sutures (Table 14.3; Figures 14.10–14.13 and 14.18) are commonly used to close hollow viscera in gastric and urogenital surgery. Inversion decreases exposure of the suture when properly tightened and, therefore, may decrease contamination and adhesion formation. The Lembert suture can also be used for fascial imbrications such as done during correction of patellar luxation and for closure of muscle stumps when a limb is amputated. Tension-relieving suture patterns (Table 14.4; Figures 14.14–14.16, 14.19, and 14.20) are used to decrease stress on suture lines, such as in reconstructive skin surgery and herniorrhaphy. Tension-relieving sutures are also used in tissues where gain of wound strength is protracted, such as in nerves and tendons. In reconstructive surgery, skin edges are often advanced using

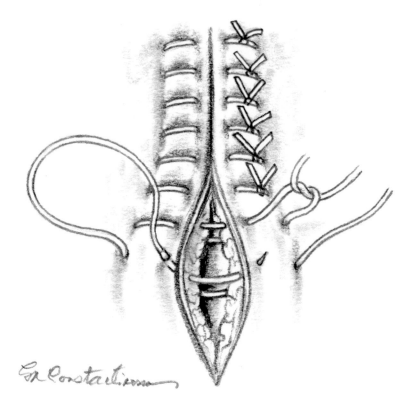

Figure 14.14   Interrupted vertical mattress.

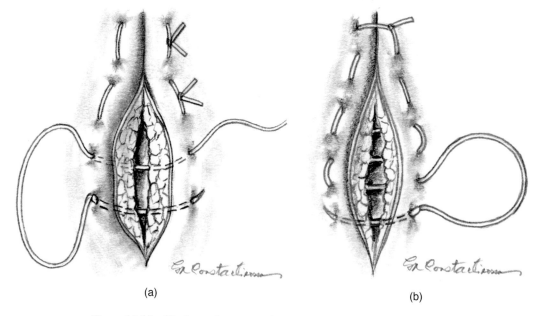

(a)   (b)

Figure 14.15   Horizontal mattress: (a) interrupted and (b) continuous.

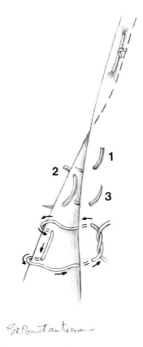

Figure 14.16 Mayo mattress (vest over pants) suture pattern.

Table 14.2 **Appositional suture patterns**

Pattern	Features	Uses
Simple interrupted (Figure 14.2)	Easy to perform. Provides secure closure. Equal tension throughout the wound. Can cause eversion of edges if excessive knot tightening is applied.	Skin, muscle fascia, gastrointestinal tract
Interrupted cruciate and figure-of-eight sutures (Figures 14.3 and 14.4)	Stronger closure compared to simple interrupted. Less skin eversion compared to simple interrupted.	Skin, muscle fascia
Interrupted intradermal (subcuticular) (Figure 14.5)	Deep superficial-superficial deep pattern.	Skin apposition (with buried knots)
Simple continuous (Figure 14.6)	Fast and economical pattern. Leads to air/water tight seals. Knot/suture failure may lead to complete dehiscence.	Subcutis, linea alba, stomach, and small intestine
Continuous intradermal (subcuticular) (Figures 14.7 and 14.8)	Horizontal or vertical pattern. Results in excellent apposition and aesthetics if carefully and correctly applied.	Meticulous skin apposition, especially when skin sutures are not performed
Ford interlocking (Figure 14.9)	Greater security in case of a broken suture (dehiscence usually incomplete).	Skin
Gambee (Figure 14.17)	Modified simple interrupted. Prevents mucosal eversion.	Small intestinal apposition

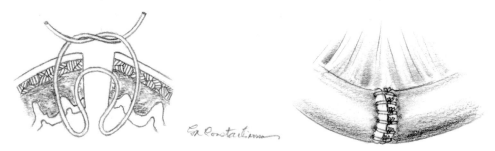

Figure 14.17 Gambee suture.

a tension-relieving technique called walking sutures (Figure 14.20). Walking sutures are simple interrupted sutures placed in the sub-cutaneous space that engage (1) the dermis (intradermal), beginning some distance back from the skin edge, and (2) the underlying muscle fascia toward the center of the wound. As each suture is tied (requires a surgeon's knot), the skin advances because the fascial suture bite is taken closer to the eventual wound edge than the suture bite in the dermis. Staggered rows of walking sutures are placed until the skin edges can touch each other without tension. Synthetic absorbable suture material (such as polydioxanone) is used for walking sutures.

Table 14.3 Inverting suture patterns

Pattern	Features	Uses
Lembert (Figure 14.10)	Similar to a vertical mattress except it inverts tissue. Interrupted or continuous.	Closure of hollow viscera. Imbrication of fascia.
Cushing (Figure 14.11)	Suture bites parallel to incision. Does not penetrate mucosa.	Closure of hollow viscera.
Connell (Figure 14.12)	Same as Cushing pattern, but penetrates the mucosa.	Closure of hollow viscera.
Halsted (Figure 14.13)	Variation of interrupted Lembert (looks like a combination of Lembert and horizontal mattress that results in tissue inversion).	Fascia imbrication.
Purse-string (Figure 14.18)	Variation of Lembert. Suture bites progress in a circle.	Closure around ostomy tubes. Temporary anal closure to prevent fecal contamination during surgery and to treat rectal prolapse.

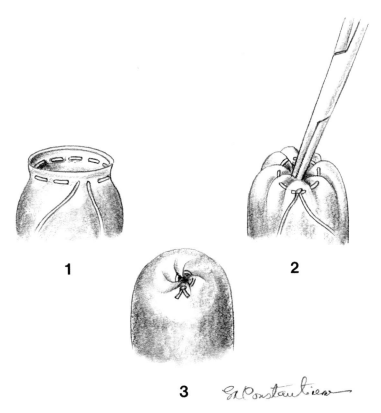

1

2

3   *ElConstautien*

Figure 14.18   Purse-string suture pattern.

Table 14.4   **Tension-relieving suture patterns**

Type	Features	Uses
Interrupted vertical mattress (Figure 14.14)	Everting, but can be appositional if carefully placed.	Skin, oral mucosa, and fascia
Horizontal mattress (Figure 14.15)	Everting. Can potentially cause decrease blood supply of the incorporated tissue. Usually interrupted, but can be continuous.	Skin, subcutis, and fascia
Mayo mattress (vest over pants) (Figure 14.16)	Overlaps one tissue edge over the other.	Herniorrhaphy, such as repair of linea alba dehiscence
Near and far variations (Figure 14.19)	May cause eversion. Diminish tension on the wound edges.	Skin and fascia
Walking sutures (Figure 14.20)	Placed in staggered rows. Advance skin edges toward each other.	Closure of large skin defects

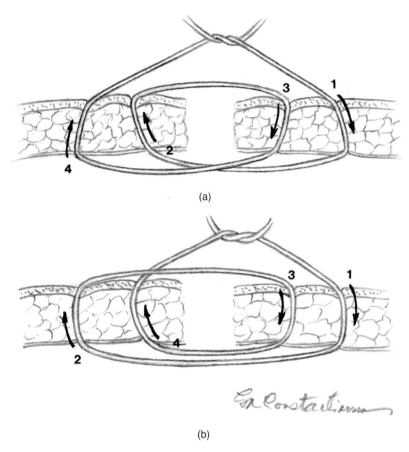

(a)

(b)

Figure 14.19 Near and far variations: (a) far-near, near-far and (b) far-far, near-near.

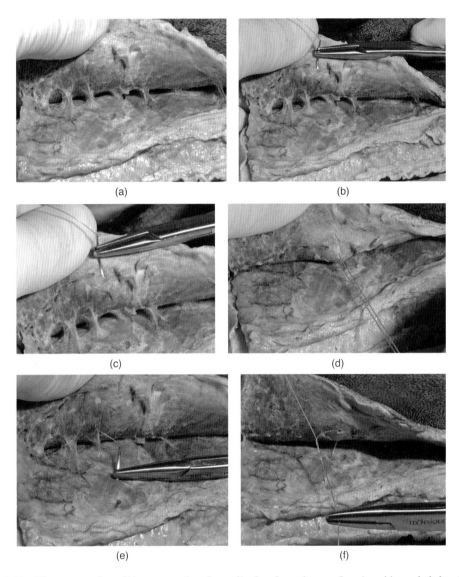

(a)   (b)

(c)   (d)

(e)   (f)

Figure 14.20   Placement of a walking suture in a formalin-fixed specimen of canine skin and abdominal wall: (a) The skin to be advanced is undermined judiciously leaving islands of loose connective tissue attaching the dermis to the underlying fascia in order to preserve blood supply to the skin. (b) A suture bite is taken in the dermis with a finger of the nondominant hand (not seen) serving as a backstop to ensure that the needle does not penetrate the epidermis. [Note: fluorescent polypropylene suture is used here for purposes of demonstration, whereas synthetic absorbable suture would be used clinically.] (c) This close-up view demonstrates proper needle passage in the dermis. (d) Pulling the strands of suture in the dermal suture bite confirms adequate engagement of the dermis and assists in determining how far to stretch the skin for the muscle fascia engagement. (e) The needle engages the muscle fascia toward the center of the wound closer to the proposed wound edge than the dermal bite so that the skin will advance when the knot is tied. (f) A surgeon's knot (followed by a square knot) is necessary because the tendency of the dermis to retract will make it difficult to maintain tightness of the first throw of a square knot while the second throw is being tied.

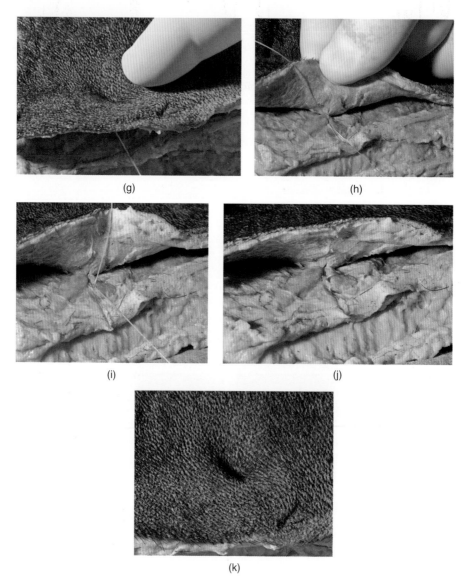

Figure 14.20 (*Continued*) (g) As the surgeon's throw is tightened, a dimple will occur in the epidermis at the point of dermal engagement. The suture must not be visible in this dimple when viewed on the skin surface. (h) The dimple may be pushed by an assistant's finger toward the muscle fascia engagement site to make tying the knot easier. With this maneuver, the assistant may roll the skin edge back as demonstrated here to allow the surgeon to visualize the knot as it is tied. (i) The completed knot advances the skin edge as is demonstrated here. (j) When the suture strands are cut the free portion of the skin typically obscures the knot, but the knot remains visible in this fixed specimen. (k) A dimple should be present in the skin at the position of each walking suture, but the suture should not penetrate the epidermis and, therefore, should not be visible on the skin.

REFERENCES

1. Rochat MC, Pope ER, Carson WL, Wagner-Mann CC, et al. Comparison of the degree of abdominal adhesion formation associated with chromic gut and polyprolylene suture materials. *Am J Vet Res* 1996;57:943–947.
2. Kirpensteijn J, Maarschalkerweerd RJ, Koeman JP, Kooistra HS, et al. Comparison of two suture materials for intradermal skin closure in dogs. *Vet Q* 1997;19:20–22.
3. Runk A, Allen SW, Mahaffey EA. Tissue reactivity to polyglecaprone in the feline linea alba. *Vet Surg* 1999;28:466–471.
4. Molea G, Schonauer F, Bifulco G, D'Angelo D. Comparative study on biocomapatibility and absorption times of three absorbable monofilament suture materials (polydioxanone, poliglecaprone, glycomer 631). *Br J Plast Surg* 2000; 53:137–141.
5. Nary Filho H, Matsumoto MA, Matista AC, Lopes LC, et al. Comparative study of tissue response to polyglecaprone 25, polyglactin 910, and polytetrafluoroethylene suture materials in rats. *Braz Dent J* 2002;13:86–91.
6. Tan RHH, Bell RJW, Dowling BA, Dart AJ. Suture materials: composition and applications in veterinary wound repair. *Aust Vet J* 2003;81: 140–145.
7. Greenberg CB, Davidson EB, Bellmer DD, Morton RJ, et al. Evaluation of the tensile strengths of four monofilament absorbable suture materials after immersion in canine urine with or without bacteria. *Am J Vet Res* 2004;65:847–853.
8. Ribeiro CMB, Silva Jr VA, Silva Neto JC, Vasconcelos BCE. Estudo clinico e histopatologico da reacao tecidual interna e externa dos fios monofilamentos de nylon a poliglecaprone 25 em ratos. *Acta Cir Bras* 2005;20:284–291.
9. Al-Qattan MM. Vicryl Rapide® versus Vicryl® suture in skin closure of the hand in children: a randomized prospective study. *J Hand Surg* 2005;30B:90–91.
10. Hochberg J, Meyer KM, Marion MD. Suture choice and other methods of skin closure. *Surg Clin North Am* 2009;89:627–641.

ADDITIONAL RESOURCES

Additional information about suture materials and suture patterns in small animal surgery can be found in the following textbooks:

1. Fossum TW, ed. *Small Animal Surgery*, 3rd ed. St. Louis, Missouri: Mosby Elsevier, 2007.
2. Slatter D, ed. *Textbook of Small Animal Surgery*, 3rd ed. Philadelphia, Pennsylvania: Saunders, 2003.
3. Edlich RF, Long WB. *Surgical Knot Tying Manual*, 3rd ed. Norwalk, Connecticut: Covidien, 2008.
4. Ethicon, Inc. *Knot Tying Manual*. Somerville, New Jersey: Ethicon, Inc., 2005.

Chapter 15

BASIC WOUND HEALING AND WOUND CLOSURE

Carlos H. de M. Souza and Fred Anthony Mann

A wound can be defined as the loss of continuity of the structure of the body resulting from an injury. Wound healing is the reestablishment of tissue continuity. Healing of wounds occurs through well orchestrated cellular and biochemical events. For the purpose of teaching, these events can be explained by phases where activation of different cellular elements and specific signaling molecules takes place. In living organisms, the processes of wound healing are interwoven and a clear demarcation between phases does not occur. The three broad phases of wound healing are (1) inflammation and debridement, (2) repair (also called proliferation), and (3) maturation.

INFLAMMATION AND DEBRIDEMENT PHASE

The wound is filled with blood immediately after injury. After clotting, the blood becomes the first barrier to the outside environment. Transient vasoconstriction of local blood vessels,

which lasts 5–10 minutes, occurs in response to catecholamines and local mast cell products (serotonin and bradykinin) to temporarily decrease blood loss from small vessels. Local vasodilatation follows, in response to histamine and interleukin-8 (IL-8), which allows plasma and intravascular cellular components to reach the extravascular space. By the action of the damaged blood vessels, platelets, and clotting factors contained in the blood, fibrin is generated and a blood clot is formed. Fibrin in association with fibronectin and activated factor XIII generate the provisional extracellular matrix, creating a scaffold for cell migration and early collagen deposition.

The inflammation that occurs after creation of a wound is characterized by migration of leukocytes from the intravascular space into the wound bed. Initially, neutrophils constitute the majority of leukocytes in the wound, but their numbers are soon exceeded by macrophages. Tissue macrophages and mast cells are activated at the time of injury and are responsible for the release of prostaglandins and leukotrienes, which attract neutrophils to the wound. Macrophages also produce interleukin-1 (IL-1), which stimulates endothelial cells to produce IL-8, also important for neutrophil

Fundamentals of Small Animal Surgery, 1st edition.
By Fred Anthony Mann, Gheorghe M. Constantinescu and Hun-Young Yoon.
© 2011 Blackwell Publishing Ltd.

chemotaxis. The neutrophils and macrophages reach the affected area by margination, attachment, and diapedesis. Once at the wound site, neutrophils release proteinases and superoxide radicals that degrade necrotic tissue and kill bacteria, respectively. Although important, neutrophils are not essential for wound healing. The short-lived neutrophils degenerate and die, and together with degraded tissue and wound fluid, form the wound exudate known as pus.

Blood monocytes differentiate into macrophages in the wound. Macrophages are essential for wound healing. They produce a variety of cytokines that potentiate the immune response. Macrophages also produce fibronectin and a variety of growth factors, such as vascular endothelial growth factor (VEGF), platelet-derived growth factor (PDGF), epidermal growth factor (EGF), and fibroblast growth factor (FGF). These growth factors stimulate mitosis and are essential for cell proliferation to occur. Macrophages are capable of phagocytosis of large particles and are vital to the debridement process of the wound. Their presence in the wound decreases as the wound becomes free of necrotic tissue and bacteria.

As the production of prostaglandins, leukotrienes, and cytokines decrease, fewer cells are attracted to the wound bed. However, chronic wounds, especially those containing foreign matter, usually continue to feature increased numbers of macrophages, which can coalesce and become very large and multinucleated (epithelioid macrophages). Growth factors and cytokines produced by macrophages stimulate fibroblasts to produce and eventually modify the provisional matrix, which becomes granulation tissue.

REPAIR (PROLIFERATIVE) PHASE

The repair phase of wound healing includes angiogenesis, fibroplasia, epithelialization, and wound contraction. The appearance of increased numbers of fibroblasts, which leads to accumulation of collagen in the wound, separates the repair phase from the inflammatory phase. The combination of large numbers of fibroblasts and the formation of new capillaries gives the granulation tissue its red fleshy and granular appearance. The transition from provisional extracellular matrix to granulation tissue is usually evident by 3–5 days after initial wounding. The period prior to granulation tissue formation is also called the lag phase due to the lack of gain in wound strength. The presence of granulation tissue markedly increases the wound's resistance to infection. Granulation tissue also serves as a surface for epithelial cell movement and provides myofibroblasts for wound contraction.

Angiogenesis is the formation of new capillaries from vessels present at the limits of the wound. Angiogenesis results from the migration and proliferation of endothelial cells in response to growth factors produced by macrophages, such as VEGF, FGF, transforming growth factor beta (TGFβ), angiogenin, and angiopoetin. The migration of endothelial cells and the proliferation of endothelium from the wound margins are regulated by the extracellular matrix (ECM). As wound healing progresses, proteins also present in the ECM (i.e., trombospondin and angiostatin) are responsible for apoptosis of endothelial cells and decrease in the number of capillaries. Capillary death gives the wound a pale appearance characteristic of old granulation tissue.

Fibroplasia is the proliferation of wound fibroblasts and the consequent production of collagen. Growth factors (including PDGF, FGF, and TGFβ) and proteins called integrin receptors present in the ECM are responsible for the attraction and migration of fibroblasts into the wound, respectively. Fibroblasts and epithelial cells express integrins on their surface. Binding to the integrin receptors stimulates and guides the movement of both fibroblasts and epithelial cells to cover the wound. The migration of fibroblasts into the wound leads to increased production of collagen and change in the predominant type of collagen in the wound. Initially, collagen type III predominates, but collagen type I becomes the most common type of collagen as the wound is filled with fibroblasts. The greatest increase in collagen content occurs between 7 and 14 days after wounding. After this period, the numbers of fibroblasts and new capillaries decrease, the collagen content stabilizes, and the granulation tissue changes into a relatively acellular scar. Gaining of strength continues slowly over several months, although the scar tissue never achieves the strength of the original intact tissues.

Epithelialization is the covering of the wound with new epithelial cells. The early events of epithelialization include mobilization and migration of epithelial cells from the wound edges. In partial-thickness skin wounds, epithelialization occurs almost immediately, with mobilization of epithelial cells from the wound edges and skin appendages. In full-thickness wounds, formation of granulation tissue is necessary before epithelialization can occur. In order to migrate, the epithelial cells at the edges of the wound must change their phenotype and disconnect from neighboring cells. Up-regulation of matrix metalloproteinases to act on the basement membrane, change in the pattern of surface integrins, and up-regulation of microtubules and other contractile proteins, are some of the changes necessary for movement of epithelial cells. Once cells come in contact with each other, their movement ceases (contact inhibition), the phenotypic changes reverse, and a new basement membrane is formed. In large open wounds, where complete contraction does not occur, epithelialization continues. A thin layer of epithelial cells covers the wound in such cases. This thin layer is easily traumatized, and repetitive trauma may prevent epithelialization from being complete.

Wound contraction is a process that decreases the size of a wound. Wound contraction is achieved by the migration of myofibroblasts toward the center of the wound. As the wound contracts, the surrounding skin stretches and the wound becomes stellate in appearance. Contraction of the wound ceases as the tension on the surrounding skin equals contracting forces. The end result of contraction is usually beneficial by decreasing the diameter of the wound. Around tubular structures and joints, excessive contraction may lead to strictures and gait abnormalities, respectively, a process referred to as contracture.

MATURATION PHASE

Maturation is the phase of wound healing characterized by progressive gain of tissue strength. As the wound matures, the ECM progressively becomes scar. Collagen deposition and gain in tissue strength are marked in the first 7–14 days and then decrease. Despite the initial rapid gain in strength, wounded tissues attain only 20% of their final strength in the first three weeks after wounding. Tissue strength continues to improve as collagen fibers rearrange and cross-linkage of collagen fibers increases. Equilibrium between ECM degradation by matrix metalloproteinases and inhibition of degradation by tissue inhibitors of metalloproteinases is slowly achieved. Maturation may take months or years, but still, the final tensile strength of the scar is only 70–80% of normal tissue. In fact, the process of wound maturation continues for the life of the animal, with only two tissues capable of returning to 100% of the tissue's unwounded strength: urinary bladder and bone.

WOUND CLOSURE

Local wound factors, additional injuries, and time elapsed since the creation of the wound must be considered prior to wound closure in order to increase the chances of uncomplicated healing. Knowledge of how the wound was created (incision by a sharp blade, gunshot, car accident, etc.) is of extreme importance to determine the expected amount of tissue trauma and chances of wound contamination and necrosis. Wounds can be managed by primary closure, delayed primary closure, secondary closure, and second intention healing. First-intention healing refers to surgical closure of a wound with the intent of having the apposed wound edges heal to each other without a need for epithelium to migrate across a granulation bed. All three of the above mentioned *closures* are performed to achieve first-intention healing, whereas second-intention healing does not involve surgical apposition of wound edges.

Primary closure is closure of a wound soon after it is created. A planned surgical incision is the most obvious example of a wound suitable for primary closure. Clean wounds can be managed by wound cleaning and primary closure if within a few (preferably 6) hours of wound creation. In such wounds, there should be minimal, if any, need for debridement. At wound evaluation, the surgeon must decide that the chances of additional loss of tissue viability and infection will be minimal after closure. In addition, primary closure should result in minimal tension on wound edges in order to minimize the chances for dehiscence.

Delayed primary closure is closure of a wound after a delay to determine wound viability, but before the onset of granulation tissue. Delayed primary closure is employed when there is minimal to moderate tissue damage, but the chances of contamination progressing to infection are significant. Cleaning, debridement, and bandaging are performed until the wound is suitable for closure. Delayed primary closure is performed within 3 days after wound creation, prior to the presence of granulation tissue. Local or distant tissue (tissue flaps) may be required for wound closure.

Secondary closure is wound closure after the onset of granulation tissue. Wounds with extensive tissue loss or necrosis, severe contamination, or marked presence of debris are good candidates for secondary closure. In such wounds, extensive cleaning is usually necessary due to the presence of large amounts of foreign material (dirt, asphalt, feces, etc.). Debridement of necrotic tissue should be performed daily until additional necrosis is not detected and a healthy bed of granulation tissue covers the wound (longer than 5 days). Advancement of local skin with walking sutures, skin flaps, or skin grafts may be required for closure.

Second intention healing is nonclosure of a wound. Closure is achieved naturally as previously described in this chapter. Second intention healing is dependent on wound contraction and epithelialization. Small uncomplicated wounds or wounds where local or distant tissues are not available for closure may be suitable for second intention healing. Second intention healing should be avoided in wounds adjacent to tubular structures (perianal wounds), or in periarticular wounds, due to the risk of stricture and decrease in range of motion, respectively.

MANAGEMENT OF ACUTE TRAUMATIC WOUNDS AND DECIDING WHEN AND HOW TO CLOSE THEM

General practitioners and veterinarians who practice emergency medicine are often presented with wounds that have just occurred, and what veterinarians do to initially manage these wounds may dictate the ultimate outcome of the definitive treatment. The remainder of this chapter is written to stimulate the reader to think about the decisions involved in acute wound management and accompanying antibiotic therapy that may (or may not) be indicated. Answers to the questions posed below are incomplete or absent in order to promote an active thought process when managing any particular wound.

Initial Wound Care

Early management of acutely inflicted wounds greatly influences healing and ultimate outcome. Prompt and efficient wound inspection, lavage, appropriate debridement, and aseptic bandaging of wounds are the predecessors of optimal results. It is debatable whether topical medications are indicated and, if indicated, what topical medications should be used. A "cook book" approach to the steps in wound management discussed below will inevitably result in an undesirable outcome at an unexpected time. Thoughtful consideration of the questions below should be part of the wound management process each time a veterinarian is presented with an acute wound to manage.

Wound Inspection

A thorough examination of the wound is essential for determining the immediate course of action, the possibilities for closure, and initial prognosis for success of treatment. Consider the necessity of the various components of wound inspection. Why is adequate clipping of hair around the wound important? How does one protect the wound from clipped hair during the process of clipping, and why is it important to provide this protection? Why are sterile gloves and sterile instruments used to inspect acute traumatic wounds? Is it really necessary that the gloves and instruments are sterile given that these wounds are already contaminated?

Here are some answers: Generous hair removal is important for adequate visualization, optimal decontamination, and general hygiene. Protection of the wound from clipped hair is accomplished by packing the wound with sterile gauze and/or sterile jelly. This protection is necessary to avoid foreign body (hair) contamination of the wound. Sterile gloves and instruments are used to avoid iatrogenic contamination. The wound needs to be protected from contamination by microorganisms in the hospital environment that could lead to serious nosocomial infection by resistant bacteria.

Lavage

It is generally accepted that wounds should be irrigated (lavaged) during inspection and treatment, but why should wounds be lavaged? And, what solutions are appropriate for wound lavage? List one advantage and one disadvantage of pressurizing the lavage. What is the optimal lavage pressure and how can this pressure be achieved? Should puncture wounds be lavaged? Why or why not?

Here are some answers: Wounds are lavaged to hydrate them. Remember the old adage that "moist tissues are happy tissues." Also, another old adage states that "dilution is the solution to pollution." As such, lavage is performed to remove small debris and to "dilute" the bacteria that are likely present. Removal of all foreign matter, even the particulate variety, will make the wound environment less conducive to bacterial growth, and copious lavage will help "wash away" bacteria as well. Depending on the solution used for lavage, some bacteria may even be killed. A number of solutions have been used to lavage acute traumatic wounds. A balanced electrolyte solution with a physiologically acceptable pH (such as lactated Ringer's solution) is ideal. Other solutions that have been successfully used for wound lavage include normal saline, 0.05% chlorhexidine, and tap water, the latter typically reserved for wounds that are excessively covered with environmental dirt and grime. When antiseptics are used, solutions should be used; scrubs (detergents) should not be applied to wounds. Some prefer to pressurize the lavage to facilitate removal of foreign matter in the wound. A disadvantage to pressurized lavage is the potential to drive bacteria into the tissues rather than washing them away. The optimal lavage pressure has been taught to be 9 psi achieved using an 18- or 19-gauge hypodermic needle attached to a 35-mL syringe. However, in one study (Gall T, Monnet E. Pressure dynamics of common techniques used for wound flushing. Abstract. In: *Proceedings of the 2008 American College of Veterinary Surgeons Veterinary Symposium*, San Diego, CA, October 23–25, 2008, p. 13.), a 35-mL syringe and 18-gauge hypodermic needle produced nearly double that amount of pressure. Lavage of puncture wounds can be detrimental. Doing so could introduce fluid into the subcutaneous tissues, and it is likely that all of the introduced fluid cannot be retrieved, ultimately resulting in "iatrogenic" edema. Therefore, it is recommended not to lavage puncture wounds, but rather to surface cleanse them.

Surgical Debridement

Debridement is the "removal of debris," the removal of dead tissue and foreign material. The proper English pronunciation (dĭ-brēd'mənt) is recommended to emphasize that debris, not living tissue, is being removed. How does debridement differ from "freshening wound edges"? Why would "freshening edges" ever be indicated? Describe appropriate anesthesia/restraint for surgical debridement. Why are sterile drapes, instruments, and gloves important for debridement?

Here are some answers: The technique of freshening wound edges involves incision until bleeding is witnessed; therefore, freshening removes viable tissue. Debridement does not remove viable tissue. Freshening edges has no role in surgical debridement of wounds. Freshening is occasionally done during wound closure (see "Freshening wound edges" below), but only when necessary for cosmesis or to avoid burying epithelium. The most appropriate restraint for surgical debridement is general anesthesia. The actual protocol should be tailored to the individual patient, but in most cases, thorough debridement is best done with an intubated patient and inhalant anesthesia. Sterile drapes, instruments, and gloves are important for surgical debridement to avoid iatrogenic contamination.

Aseptic Bandaging

Bandaging a wound after surgical debridement can be beneficial if appropriately applied, or detrimental if errantly applied. What wounds require bandaging? What wounds require splinted bandaging? What wounds do not require bandaging? Why is it important for the contact layer of the bandage to be sterile? What is the purpose of a wet-to-dry dressing? When is a dry-to-dry dressing used? When is it appropriate to switch from an adherent to a nonadherent dressing?

Here are some answers: Ideally, all wounds should be bandaged after surgical debridement. Unfortunately, bandaging is not always practical. Essentially, all wounds in hospitalized patients should be bandaged if at all possible in order to minimize the chance of nosocomial wound infection. Splinted bandages are required for wounds around joints or wounds that are otherwise subjected to excessive movement. Wounds that can be safely left unbandaged are those that are covered by healthy granulation tissue and are going to be managed at home and not in the hospital environment. The contact layer of bandages is sterile in order to protect against iatrogenic contamination. Wet-to-dry dressings are used when continued debridement is required. A dry-to-dry dressing is used when the wound is already wet due to exudation, and, like the wet-to-dry dressing, the dry-to-dry dressing is used for debridement. Wet-to-dry and dry-to-dry dressings are adherent to the wound. A switch from adherent to nonadherent dressing is done once there is a granulation bed to protect the granulation tissue from being disrupted during bandage changes.

Topical Medications/Ointments

There seems to be an innate tendency for veterinarians to apply medications to wounds, and wound care products seem to be widely available. What ointments are appropriate for application to wounds? What ointments may delay wound healing? What ointments may enhance wound healing? List the reason(s) for using any justifiable ointment. [Is the ointment used for antimicrobial effect, enzymatic debridement, and/or direct enhancement of healing?]

Here are some answers: Any of a number of available topical wound medications may be deemed appropriate. Some for which the author has found appropriate use include triple antibiotic ointment, gentamicin ointment, silver sulfadiazine cream, trypsin with balsam of peru and castor oil spray or ointment (Granulex V, Pfizer Animal Health, Exton, PA), sugar, and unpasteurized honey. However, the author typically avoids topical wound treatments unless a specified purpose is desired and likely to be achieved with the ointment. Further, one must consider potential detrimental effects of ointments. For example, some ointments will trap exudates in the wound thereby contributing to bacterial growth rather than combating it. And, many ointments will have some negative effect on wound healing. Petrolatum, a base found in some ointments, delays the epithelial stage of wound healing. On the other hand, some topical wound medications enhance wound healing. Notable examples of products that optimize wound healing are trypsin (because of enzymatic debridement), sugar, and unpasteurized honey. Whenever a topical agent is applied to a wound a justifiable reason (antimicrobial effect, enzymatic debridement, and/or direct enhancement of healing) should be evident.

Deciding on Wound Closure

Options for wound closure (as detailed above) are primary closure, delayed primary closure, secondary wound closure, and second intention healing. Primary wound closure is closure performed immediately after wounding (within the first few hours). Delayed primary closure is closure of the wound after allowing enough time to ascertain vascular compromise (usually 18–24 hours, but definitely before the onset of granulation tissue). Secondary wound closure is closure after the appearance of granulation tissue within the wound. The presence of granulation tissue signals that the wound is reasonably resistant to infection and, therefore, safe to

close. Second intention healing is nonclosure. Instead of closing the wound, the processes of contraction and epithelialization are allowed to progress naturally to afford eventual closure. Deciding which method of closure is best for any individual patient requires analysis of multiple factors, such as wound classification, timing of the injury, cause of the injury, and the owner's financial limitations. Relying only on any one of these four factors for determining the method of wound closure is flirting with failure. Following is an outline of the four factors used to determine the most appropriate type of wound closure and discussion of each factor.

Wound classification

1. Clean
2. Clean-contaminated
3. Contaminated
4. Dirty/Infected

Timing of injury

1. Within 6 hours of injury
2. Beyond 6 hours of injury

Cause of injury

1. Puncture wound
2. Sharp laceration
3. Sharp laceration with tissue loss (anatomic degloving)
4. Blunt injury (physiologic degloving)

Owner's financial limitations

1. Is second intention closure really more economical than surgical closure?
2. Is primary closure ever warranted if dehiscence is likely?

Wound Classification

Clean wounds are rare with acute injury. The best example of a clean wound is a surgical incision in aseptically prepared skin that does not penetrate a contaminated lumen, such as the alimentary or respiratory tract. Clean-contaminated wounds are wounds with minimal contamination. The best example of a clean-contaminated wound is a surgical incision in an aseptically prepared patient in which the alimentary or respiratory tract is entered. Acute traumatic wounds with minimal environmental debris and absence of necrotic tissue may also be considered to be clean-contaminated wounds. Primary wound closure can be performed with minimal risk of ensuing infection in clean and clean-contaminated wounds (after appropriate wound inspection and lavage). Contaminated wounds are nonsurgical wounds (or surgical wounds with major breaks in aseptic technique) where presence of bacteria is likely, but there are no gross signs of infection. Contaminated wounds can be closed by primary wound closure if they are converted to clean-contaminated wounds through the process of lavage. Dirty/infected wounds are wounds with foreign debris and/or gross evidence of infection (such as purulent exudate). Dirty/infected wounds might also contain necrotic tissue. For a wound to be infected, enough time must have passed to allow proliferation of bacteria to the concentration of 10^5 bacteria per gram of tissue (or per mL of tissue fluid). Primary wound closure is rarely performed for dirty/infected wounds, but theoretically could be done if the wound can be converted to a clean-contaminated state through the processes of lavage and debridement.

Timing of Injury

Assuming all other factors support primary wound closure, such closure is safer if performed within 6 hours of the injury, because by 6 hours, bacteria have had enough time to multiply to numbers capable of causing infection (10^5 bacterial organisms per gram of tissue or per mL of tissue fluid for most bacteria). Wounds older than 6 hours would ideally be managed as open wounds and have delayed primary or secondary wound closure once it is certain that infection is not developing or after an infection that develops is eliminated.

Cause of Injury

Puncture wounds are not typically closed because the amount of subcutaneous trauma is difficult to determine, and the punctures allow for drainage. In general, puncture wounds are not surgically explored unless there is a known foreign object that must be retrieved. Sharp lacerations offer the best opportunity for primary wound closure, whereas sharp laceration with tissue loss (anatomic degloving) and open wounds due to blunt injury (physiologic degloving) require some time to determine the health of the tissue. Delayed primary closure is more appropriate than primary closure for anatomic and physiologic degloving wounds. In some cases, secondary wound closure is best for degloving wounds.

Owner's Financial Limitations

The owner's desire for a fiscally conservative approach may make second-intention healing or primary wound closure more appealing than delayed primary or secondary wound closure. However, the wrong closure choice could result in more financial burden than if the wound was managed most appropriately in the first place. Second-intention healing may necessitate wound management and bandaging for a protracted period of time resulting in accumulation of more financial investment than if surgical closure (at the appropriate time) was performed. Likewise, closing a wound before it is ready could result in infection and/or dehiscence and the added costs of dealing with those complications.

"Freshening Wound Edges"

During wound closure, one is often tempted to "freshen the wound edges." "Freshening wound edges" is contraindicated because it offsets the advantage of the secondary wound phenomenon (i.e., accelerated healing due to already present and active fibroblasts). When might one justify "freshening the edges" of a wound? Perhaps edges should be trimmed if an exquisite cosmetic effect is desired (and in the best interests of the patient). During secondary wound closure epithelium that has begun migration over the granulation bed may require excision to prevent its burial under the surgically advanced skin edges. One might consider excision of this advancing epithelium to be "freshening of the wound edge."

Managing Wound Drainage

Wound drainage can be expected in most traumatic wounds. How is wound drainage managed in open wounds? Drainage must be controlled in wounds that are surgically closed. Methods for drainage control include obliteration of dead space and incorporation of a passive or active wound drain. Describe a wound in which no surgical drain is necessary. Describe the proper method of dead space obliteration. When would a passive or active wound drain be indicated? Identify some particular types of passive drains. Identify some particular types of active drains. What are the advantages and disadvantages of a passive wound drain? What are the advantages and disadvantages of an active wound drain?

Here are some answers: Drainage in open wounds is achieved through the wounds themselves. Ideally, open wounds are bandaged so that wound fluids are absorbed into the bandage and removed during bandage changes. Drains can be omitted in surgically closed wounds if dead space is obliterated. Dead space is obliterated with careful placement of sutures similar to "walking sutures." Dead space can also be obliterated with bandaging, but bandage obliteration of dead space is more readily achieved on limbs than on other areas of the body. When it is not possible to effectively obliterate dead space with suture or bandage, a passive or active wound drain is recommended

(see also Chapter 17). A commonly used passive drain is the Penrose drain (Figures 17.8a and 17.8b). A commonly used active drain is the Jackson-Pratt drain (Figures 17.8c and 17.8f through 17.8k). Passive drains are economical and easily placed, but ideally should be bandaged to collect drainage and protect from ascending infection. Also, passive drains must be maintained for 5 days before removal to ensure that the tissues have sealed to obliterate dead space. A passive drain that can be removed prior to 5 days was probably unnecessary. Active drains pull tissues together causing early obliteration of dead space and permitting early drain removal (typically 2–3 days after surgery). Further, active suction and the closed nature of the drain help protect against ascending infection. The major disadvantage of active drains is that they are more expensive than passive drains; however, their effectiveness may offset the expense.

Antibiotic Therapy in Wound Management

There is a tendency to prescribe antibiotic therapy for animals with wounds to provide a "cover" for infection, even when there is no evidence that infection is present or likely. However, indiscriminate use of antibiotics is potentially harmful. And, as a profession, if we do not curtail inappropriate use of antibiotics, governmental restrictions could limit, or prevent altogether, access to certain antimicrobial drugs for veterinary use. When managing a wound, certain questions should come to mind regarding antibiotic therapy. Answering these questions is much preferred to the simpler "knee jerk" response of prescribing an antibiotic or applying an antimicrobial ointment. The reader is encouraged to carefully consider the following questions before prescribing systemic or topical antibiotics in the treatment of wounds.

Acute Wounds

The mere presence of a laceration is not an indication for emergency administration of antibiotic therapy. However, the acutely traumatized patient may require antibiotic therapy for other reasons. List some potential indications for antibiotic therapy in acutely traumatized patients. How might antibiotic administration affect the wound?

Infected Wounds

Most clinicians feel that antibiotic therapy is indicated for infected wounds. If that is the case, what antibiotic should be used? The antibiotic should be given by what route? How long should the antibiotic be administered? What factors guide the choice of antibiotic? Should antibiotic therapy be guided by culture and susceptibility? If so, when and how should the bacteriology sample be obtained? What would be some disadvantages of antibiotic administration in the management of open wounds?

See Chapter 4 for discussion of antibiotic use in surgery.

ADDITIONAL RESOURCES

For detailed descriptions of wound management and discussion of the issues represented in the questions posed in this chapter, the reader is referred to the following references:

1. Brown DC, Conzemius MG, Shofer F, Swann H. Epidemiologic evaluation of postoperative wound infections in dogs and cats. *J Am Vet Med Assoc* 1997;210:1302–1306.
2. Buffa EA, Lubbe AM, Verstraete FJM, Swaim SF. The effects of wound lavage solutions on canine fibroblasts: an in vitro study. *Vet Surg* 1997;26:460–466.
3. Davidson EB. Managing bite wounds in dogs and cats: part I. *Compend Contin Educ Pract Vet* 1998;20:811–821.
4. Davidson EB. Managing bite wounds in dogs and cats: part II. *Compend Cont Educ Pract Vet* 1998;20:974–991, 1006.
5. Devitt CM, Seim HB, Willer R, et al. Passive drainage versus primary closure after total ear canal ablation-lateral bulla osteotomy in dogs: 59 dogs (1985–1995). *Vet Surg* 1997;26:210–216.
6. Dunning D. Surgical wound infection and the use of antimicrobials. In: Slatter D, ed. *Textbook of Small Animal Surgery*, 3rd ed. Philadelphia, Pennsylvania: Saunders, 2003:113–122.
7. Eron LJ. Targeting lurking pathogens in acute traumatic and chronic wounds. *J Emerg Med* 1999;17:189–195.
8. Fossum TW, Willard MD. Surgical infections and antibiotic selection. In: Fossum TW, ed. *Small Animal Surgery*, 3rd ed. St. Louis, Missouri: Mosby, 2007:79–89.
9. Gall T, Monnet E. Pressure dynamics of common techniques used for wound flushing. Abstract. In: *Proceedings of the 2008 American College of Veterinary Surgeons Veterinary Symposium, San Diego, CA*, October 23–25, 2008, p. 13.
10. Hedlund C. Surgery of the integumentary system. In: Fossum TW, ed. *Small Animal Surgery*, 3rd ed. St. Louis, Missouri: Mosby Elsevier, 2007:159–176.
11. Holt DE, Griffin G. Bite wounds in dogs and cats. *Vet Clin North Am Small Anim Pract* 2000;30:669–679.
12. Jang SS, Breher JE, Dabaco LA, Hirsh DC. Organisms isolated from dogs and cats with anaerobic infections and susceptibility to selected antimicrobial agents. *J Am Vet Med Assoc* 1997;210:1610–1614.
13. Janis JE, Kwon RK, Lalonde DH. A practical guide to wound healing. *Plast Reconstr Surg* 2010;125:230e–244e.
14. Marberry KM, Kazmier P, Simpson WA, et al. Surfactant wound irrigation for the treatment of staphylococcal clinical isolates. *Clin Orthop Relat Res* 2002;403:73–39.
15. Mathews KA, Binnington AG. Wound management using sugar. *Compend Cont Educ Pract Vet* 2002;24:41–50.
16. Mathews KA, Binnington AG. Wound management using honey. *Compend Cont Educ Pract Vet* 2002;24:53–60.
17. Miller CW. Bandages and drains. In: Slatter D, ed. *Textbook of Small Animal Surgery*, 3rd

ed. Philadelphia, Pennsylvania: Saunders, 2003: 244–249.

18. Nicholson M, Beal M, Shofer F, Brown DC. Epidemiologic evaluation of postoperative wound infection in clean-contaminated wounds: a retrospective study of 239 dogs and cats. *Vet Surg* 2002;31:577–581.

19. Noble WC, Lloyd DH. Pathogenesis and management of wound infections in domestic animals. *Vet Dermatol* 1997;8:243–248.

20. Vasseur PB, Levy J, Dowd E, Eliot J. Surgical wound infection rates in dogs and cats: data from a teaching hospital. *Vet Surg* 1988;17:60–64.

21. Waldron DR, Zimmerman-Pope N. Superficial skin wounds. In: Slatter D, ed. *Textbook of Small Animal Surgery*, 3rd ed. Philadelphia, Pennsylvania: Saunders, 2003:259–273.

22. Weston C. The science behind topical negative pressure therapy. *Acta Chir Belg* 2010;110:19–27.

Chapter 16

SURGICAL HEMOSTASIS

Elizabeth A. Swanson and Fred Anthony Mann

Achieving hemostasis in surgery is essential for prevention of severe hemorrhage and for provision of adequate visualization of the surgical field. Maintaining hemostasis in the surgical patient is aided by proper surgical technique including gentle tissue handling, the use of appropriate instruments, and a thorough knowledge of both the anatomy and the procedure to be performed. Despite proper attention to hemostasis, hemorrhage inevitably occurs during surgery, and a working knowledge of the hemostatic measures available to the veterinary surgeon is invaluable. Multiple options available to help control surgical hemorrhage are discussed in this chapter, the selection of which is greatly enhanced by a basic understanding of the biology of hemostasis. The reader is referred to internal medicine and hematology textbooks for more in-depth discussions of hemostasis, but an overview is provided here.

HEMOSTASIS

Hemostasis is a complex process that involves multiple interactions between the vascular wall,

Fundamentals of Small Animal Surgery, 1st edition.
By Fred Anthony Mann, Gheorghe M. Constantinescu and Hun-Young Yoon.
© 2011 Blackwell Publishing Ltd.

platelets, and the coagulation cascade to initiate the formation of a temporary platelet plug followed by a more stable fibrin clot. Following injury to a vessel, transient vasoconstriction occurs in response to endothelin release by damaged vascular endothelium. Thromboxane A_2 (TXA_2), bradykinin, and fibrinopeptide B are also released and may contribute to vasoconstriction. The extent of vasoconstriction and its effect on bleeding depends on the amount of smooth muscle present in the vessel wall (i.e., arteries have more smooth muscle than veins; capillaries have no smooth muscle), the size of the vessel, and the size and location of the defect in the endothelium.

The endothelium of a blood vessel is an active component of hemostasis. In health, the endothelium functions to maintain vascular tone, to provide a semipermeable barrier, and to prevent inappropriate thrombus formation via the release of prostacyclin (prostaglandin I_2), thrombomodulin, heparin-like molecules, and tissue plasminogen activator. *Primary hemostasis* (Figure 16.1) is initiated by contact of the circulating blood with exposed extracellular matrix at the site of the injury. This matrix is primarily composed of subendothelial type II collagen, which can bind and activate platelets. The damaged endothelium releases von Willebrand's factor (vWF), an adhesive protein that

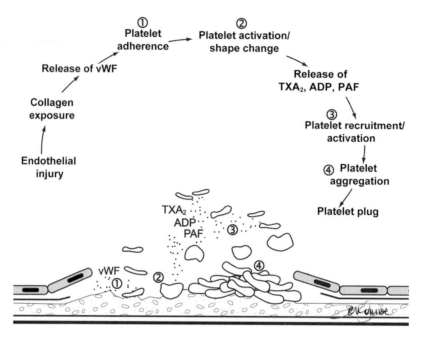

Figure 16.1   The primary hemostasis pathway. Damage to the endothelium exposes collagen which releases vWF and causes platelets to adhere to the damaged area (1). Once adhered, the platelets activate and change shape (2). The activated platelets release granules containing TXA_2, ADP, and PAF, which act to recruit and activate additional circulating platelets (3). The activated platelets aggregate (4) to form a platelet plug over the damaged vessel wall. *vWF*, von Willebrand's factor; *TXA₂*, Thromboxane A_2; *ADP*, Adenosine diphospate; *PAF*, Platelet activating factor.

allows the platelets to adhere to the damaged vessel wall. Once they adhere, the platelets become activated, change shape, and release TXA_2, adenosine diphosphate and platelet activating factor to recruit additional platelets from the circulation and form a platelet aggregate. The platelet aggregate serves to plug the injured site while a more stable fibrin clot forms.

The activated platelets change their phospholipid profile to increase phosphatidyl serine (also known as platelet factor 3) and procoagulant activity. This procoagulant activity is an essential link between primary hemostasis and secondary hemostasis, as it provides the phospholipid surface needed to bind calcium to prothrombin and factors VII, IX, and X of the coagulation cascade and serves to localize secondary coagulation to the site of vessel injury. The size of the platelet plug is limited by prostacyclin secreted by normal, intact endothelial cells and by endothelium-dependent relaxing factor-nitric oxide released from venous endothelium. Both substances inhibit platelet function and cause vasodilation, which increases blood flow and dilutes other platelet activators.

The initial platelet plug is stabilized by a series of enzymatic reactions that result in the cleavage of fibrinogen into fibrin, which crosslinks on the surface of the activated platelets and traps platelets, red blood cells, leukocytes, and plasma into a fibrin clot. This process is known as *secondary hemostasis* (Figure 16.2). Traditionally, the coagulation cascade is taught as two pathways, extrinsic and intrinsic, of cascading reactions that result in the formation of a fibrin clot. In actuality, these pathways interact

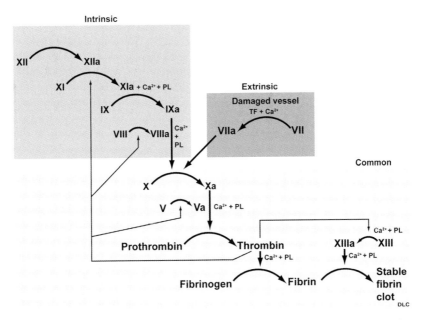

Figure 16.2 The secondary hemostasis pathway. The extrinsic pathway is initiated when tissue factor from damaged endothelium combines with calcium and activates factor VII. The intrinsic pathway is initiated when thrombin activates factor XI and, to a lesser extent, when blood contacts damaged endothelium, which activates factor XII. Both pathways intersect at the common pathway, and activate factor X which leads to the formation of a fibrin clot. Prothrombin is also known as factor II, and fibrinogen is also known as factor I. Factors are indicated as Roman numerals, activated factors are denoted by the letter *a*. Ca^{2+}, Calcium ion; *PL*, Phospholipid; *TF*, Tissue factor. Each branch of the pathway is shaded and labeled.

at many different levels, and the extrinsic pathway is now considered the initiator of coagulation while the intrinsic pathway sustains and amplifies the reaction.

The extrinsic pathway (also known as the initiation pathway) begins with damage to the endothelium and surrounding tissues. The damaged tissues release tissue factor which in the presence of ionized calcium forms a complex with factor VII. This activated factor VII complex, then activates factor X to begin the common pathway.

The intrinsic pathway (also known as the amplification pathway) was previously thought to be solely initiated in the blood by contact between the blood and the damaged subendothelial collagen, resulting in activation of factor XII, which in turn activates factor XI. While this

initiation mechanism does occur, *in vivo* studies have now shown that the majority of the factor XI activation is provided by thrombin produced by the extrinsic pathway and explains why factor XII deficiencies are clinically silent. Activated factor XI activates factor IX in the presence of ionized calcium. Factor IX combines with activated factor VIII in the presence of platelet or tissue phospholipids and ionized calcium and activates factor X.

At this point, a common pathway is described in which activated factor X forms a complex with tissue or platelet phospholipids, ionized calcium, and activated factor V, which cleaves prothrombin (also called factor II) into thrombin. Thrombin cleaves fibrinogen (also called factor I) into fibrin monomers that polymerize into fibrin chains and form a weak clot.

Thrombin further activates factor XIII, catalyzed by ionized calcium, which promotes cross-linking between the fibrin fibers and the formation of a stable clot. Thrombin also acts to cleave prothrombin to activate factors V, VIII, and XI and to activate platelets in an excellent model of biological amplification.

The coagulation cascade is primarily inhibited by two pathways: the antithrombin-heparin pathway and the thrombomodulin-protein C-protein S pathway. Antithrombin provides 80% of the thrombin inhibitory capacity of plasma. Combined with heparin-like molecules on the endothelium, antithrombin binds to thrombin and neutralizes its activity. Antithrombin also inactivates active factors XII, XI, X, and IX. Endogenous heparin-like molecules are also believed to enhance the release of tissue factor pathway inhibitor from endothelial cells, and in a high shear stress environment will interfere with platelet-vWF binding. Protein C, activated by the thrombin–thrombomodulin complex, inhibits the coagulation system and activates the fibrinolytic system. Fibrinolysis acts to limit the size of the developing thrombus. Activated protein C, in combination with calcium and cofactor protein S, inactivates membrane phospholipid-bound activated factors V and VIII, preventing the activation of factor X and the cleavage of fibrinogen into fibrin. Thrombomodulin complexes with and neutralizes thrombin, thereby inhibiting fibrinogen cleavage, activation of factor V, and activation of platelets.

The fibrinolytic system serves to enzymatically degrade fibrin clots and to maintain a patent vascular system. Plasminogen can be activated into plasmin by activated factor XII, tissue plasminogen activator, urinary plasminogen activator, urokinase, and streptokinase. Plasmin causes the breakdown of fibrin into fibrinogen degradation products, which are cleared by mononuclear cells via phagocytosis. Fibrinolysis is inhibited by α2-antiplasmin, α2-macroglobulin, and plasminogen activator inhibitor types one and two.

The primary and secondary hemostatic pathways, the inhibitory pathways, and the fibrinolytic system all work together with the ultimate goal to restore vascular wall integrity with minimal blood loss and prevention of coagulation beyond the injured area.

CONTROL OF SURGICAL HEMORRHAGE

Hemorrhage during surgery occurs when an incision made into a tissue disrupts blood vessels. It is desirable to minimize blood loss to avoid detrimental effects to the patient and to maintain visualization of the surgical field. Bloodless fields save valuable surgical time. The type of hemostatic method used depends on the tissue type, nature of the hemorrhage, and size of the bleeding vessel. The following section will introduce the hemostatic methods currently available in veterinary medicine.

DIRECT PRESSURE AND HEMOSTATIC FORCEPS

Applying direct pressure to a bleeding vessel is a rapid method of staunching blood loss. This may be done with gentle digital pressure or by compression or blotting with a gauze sponge (Figure 16.3). Excessive pressure may inhibit coagulation by preventing platelets and coagulation factors from reaching the site of transection. When using a gauze sponge, gentle pressure over the area of hemorrhage should be applied for a length of time sufficient for coagulation and then lifted, being careful not to disrupt the clot that has formed. A wiping motion should be avoided. Using a moistened sponge may help minimize disruption of the clot when the sponge is removed, but too much moisture in the sponge will result in less effective hemostasis. Direct pressure provides permanent hemostasis for small vessels (capillaries)

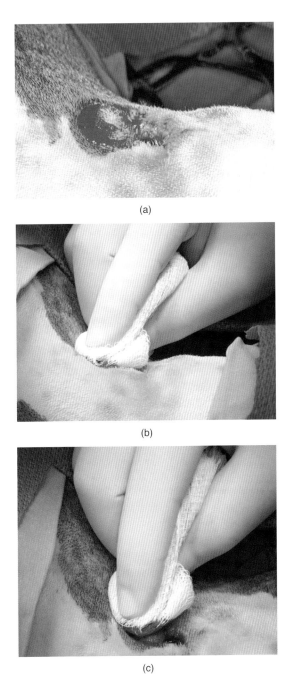

(a)

(b)

(c)

Figure 16.3 Application of pressure with a dry gauze sponge for hemostasis during a skin biopsy: (a) Hemorrhage from the scalpel incision obscures the subcutaneous tissues that still must be incised to remove the segment of skin. (b) Direct pressure is being applied to the skin incision with a dry gauze sponge. (c) The gauze sponge is gently lifted to ascertain if hemostasis has been achieved.

with low-pressure hemorrhage and is atraumatic when used properly. Direct pressure also provides temporary hemostasis for large or high-pressure vessels until permanent hemostasis can be performed by electrocoagulation or ligature placement.

Large vessels can be clamped with hemostatic forceps. Hemostats crush the tissue and stimulate coagulation. Small, low-pressure vessels can be sealed this way without the need for ligation. Hemostats may be placed on large vessels to stop bleeding until the vessel can be ligated or electrocoagulated. Grasp as little of the surrounding tissue as possible to avoid tissue damage and impaired healing. When using hemostats, the size of the instrument should be matched to the vessel being clamped. The tips of the instrument should be used to grasp the cut end of small vessels. Larger vessels and vascular pedicles should be clamped in the jaws of the instrument with the curved tips pointing up (Figure 16.4).

ELECTROSURGERY

Electrosurgery is the application of a high-frequency electrical current to tissue for the purpose of incision, coagulation, dessication, or fulguration. The characteristics of the waves in the current determine the degree of incision and coagulation. Continuous waves produce cutting while interrupted waves produce coagulation. A fully rectified current allows for both incision and coagulation. The electrosurgical generator (Figure 16.5) has settings for both incision (cutting mode) and coagulation. The choice of mode (cutting versus coagulation) is made by a switch on the generator or on the monopolar hand piece (Figure 16.6). Electrodessication is performed by choosing the coagulation mode and touching the electrode tip to the tissue to allow radial spread of the heat-generating current to dry the tissues. Electrodessication is not commonly indicated, but has been used to ablate chronic inflammatory

tissue when electrofulguration is not available. Another use for electrodessication is to dry the surface of an ulcerated tumor prior to its excision, thus minimizing the potential for contamination of the surgical wound during excision of the mass. Some electrosurgical units have a fulguration setting that allows for the destruction of living tissue by delivering electrical sparks to the tissue without touching the electrode tip to the tissue. The primary use of electrofulguration is for ablation of chronic inflammatory tissue. Electrofulguration offers the capability of more tissue destruction than electrodessication, and the amount of that destruction is controlled by the power setting. Electrofulguration is used without a ground plate, and electrodessication can be performed without a ground plate, but care must be taken to avoid excessive tissue damage from currents dissipating into surrounding tissues. Ground plates (Figure 16.5) with adequate patient contact are mandatory for electroincision and electrocoagulation to ensure a proper circuit and prevent patient injury.

Electrosurgery is rarely used to incise skin because collateral thermal necrosis may result in delayed wound healing and possibly dehiscence. However, the combination of cutting and coagulation provided by electroincision is advantageous and effective in vascular tissues, such as muscle. As the tip incises the muscle belly, it coagulates the tissue and minimizes bleeding. Subcutaneous fat and fascia are also amenable to electroincision for hemorrhage control and visualization of tissue planes, making electrosurgery an excellent tool for cutting tissues deep to masses that are being excised. Short, brush-like strokes are used to reduce lateral heat production and tissue damage during electrosurgical incision.

Electrocoagulation is often erroneously called electrocautery. Electrocautery (Figure 16.7) heats a metal tip or blade by low voltage, high amperage, direct or alternating current that coagulates the vessel without passing a current through the patient.[1] With electrocautery, heat is applied directly to the tissue. True

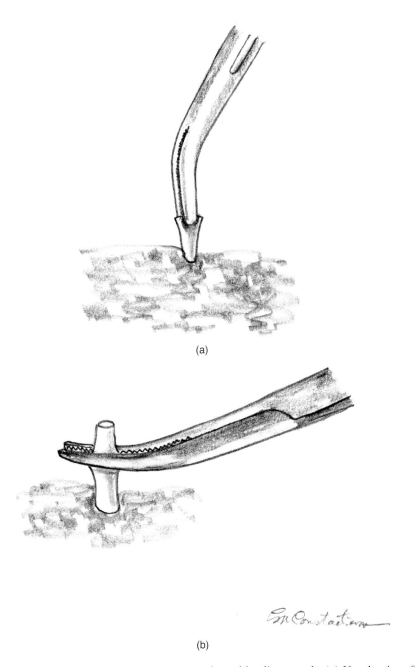

(a)

(b)

Figure 16.4 The proper use of hemostatic forceps to clamp bleeding vessels: (a) Use the tips of a mosquito or Kelly hemostatic forceps to grasp the end of a small vessel. Grasping with the tip parallel to the vessel as demonstrated here is ideal, because this grasp orients the forceps serrations perpendicular to the vessel, making the vessel less likely to slip from the forceps. (b) The jaws (serrated portion) of the hemostatic forceps may be placed perpendicular to the vessel or pedicle with the curved tip pointing upward for large vessels and vascular pedicles.

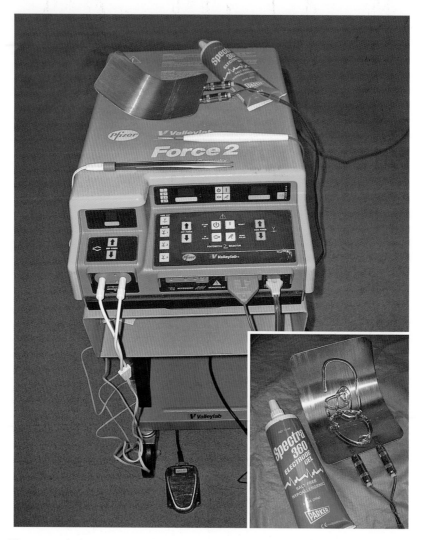

Figure 16.5 Electrosurgical generator with monopolar (white hand piece) and bipolar (forceps hand piece with white cord) capabilities. The bipolar forceps electrode is activated by pressing the foot switch located on the floor, and the current flows from one tip of the forceps to the other. The monopolar electrode requires generous patient contact of the ground plate with conductive gel (inset) for safe and effective current that runs through the patient's body. Metal ground plates as demonstrated here have given way to safer adhesive conductive ground plates.

electrocoagulation passes electrical current from a metal tip to the blood vessel as described above. Heat is produced in the tissue itself by absorption of the electrical energy and conversion into thermal energy that seals the vessel. The tip of the electrosurgery hand piece does not become hot. Electrocoagulation is best used on arteries 1 mm or less in diameter and on veins 2 mm or less in diameter.

Monopolar electrocoagulation (Figure 16.6) is the most commonly employed form of electrosurgery. Alternating electrical current passes from the hand piece, through the patient's body, and into a ground plate. The metal tip

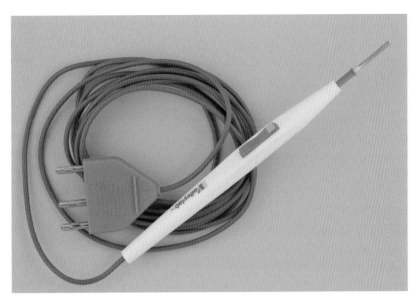

Figure 16.6   Monopolar electrosurgical hand piece. This hand piece can be used with either a flat blade (shown here) or a needle tip. The toggle switch is used to activate the electrical current. One side of the toggle activates electrocoagulation and the other side activates electroincision.

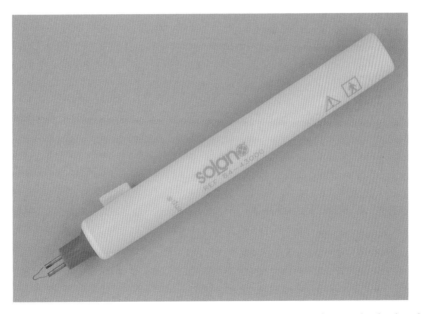

Figure 16.7   Electrocautery unit. An electrical current generated from a battery in the handle heats the metal filament. The heated metal is then applied directly to the bleeding source to burn (i.e., cauterize) the tissue to control bleeding.

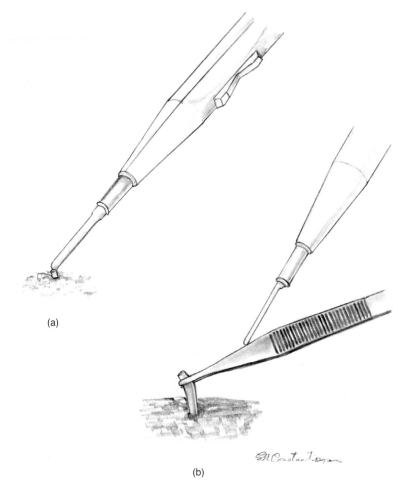

(a)

(b)

Figure 16.8 Monopolar electrocoagulation comparing direct and coaptive methods: (a) Direct electrocoagulation is performed by touching the tip of the hand piece directly to the vessel to be coagulated. (b) Coaptive electrocoagulation is performed by grasping the vessel with a hemostat or thumb forceps and then touching the tip of the hand piece anywhere on the metal instrument to transmit electrical current through the instrument to the vessel. During coaptive electrocoagulation caution must be exercised to prevent touching any other tissues with the metal instrument, because those tissues will also be coagulated.

of the hand piece should contact a very focal area of tissue, ideally, only the blood vessel to be coagulated; however, the ground plate must maximize contact surface area with the patient's body to prevent thermal burns. The surgical field must be dry for monopolar electrocoagulation to work, as the accumulated blood will limit direct application of energy to the point of interest. A monopolar tip can be applied directly to the tissue to be coagulated (direct electrocoagulation; Figures 16.8a and 16.9a), or the current can be transmitted along a metal instrument to the vessel (coaptive electrocoagulation; Figures 16.8b and 16.9b). To prevent collateral burns, the instrument should be held perpendicular to the surface to be coagulated so that the metal tip does not touch unintended tissue.

Bipolar electrocoagulation (Figure 16.10) uses electrode forceps to pass the electrical current from one tip to the other through

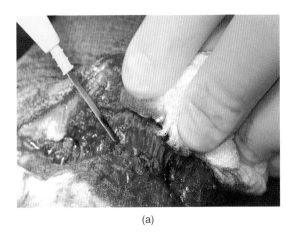 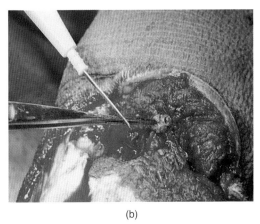

(a)   (b)

Figure 16.9   Monopolar electrocoagulation in a clinical case: (a) Direct electrocoagulation is being applied to control muscular bleeding during an amputation. (b) Coaptive electrocoagulation is being applied through a DeBakey tissue forceps to control a bleeding vessel during an amputation.

the vessel to be coagulated. Since no current passes through the rest of the patient's body, no ground plate is necessary. The tips of the forceps must be held about 1 mm apart when grasping tissue to allow the current to flow. Advantages of bipolar over monopolar electrocoagulation include requiring a lower current, having a minimal effect on surrounding tissues, and allowing coagulation to occur in a wet surgical field. The lower risk of causing thermal injury to nearby tissues makes bipolar electrocoagulation particularly advantageous for neurologic procedures, such as hemilaminectomy. Unlike monopolar electrocoagulation which can be activated by a

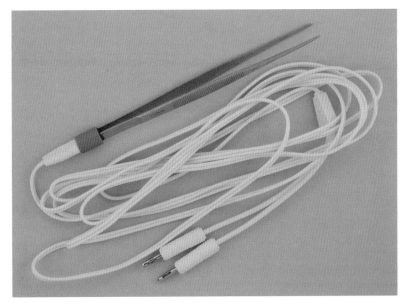

Figure 16.10   Bipolar electrocoagulation hand piece. A 1 mm gap must be maintained between the tips of the hand piece to allow electrical current to flow.

switch on the hand piece (Figure 16.6), a foot pedal (Figure 16.5) is required to activate the bipolar current.

Both forms of electrocoagulation require that the hand piece tips be kept clean of debris and char to maximize direct current transmission to the vessel. Improper use may allow arcing of the electrical current and sparks, which can result in severe burns, tissue channeling (current passing through a narrow channel of tissue causing thermal injury distant from the electrode tip), secondary hemorrhage due to a lack of a good seal, delayed wound healing, and operating room fires.

RADIOSURGERY

Radiosurgical devices (Surgitron Dual Frequency RF/120 Device and Surgitron EMC – Vet Surg, Ellman International, Oceanside, NY) function in a similar manner as standard electrosurgery with both cutting and coagulating settings. The source of energy for these units is ultra high-frequency (e.g., 4 MHz) radio waves that pass from a fine wire tip (active electrode) into the tissue to be cut or coagulated, depending on the waveform setting chosen, and on to a flat antenna (passive electrode) located in a plate placed underneath the patient (Figure 16.11). There is no need for conductive gel on the passive electrode, because it is not a grounding terminal and does not need to be in direct contact with the skin. The patient is not part of an electrical circuit, and the wire electrode remains cold at all times. Incision and coagulation occur when tissue resistance to the high-frequency radio energy induces localized heat that vaporizes individual cells. Fine soft tissue incisions are possible with this technology.

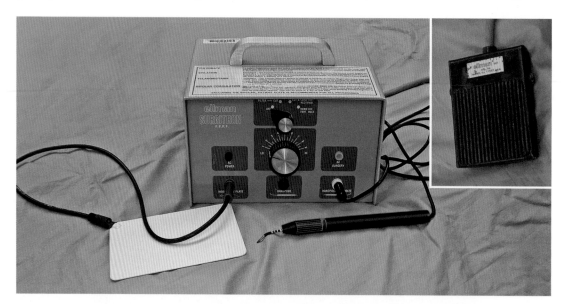

Figure 16.11   Radiosurgery unit. Multiple tip styles are available for the handle. A curved tip is demonstrated here. The handle is plugged into the white fulguration port in this photo, but would be plugged into the black center hand piece port for the more commonly used modes of cutting and coagulation. The white passive electrode is an antenna that receives the radio waves to complete the circuit running through the patient. The white plate is not a grounding terminal and does not need to be in direct contact with the skin. As such, there is no need for conductive gel. The white plate is not necessary for fulguration, but is necessary for cutting and coagulation. The current is activated by stepping on the foot switch (inset).

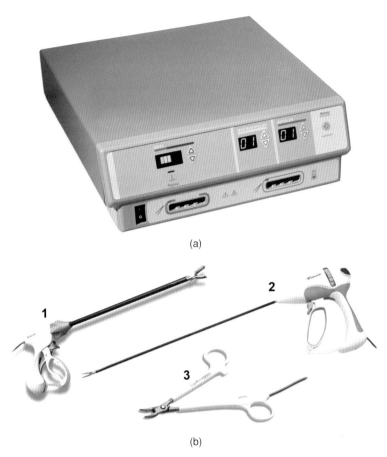

Figure 16.12 LigaSure™ Vessel Sealing System (photos courtesy of Covidien Animal Health and Dental Division, Mansfield, MA): (a) The LigaSure™ Vessel Scaling Generator provides the energy that is delivered to the hand pieces. (b) Some commonly employed LigaSure hand pieces include: (1) the LigaSure Atlas™ Hand Switching Laparoscopic Instrument, (2) the LigaSure™ V Sealer/Divider Laparoscopic Instrument, and (3) the LigaSure Precise™ Sealer/Divider Instrument.

FEEDBACK-MONITORED BIPOLAR FORCEPS

Newer forms of electrosurgical devices have been developed as feedback-monitored bipolar forceps. These devices are very useful in open celiotomy procedures, such as splenectomy and liver lobectomy, and in laparoscopic procedures. Both the LigaSure Vessel Sealing System (Covidien Animal Health and Dental Division, Mansfield, MA; www.ligasure.com;

Figure 16.12) and the EnSeal Tissue Sealing and Hemostasis System (Ethicon Endo-Surgery, Cincinnati, OH; www.surgrx.com) seal vessels and tissue bundles up to and including 7 mm diameter. Feedback-monitored devices are able to produce a more reliable seal on large vessels with less lateral thermal energy than traditional monopolar or bipolar electrosurgical units. The grasping end of the forceps crushes the incorporated tissues and completes a bipolar circuit. High-voltage, low-current energy passes through the tissue and produces heat that denatures collagen and elastin in the tissue. Collagen bundles form across the vessel lumen in the crushed area and seal the vessel.[2] Both devices possess a feedback control system that senses the amount and conductivity of the tissues within the instrument's grasp and adjusts the strength of current delivered. Once the endpoint is reached, the current is discontinued and the machine emits a signal indicating the process is complete.

ULTRASONICALLY ACTIVATED SCALPEL

Another type of energy-based vascular sealing and cutting instrument is the ultrasonically activated scalpel (Harmonic Scalpel, Ethicon Endo-Surgery, Cincinnati, OH; www.harmonic.com; Figure 16.13). An electromagnetic current produced by the generator is passed through a piezoelectric transducer in the hand piece. The transducer converts the current into mechanical energy by causing the blade to vibrate at a frequency of 55.5 kHz. Friction caused by the vibrating jaws of the instrument creates thermal energy in the tissues that heats and vaporizes water.[3,4] The proteins within the tissues are denatured and form a coagulum that seals the vessels and tissues in the instrument's grasp. The temperatures in the tissues are lower than those produced by other electrosurgical devices; therefore, less smoke and char are produced.[4] The Harmonic Scalpel is approved to seal vessels up to 5 mm in diameter.

SURGICAL LASERS

The use of surgical lasers for soft tissue surgeries of various complexities has become popular in small animal practice. The most popular laser in general practice is the carbon dioxide laser (Figure 16.14),[5] which produces a focused, 10,600 nm wavelength that is highly absorbed by water. Water in cells and tissues is heated on contact with the beam. Tissues coagulate as the temperature reaches 50–100°C and vaporize when the temperature rises above 100°C.[5] Laser surgery provides hemostasis of small vessels during incision, maintaining a dry surgical field. Larger vessels can be ablated by increasing the distance between the tip of the hand piece and the tissue to defocus the laser beam. The beam is then moved in a sweeping motion over the vessel.

VESSEL LIGATION

Large vessels should be ligated with suture to provide adequate hemostasis (Figure 16.15). Ligatures can be placed before or after a vessel is transected. If ligating after transection, usually a hemostat is placed on the vessel as previously described to provide temporary hemostasis. The vessel should be cleared of as much surrounding tissue as possible to help prevent slipping of the ligature. Double ligation is recommended, especially for large arteries. Arteries and veins should be ligated separately to avoid formation of arteriovenous fistulas.

Acceptable materials for routine vessel ligation are monofilament or braided absorbable sutures (poliglecaprone 25, polyglactin 910, chromic gut). Long-lasting suture is usually not necessary for ligation because vessels seal quickly. Some surgeons, however, prefer silk because of its handling characteristics and knot security. Suture size is matched to the size of the vessel to be ligated, keeping in mind that using the smallest appropriate size of suture will improve knot security. Ligatures should be tied with square knots because of the dependable security of square knots. A surgeon's throw may be used for the first knot when ligating vascular pedicles if tissue tension does not allow adequate tightening of a simple throw. It should be remembered that surgeon's knots are bulky and may provide less knot security.

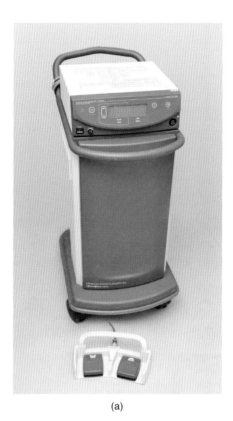

(a)

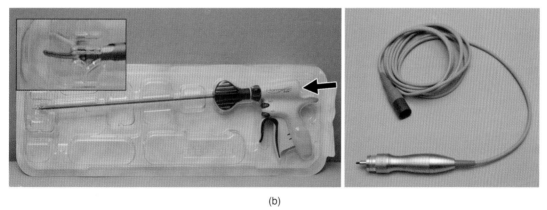

(b)

Figure 16.13   The Harmonic Scalpel (Ethicon Endo-Surgery, Cincinnati, OH): (a) The Harmonic® Generator 300 produces an electromagnetic current that passes through a piezoelectric transducer in the hand piece. (b) The Harmonic ACE® 36 cm Ergonomically-Enhanced Curved Shear disposable blade (left) is interfaced with the generator by a cable (right). The metal portion of the cable (called the hand piece) attaches to the disposable blade at the location indicated by the arrow. The inset is a closeup of the blade tip. Electromagnetic energy from the generator stimulates vibration of the piezoelectric transducer located between two metal cylinders in the hand piece. The sine waves that are produced travel to the blade and cause the blade to vibrate at 55.5 kHz.

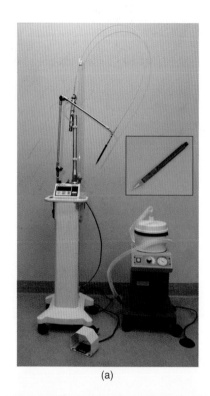

(a)

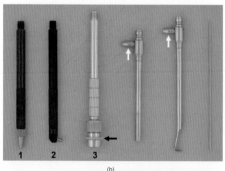

(b)

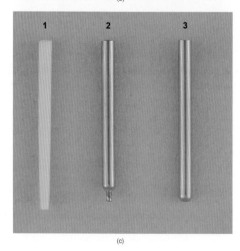

(c)

Figure 16.14

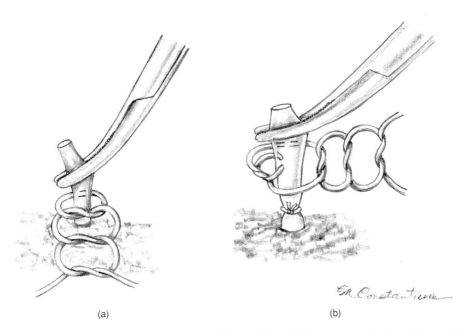

(a)   (b)

Figure 16.15   Suture ligation of a blood vessel: (a) A circumferential ligature may be placed around the vessel under the tips of a hemostatic forceps. The first (simple) throw is tightened to securely occlude the blood vessel. Then, three additional throws are added to result in two square knots. When there is a surrounding tissue along with the vessel in the jaws of the forceps, the forceps is flashed as the first throw is secured. Specifically, flashing refers to rapid loosening and tightening of the hemostatic forceps as the first throw of the ligature is secured. The flashing maneuver is done such that one does not actually see the forceps loosening and the jaws do not move off of the tissue/vessel pedicle. (b) A transfixation ligature is used for large vessels and pedicles. The transfixation is performed after a more proximally located circumferential suture is placed. The needle of the suture is passed through a small section of the wall of the vessel and secured with a simple throw. Then, the rest of the suture is passed around the circumference of the vessel, tightened, and secured with two square knots. [See Chapter 18 for the method of transfixation for vascular pedicles.]

Figure 16.14   Carbon dioxide laser: (a) A common veterinary laser (The Luxar AccuVet Novapulse LX-20SP surgical CO_2 laser, Lumenis, Inc., Santa Clara, CA; left side of photograph) employs a hollow wave guide to deliver the laser beam to the hand piece and tip (inset). An evacuation system (right side of photograph) is used to remove plume that is generated when the laser interacts with tissue. (b) Different laser hand pieces available for various applications include: (1) the standard hand piece which is held as a pencil, (2) an angled hand piece that is useful for work in the oral cavity, and (3) LAUP attachments. LAUP stands for laser-assisted uvuloplasty, a soft palate surgery performed in people. The LAUP attachments are useful for resection of canine elongated soft palates. The LAUP handle (to right of angled hand piece) has a quick release mechanism (black arrow) to which can be attached an extension without a backstop (to right of LAUP handle) or with a metal backstop (to right of the extension without a backstop). Both extensions are equipped with exhaust ports (white arrows) that can be connected to suction tubing. These extensions require a long 0.8 mm tip (far right). (c) Some optional tips for use in the standard hand piece are (1) a 0.25 mm ceramic tip, (2) a 0.3 mm metal tip, and (3) a 0.4 mm fine metal taper tip.

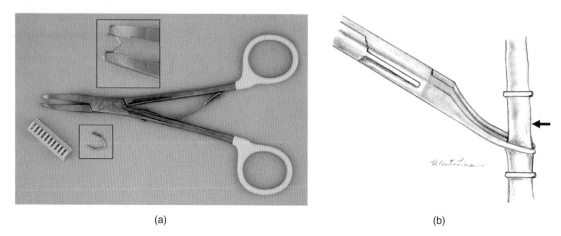

(a)   (b)

Figure 16.16   Stainless steel hemostatic clips: (a) This photo demonstrates the Hemoclips (Weck Closure Systems, Research Triangle Park, NC) applicator and clips in the cartridge. The insets show closeups of a metal Hemoclip alone and loaded in the applicator tip. (b) Hemoclips may be placed on an isolated blood vessel where a hemostatic forceps would ordinarily be placed, followed by transection of the vessel in the appropriate location (arrow). Hemoclips may also be applied after a vessel has been cut and occluded with a hemostatic forceps. The diameter of the blood vessel should measure 1/3 to 2/3 the length of the clip arm.

Metal vascular clips (Hemoclips, Weck Closure Systems, Research Triangle Park, NC) can also be used to ligate vessels up to 5 mm in diameter (Figure 16.16). Vascular clips are applied with a special applicator after a vessel has been cleared of surrounding tissue. Clip size is based on the size of the vessel; the vessel diameter should be between one-third and two-thirds the length of the clip. Vascular clips are quicker to apply than traditional ligatures, but may be more likely to be dislodged from the vessel end, especially if they are applied inappropriately. Disposable multifire vascular clips (Auto Suture Premium Surgiclip II, Covidien Animal Health and Dental Division, Mansfield, MA) are also available.

HEMOSTATIC AGENTS

Low pressure, diffuse hemorrhage, such as that seen from the liver or spleen, is often not controllable by the methods described above. For these instances, topical hemostatic agents can assist in achieving hemostasis and improving visibility. Topical hemostatic agents are also useful in areas where pressure or heat injury is detrimental to function of an organ, as in surgery of the central nervous system. Topical hemostatic agents are not appropriate for control of active arterial hemorrhage. The exact method of action varies from one material to the next, but in general they work by providing a substrate for more rapid coagulation. For this reason, a functional hemostatic pathway must be present.

Bone Wax

Bone Wax (Medline Industries, Mundelein, IL; Figure 16.17) is used to tamponade bleeding from bone surfaces. Unlike other topical hemostatic agents, bone wax has no effect on the coagulation cascade. Bone wax is made of semisynthetic beeswax and a softening agent such as isopropyl palmitate so that it can be compressed into cancellous bone. Bone wax

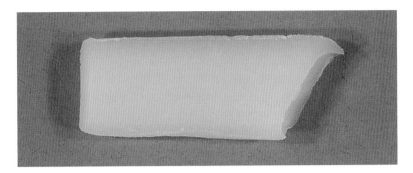

Figure 16.17   Bone Wax (Medline Industries, Mundelein, IL).

is nonabsorbable and inhibits bone healing; therefore, only a small amount should be used, and it should not be used in fractures or osteotomies where osteogenesis is required for healing. Common uses for application of bone wax are to control osseous hemorrhage from open marrow cavities during amputations and mandibulectomies. Bone wax is available in 2.5 gram sterile foil pouches.

Gelatin Sponges

Gelfoam (Pharmacia & Upjohn, New York, NY; Figure 16.18a) and Vetspon (Novartis Animal Health, Greensboro, NC; Figure 16.18b) are sterile, water-insoluble, absorbable, porcine gelatin sponges used to control low pressure capillary hemorrhage. The porous and expandable nature of gelatin sponges allows

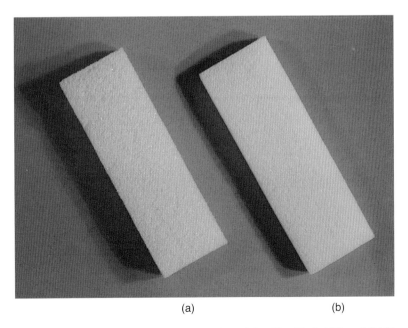

(a)   (b)

Figure 16.18   Gelatin sponges: (a) Gelfoam (Pharmacia & Upjohn, New York, NY) and (b) Vetspon (Novartis Animal Health, Greensboro, NC).

them to hold many times their weight in whole blood. As the sponge saturates with blood, it tamponades the bleeding surface and provides a mechanical matrix that promotes and supports platelet aggregation and fibrin strand formation.

Gelatin sponges are available as strips, squares, and cubes, depending on the manufacturer, and can be cut and contoured to tissue surfaces. They can be applied either dry or saturated with sterile saline solution. As with suture material, only the minimal amount needed to achieve hemostasis should be used to minimize the amount of foreign body reaction. The dry sponge should be compressed and then held in place with moderate pressure until hemostasis occurs. To use a wet sponge, the sponge should be dipped in saline, squeezed to remove excess moisture, and then immersed again to remove any air bubbles in the matrix. A wet gelatin sponge is applied to bleeding tissue in the same manner as a dry sponge.

Gelatin sponges are absorbed in four to six weeks and do not appear to inhibit wound healing. They should be removed after hemostasis is achieved in enclosed bony spaces, such as the spinal canal and calvarium to avoid inciting scar tissue formation and resultant compressive injury to neural tissues. Gelatin sponges can also

act as a nidus for infection and abscess formation, so they should never be left in a contaminated site.

Oxidized Regenerated Cellulose

Oxidized regenerated cellulose (Surgicel, Johnson & Johnson, Somerville, NJ) can be cut and easily manipulated to conform to almost any bleeding surface. Hemostasis is achieved by the formation of a gelatinous mass on contact with blood that acts as an artificial clot. Since the mechanism of action is through hemoglobin, oxidized regenerated cellulose is not activated by body fluids other than blood. It is absorbable within 7–14 days and induces minimal inflammation. Like gelatin sponges, oxidized regenerated cellulose swells after contact with blood and thus should be removed from enclosed bony spaces after hemostasis is achieved. Oxidized regenerated cellulose is available in three different forms: (1) a mesh with good flexibility and versatility (Surgicel Original, Johnson & Johnson, Somerville, NJ; Figure 16.19), (2) a mesh with a denser weave for heavier bleeding and that can hold suture (Surgicel Nu-Knit, Johnson & Johnson, Somerville, NJ), and (3) a soft, layered material with the consistency of

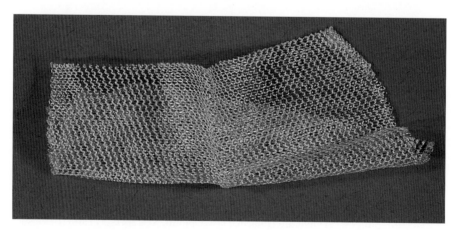

Figure 16.19   Oxidized regenerated cellulose (Surgicel Original, Johnson & Johnson, Somerville, NJ).

cotton that can be peeled off in the needed amount (Surgicel Fibrillar, Johnson & Johnson, Somerville, NJ).

ACKNOWLEDGMENT

The authors thank Linda M. Berent, DVM, PhD, Diplomate ACVP (Clinical and Anatomic Pathology), Department of Pathobiology, University of Missouri for assistance in writing the hemostasis portion of this chapter.

REFERENCES

1. Fucci V, Elkins AD. Electrosurgery: principles and guidelines in veterinary medicine. *Compend Contin Educ Pract Vet* 1991;13:407–415.
2. Harold KL, Pollinger H, Matthews BD, et al. Comparison of ultrasonic energy, bipolar thermal energy, and vascular clips for the hemostasis of small-, medium-, and large-sized arteries. *Surg Endosc* 2003;17:1228–1230.
3. Royals SR, Ellison GW, Adin CA, et al. Use of an ultrasonically activated scalpel for splenectomy in 10 dogs with naturally occurring splenic disease. *Vet Surg* 2005;34:174–178.
4. Clements RH, Palepu R. In vivo comparison of the coagulation capability of SonoSurg and Harmonic Ace on 4 mm and 5 mm arteries. *Surg Endosc* 2007;21:2203–2206.
5. Holt TL, Mann FA. Soft tissue applications of lasers. *Vet Clin North Am Small Anim Pract* 2002;32(3):569–599.

ADDITIONAL RESOURCES

Additional information about hemostasis and surgical control of bleeding can be found in the following textbooks and journal article:

1. Feldman BV, Zinkl JG, Jain NC, eds. *Schalm's Veterinary Hematology*, 5th ed. Philadelphia, Pennsylvania: Lippincott Williams & Wilkins, 2000.
2. Fossum TW, ed. *Small Animal Surgery*, 3rd ed. St. Louis, Missouri: Mosby Elsevier, 2007.
3. Slatter DH, ed. *Textbook of Small Animal Surgery*, 3rd ed. Philadelphia, Pennsylvania: Saunders, 2003.
4. Miller WW. Using high-frequency radio wave technology in veterinary surgery. *Vet Med* 2004;99:796–802.

Chapter 17

SURGICAL TUBES AND DRAINS

Fred Anthony Mann

Tubes and drains used in veterinary surgery are numerous and include intranasal tubes, thoracostomy tubes, tracheostomy tubes, cystostomy tubes, feeding tubes, wound drains, and abdominal drains. The purpose of this chapter is to introduce the reader to some common surgical tubes and drains by providing a description of each of the above-mentioned tubes, stating the indications for use of each tube, and mentioning potential complications.

INTRANASAL TUBES

Intranasal tubes are used for oxygen administration and for feeding into the esophagus or stomach (Figures 17.1a and 17.1b). The technique for placing an intranasal tube is the same for each of these uses (Figures 17.1c through 17.1o). In awake animals, ophthalmic anesthetic (Figures 17.1c and 17.1d) is instilled into the nostril and allowed to take effect while the

Fundamentals of Small Animal Surgery, 1st edition.
By Fred Anthony Mann, Gheorghe M. Constantinescu and Hun-Young Yoon.
© 2011 Blackwell Publishing Ltd.

tube and placement materials are organized. The length of tube (i.e., how far the tube is inserted) determines the usage. For oxygen administration, the tube is inserted to level of the medial canthus of the eye (Figures 17.1e and 17.1f). For nasoesophageal feeding, the tube is measured from approximately the fifth intercostal space to the lateral commissure of the nostril, and for nasogastric feeding, the tube is measured from the thirteenth rib to the lateral commissure of the nostril. Friction sutures[1] are used to anchor the tube in place. In most cases, tube anchoring may be achieved with 2–0 monofilament suture passed through a 20-gauge hypodermic needle (Figure 17.1g). The first friction suture to anchor the tube is begun at the lateral commissure of the nostril immediately before introducing the tube (Figures 17.1h and 17.1i). After tying one square knot and leaving the strands long in preparation for a surgeon's knot, the tube is lubricated (Figure 17.1j). The lubricated tube is introduced after using a thumb to elevate the nose (Figure 17.1k). Elevating the nose in this manner facilitates introduction of the tube into the ventral meatus, the desired route of passage. Passing the tube in the dorsal and/or middle meatus may result in hemorrhage and discomfort.

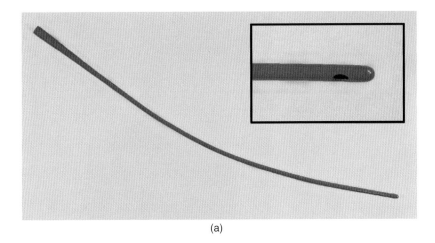

(a)

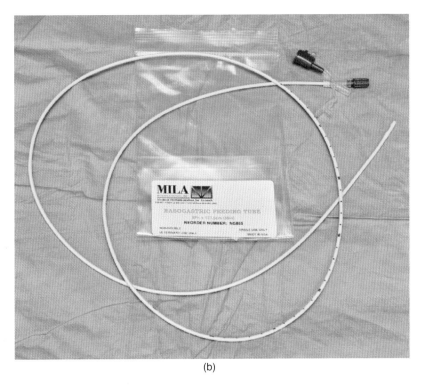

(b)

Figure 17.1 (a) Red rubber feeding tube. This tube is commonly used for intranasal oxygen administration. If long enough for the patient in question, this tube may also be used for nasogastric or nasoesophageal feeding. Common red rubber tube lengths are 41 and 56 cm. The long version of this tube can be used as a jejunostomy tube, although other tube types are preferred for that usage. (b) Nasogastric feeding tube. The tube pictured is made of polyurethane, which causes less inflammatory tissue reaction than red rubber tubes. A stylet is typically required to stiffen the tube enough for passage.

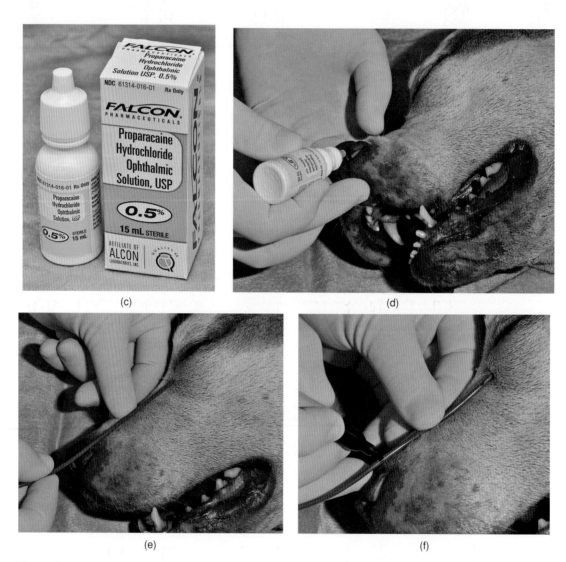

Figure 17.1 (*Continued*) (c) Topical ophthalmic anesthetic for numbing the nasal mucosa prior to introducing an intranasal tube. (d) Instilling topical ophthalmic anesthetic into the nose prior to introducing an intranasal tube. The nose is lifted to make sure anesthetic trickles down the ventral meatus. (e) Estimating the length of red rubber tube to be inserted for nasal oxygen administration. The tube is measured from the medial canthus of the eye to the lateral commissure of the nostril. (f) Marking an intranasal tube before insertion. A permanent marker is used to mark the level of the tube that should be at the lateral commissure of the nostril when the tube is inserted to its desired location.

Once the ventral meatus is entered, the nose may be allowed to fall to a normal position while the tube is advanced to the desired length (Figure 17.1l). Then, the tube is positioned over the previously tied square knot at the lateral commissure of the nostril (Figure 17.1m), and a surgeon's knot is tied to sandwich the tube between the square knot and surgeon's knot such that the tube is indented slightly by the suture (Figure 17.1n). Additional friction

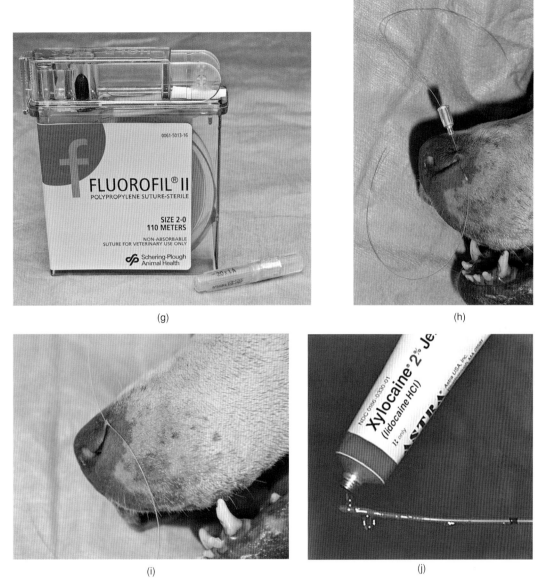

(g)   (h)

(i)   (j)

Figure 17.1   (*Continued*) (g) Suture material and needle for placing friction sutures. Suture material that is easily seen against the animal's skin and hair is desired for ease of removal when the tube is no longer needed. Most nasal tubes will require 2–0 suture material which is easily passed through a 20-gauge hypodermic needle. (h) Beginning the first friction suture for anchoring an intranasal tube. A 20-gauge hypodermic needle is inserted at the lateral commissure of the nostril, and 2–0 monofilament nonabsorbable suture is passed through the needle from the bevel to the hub. Then, the needle is withdrawn. (i) First knot in the first friction suture for anchoring an intranasal tube. One square knot is tied and the suture strands are left long enough to tie another knot once the tube is inserted into the nose and advanced to the desired location. (j) Lubricating an intranasal tube prior to insertion. The tube may be lubricated with water soluble jelly or with lidocaine jelly as demonstrated in this figure. Lidocaine jelly will provide topical anesthesia for the nasal mucosa, in case previously administered anesthetic drops are ineffective.

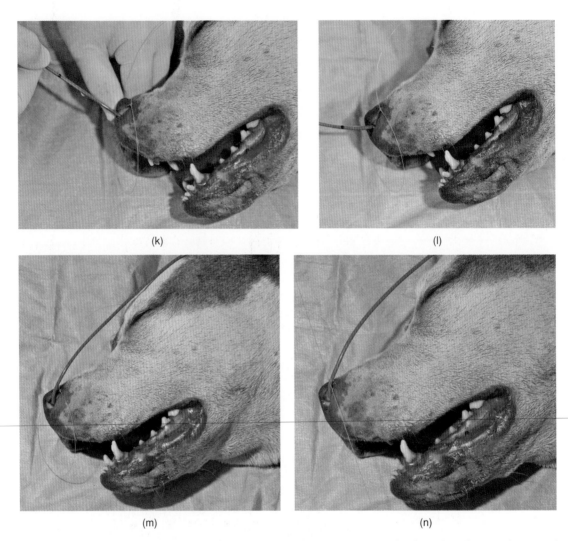

Figure 17.1 (*Continued*) (k) Thumbing the nose upward to facilitate introduction of a tube into the ventral meatus. (l) Advancement of an intranasal tube to the desired location. Once the tube is in the ventral meatus the nose is lowered to its natural position and the tube is advanced until the mark made with a permanent marker resides just out of sight within the nose. (m) Preparing to finish the friction knot at the lateral commissure of the nostril. The intranasal tube is turned upward to rest on the previously tied square knot taking care to make sure the mark made with the permanent marker does not exit the nose. (n) Completed friction suture at the lateral commissure of the nostril. The tube has been positioned onto the square knot and a surgeon knot is tied to sandwich the tube between the two knots. The surgeon, knot is tied such that there is slight indentation of the tube by the suture. Other friction sutures will be added, but this is the most crucial friction suture for maintaining position of an intranasal tube.

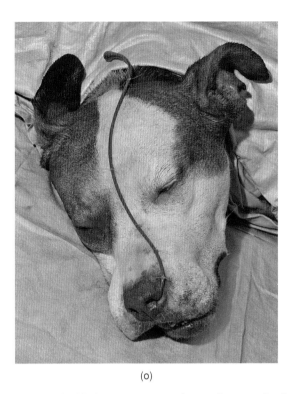

(o)

Figure 17.1 (*Continued*) (o) Multiple friction sutures securing an intranasal tube along the bridge of the nose and over the top of the head. Placing a friction suture at the external occipital protuberance prevents the tube from draping over an eye when the dog is in sternal position or standing.

sutures are placed to anchor the tube along the bridge of the nose and over the top of the head (Figure 17.1o). A friction suture placed at the external occipital protuberance will prevent the tube from hanging over the animal's eye when the animal is in sternal recumbence or standing position.

THORACOSTOMY TUBES

Thoracostomy tubes are indicated to manage traumatic or nontraumatic pneumothorax or pleural effusion when thoracocentesis is not sufficient. Thoracostomy tubes are also placed for postoperative management of thoracotomy and diaphragmatic hernia repair patients. Commercially available thoracostomy tubes are generally large bore, radio-opaque, and made of translucent polyvinyl chloride. Some are sold with an aluminum trocar-tipped insert that, when placed inside the tube, extends just past the tip of the tube and aids in penetration through the thoracic wall (Argyle Trocar Catheter, Covidien Animal Health and Dental Division, Mansfield, MA; Figures 17.2a and 17.2b). A large bore tube of red rubber, silicone (Bio-sil, Silmed Corporation, Taunton, MA; Figure 17.2c), or other biomaterial can also be used for thoracostomy; however, placement is more difficult since there is no trocar, and the possibility of air leaking around the tube is greater due to the wider tunnel created by an instrument used to facilitate introduction of the tube. Trocar tubes are suited for percutanous placement whereas nontrocar tubes are used for

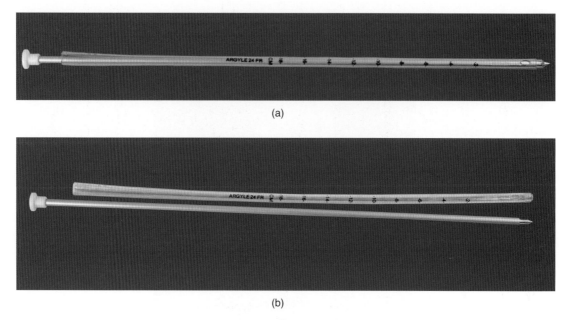

(a)

(b)

Figure 17.2 (a) Commercially available thoracostomy tube with aluminum trocar inserted into the tube. (b) Commercially available thoracostomy tube with aluminum trocar removed.

intraoperative placement during thoracotomy and diaphragmatic hernia repair. The proper size of thoracostomy tube has been said to be approximately the same diameter as the animal's mainstem bronchus. However, radiographs to make that assessment may not be available. Therefore, a thumb rule is to use the largest diameter tube that is small enough to fit comfortably between two ribs.

To prepare for percutaneous thoracostomy tube placement, ensure that the patient is under general anesthesia and is breathing supplemental oxygen through an endotracheal tube. Even in critically ill animals, thoracostomy tube placement with local anesthesia alone is not recommended, because the patient will greatly benefit from a secure airway, positive pressure ventilation, and supplemental oxygen. Patients in respiratory distress should be preoxygenated for approximately 5–10 minutes prior to beginning the procedure. Clip hair widely and aseptically prepare the skin on the side of the thorax so that the procedure can progress without

contaminating the tube or gloved hands of the surgeon with surrounding hair and skin. Barrier drapes are recommended after prepping is complete to further protect the surgical field and sterile equipment and supplies. Infiltrate local anesthetic (9 parts lidocaine mixed with 1 part sodium bicarbonate) at the proposed site of insertion through the skin, at the proposed intercostal space entry, and in the tissues that will be tunneled between these two sites. The local anesthetic placed at this time will facilitate postoperative analgesia.

Key features of percutaneous thoracostomy tube placement include a small stab incision in the skin and underlying latissimus dorsi muscle in the caudodorsal aspect of the thorax, cranioventral tunneling under the latissimus dorsi muscle[2] for a distance of at least two intercostal spaces, penetration of the intercostal space (usually, the seventh or eighth space), and continued advancement of the tube such that it rests on the dorsal portion of the sternum (Figure 17.2d). The description that follows

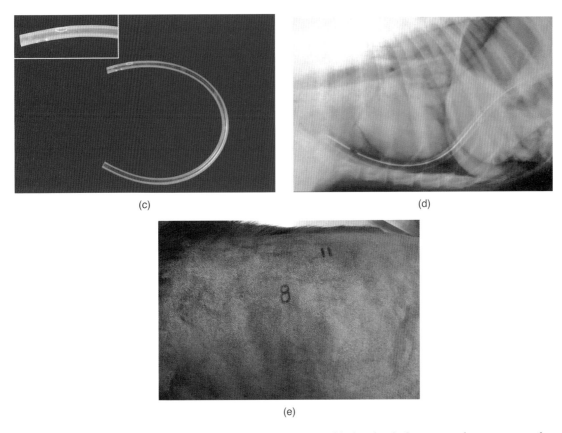

(c)

(d)

(e)

Figure 17.2 (*Continued*) (c) Silastic tubing with fenestrations added at the tip for use as a thoracostomy tube. Inset is a close-up view of the fenestrations. When making tube fenestrations care is taken to avoid making fenestrations too large, which could cause the tube to break. Ideally, a fenestration should encompass one-fourth of the tube diameter and should definitely be less than half of the diameter. [Note: Tubing modified in this manner may also be used as an esophagostomy tube.] (d) Lateral thoracic radiograph demonstrating ideal thoracostomy tube placement in a dog. (e) Left lateral canine thorax prepared for thoracostomy tube placement demonstrating the location of the eleventh rib at the point where the skin incision will be made (11) and the location of the eighth intercostal space at the point where the tube will enter the thoracic cavity (8).

details the placement of a thoracostomy tube in the left eighth intercostal space.

When using a trocar thoracostomy tube, a stab incision in the dorsal third of the left lateral thoracic wall is made through the skin and the latissimus dorsi muscle over the eleventh rib using a number 11 scalpel blade (Figures 17.2e and 17.2f). Making the stab directly over a rib allows full penetration of the latissimus dorsi mus-

cle (Figure 17.2g) without inadvertent puncture into the thoracic cavity. The stab incision should be just large enough to accommodate the tube. The trocar tube is then tunneled under the latissimus dorsi muscle from the eleventh rib to the eighth intercostal space in the middle third of the thoracic wall (Figure 17.2h). Once the tip reaches the eighth intercostal space, the trocar tube is raised perpendicular to the chest wall.

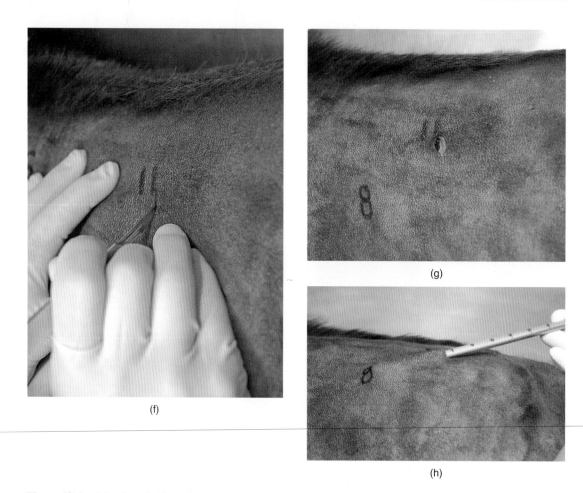

(f)

(g)

(h)

Figure 17.2 (*Continued*) (f) Stab incision with a number 11 blade over the eleventh rib in the dorsal third of a canine thorax in preparation for thoracostomy tube placement. The stab incision is made over the rib so that the entire thickness of the latissimus dorsi muscle may be cut without risk of penetrating the intercostal muscles and inadvertently entering the thoracic cavity with the blade. (g) Stab incision over the eleventh rib in the dorsal third of a canine thorax in preparation for thoracostomy tube placement demonstrating that the latissimus dorsi muscle has been incised. Incising the latissimus dorsi muscle allows the thoracostomy tube to be inserted under that muscle creating a "sublatissimal" tunnel instead of a subcutaneous tunnel, the latter which is more prone to air leakage around the thoracostomy tube. Note that the stab incision in both the skin and latissimus dorsi muscle is small, just large enough to accommodate the thoracostomy tube. (h) Advancing a trocar thoracostomy tube under the latissimus dorsi muscle from a stab incision at the eleventh rib in a cranioventral direction to the eighth intercostal space to the point of intended penetration into the thoracic cavity (8).

The trocar tube is firmly grasped with the non-dominant hand 1 to 2 cm from the body wall (or leaving just enough space between the hand and chest wall that approximates the thickness of the intercostal muscles) while the other hand is used to pop the trocar tube through the intercostal space with one rapid motion (Figures 17.2i and 17.2j). The tube is thrust carefully but briskly into the thoracic cavity by tapping with the dominant hand. Once the trocar tube is in

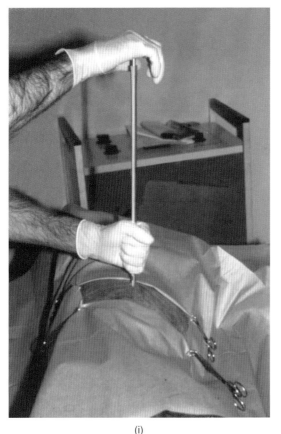
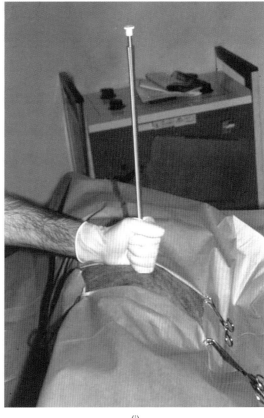

(i)   (j)

Figure 17.2   (*Continued*) (i) Positioning a trocar thoracostomy tube perpendicular to the left thoracic wall immediately prior to entering thc thoracic cavity. The latissimus dorsi muscle offers considerable resistance to this positioning. This resistance and a mound of tissue that appears at the cranial aspect of the tube when the tube is lifted to this position indicate that a tunnel deep to the latissimus dorsi muscle has indeed been achieved. The tube is grasped tightly with the nondominant hand close to the thoracic wall leaving a space between the side of the hand and thoracic skin that is approximately the same as the estimated thickness of the intercostal space through which the tube must penetrate. The palm of the dominant hand is used to hit the trocar such that the tube quickly enters the thoracic cavity without damage to underlying structures. The nondominant hand serves as a stop to prevent over penetration of the thoracostomy tube when it is hit by the dominant hand. (j) Trocar thoracostomy tube that has penetrated the intercostal space. The nondominant hand has provided a stop. The next step is to lower the tube, retract the trocar slightly, and advance the tube cranioventrally.

the pleural space, the trocar is withdrawn 1 cm (Figure 17.2k) to protect thoracic cavity contents from trocar tip trauma, and the tube is advanced in a cranioventral direction without resistance until the predetermined length of the trocar tube to be inserted from the skin incision to the thoracic inlet is inserted. The trocar is removed when the tube reaches the sternum to allow advancement to the thoracic inlet. The objective is to have the fenestrated portion of the

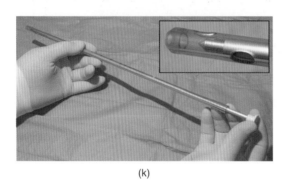

(k)

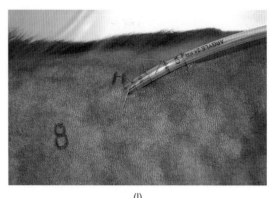

(l)

Figure 17.2 (*Continued*) (k) Withdrawal of the trocar for approximately 1 cm so that it is entirely within the tube. This maneuver is performed before the cranioventral advancement of the tube within the thoracic cavity so that the sharp tip does not injure the lungs or other intrathoracic structures during advancement. Maintaining the trocar in this manner aids in tube advancement by providing stiffness. The trocar is removed completely once the advancing tube comes in contact with the sternum, and the tube without the trocar is advanced to its final position. (l) Completed trocar thoracostomy tube placement in the left eighth intercostal space (8) of a dog. Four friction sutures of large monofilament nonabsorbable suture (size 1 polybutester in this case) anchor the tube to skin and underlying fascia. The first friction suture (the one closest to the skin incision) is placed by directing the suture needle deeply through the skin until it reflects off the closest rib (11), ensuring significant engagement of underlying fascia and minimal sliding of the tube through the skin incision.

tube just dorsal to the sternum and the tip of the tube approach (but not through) the thoracic inlet. At least one friction suture is placed to prevent dislodgement while finishing touches (such as applying a tubing clamp, connecting a tubing adaptor, and manually evacuating the thoracic cavity of air and fluid with a syringe) are performed. Then, a radiograph is taken to ensure proper placement (Figure 17.2d). Once acceptable placement is confirmed, remaining friction sutures are placed so that four friction sutures keep the tube in place (Figure 17.2l).

For a tube without a trocar, a Rochester-Carmalt forceps is used to facilitate placement. A stab incision in the dorsal third of the left lateral thoracic wall through the skin and the latissimus dorsi muscle is made with a number 11 scalpel blade as described for the trocar technique (Figure 17.2g). The incision is usually a bit larger than that made for the trocar technique in order to accommodate the forceps. A curved Rochester-Carmalt forceps is used to create a tunnel as wide as the width of the forceps under the latissimus dorsi muscle from the eleventh rib to the eighth intercostal space in the middle third of the thoracic wall, and the forceps is removed. [Note: Some clinicians prefer to penetrate the intercostal space at this point to make it easier to later get the forceps-tube combination through the space.] The tip of a thoracostomy tube is grasped in the tip of the Rochester-Carmalt forceps with the tube parallel to the body of the forceps (Figure 17.2m). The thoracostomy tube with forceps is then passed through the tunnel created under latissimus dorsi muscle from the eleventh rib to the eighth intercostal space (Figure 17.2n). Once the tip reaches the eighth intercostal space, the forceps is raised perpendicular to the thoracic wall. The thoracostomy tube with forceps is then firmly grasped 1–2 cm from the body wall with one hand while the

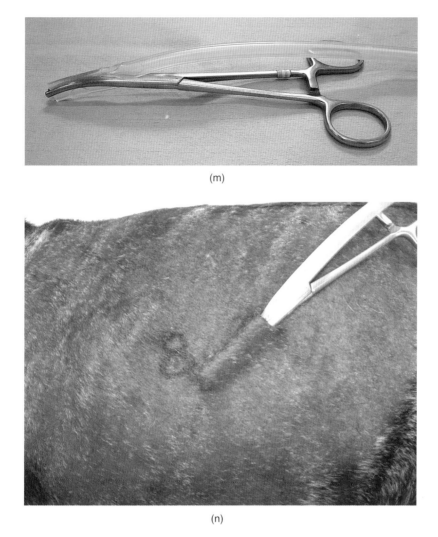

(m)

(n)

Figure 17.2   (*Continued*) (m) Grasping a thoracostomy tube in the jaws of a curved Rochester-Carmalt forceps for forceps-assisted thoracostomy tube placement. Note that the tips of the forceps extend slightly beyond the tube to facilitate penetration of the intercostal space. (n) Thoracostomy tube and forceps combination migrating cranioventrally from an incision over the eleventh rib to the eighth intercostal space.

other hand is used to pop the thoracostomy tube with forceps through the thoracic wall musculature into the pleural space (Figures 17.2o and 17.2p). [Note: If the intercostal space was previously penetrated with the forceps, the forceps-tube combination may be pushed more slowly through the intercostal space.] Once the thoracostomy tube has entered the

pleural space, the forceps is removed and the tube is advanced in a cranioventral direction without resistance until the predetermined length of the tube from the skin incision to the thoracic inlet is inserted.

After the thoracostomy tube advancement is complete for either (trocar or forceps assisted) technique, a mattress suture may be placed in

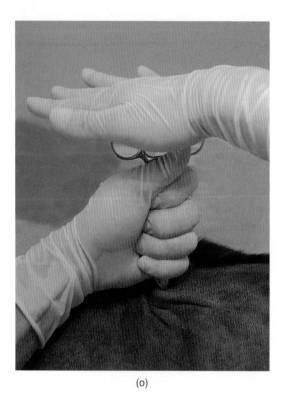

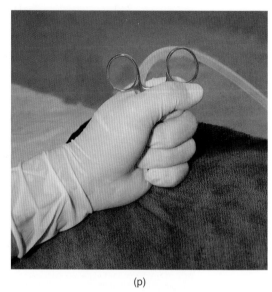

(o)   (p)

Figure 17.2   (*Continued*) (o) Positioning a thoracostomy tube and forceps combination perpendicular to the thoracic wall immediately prior to entering the left thoracic cavity. The latissimus dorsi muscle offers considerable resistance to this positioning as noted by the mound of tissue that appears at the cranial aspect of the tube-forceps combination when lifted to this position. The tube is grasped tightly with the nondominant hand close to the thoracic wall leaving a space between the side of the hand and thoracic skin that is approximately the same as the estimated thickness of the intercostal space through which the tube-forceps combination must penetrate. The palm of the dominant hand is used to hit the forceps such that the tube-forceps quickly enters the thoracic cavity without damage to underlying structures. The nondominant hand serves as a stop to prevent over penetration of the tube-forceps combination when it is hit by the dominant hand. [Note: Some prefer to advance the forceps without the tube to penetrate the intercostal space, and then remove the forceps, attach the tube, and advance the tube-forceps combination. With this method the tube-forceps combination may be pushed through the previously punctured intercostal space rather than thrust through it.] (p) Thoracostomy tube and forceps combination that has penetrated the intercostal space. The nondominant hand has provided a stop. The next step is to lower the tube, remove the forceps, and advance the tube cranioventrally.

the skin incision around the tube to provide a seal and negate the need for suturing upon tube removal. Additional interrupted sutures may be required in the skin incision on either side of the tube if the incision is markedly larger than the tube diameter. A tube clamp (Figures 17.2q and 17.2r) is placed (but left open) and

the tube is anchored with at least one friction suture[1] to secure the tube to the skin and underlying fascia while finishing touches are done. The tube is interfaced via a tubing adapter with a three-way stopcock in an "open to the patient" setting, and a syringe is used to remove air and fluid until negative intrapleural pressure

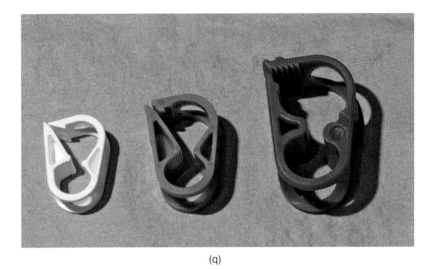

(q)

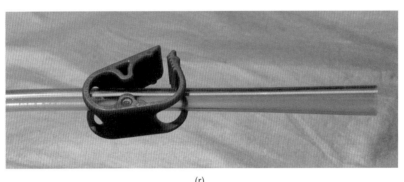

(r)

Figure 17.2 (*Continued*) (q) Plastic tube clamps, three different sizes. This clamp must be applied to a thoracostomy tube before attaching a tubing adapter and three-way stopcock or continuous suction tubing. (r) Plastic clamp applied to a thoracostomy tube. The clamp is left open until fluid and air is manually evacuated from the thoracic cavity.

is achieved (Figure 17.2s). Care is taken to avoid excessive pull on the syringe so that lung tissue is not pulled into the tube. Once negative pressure is achieved, the tube clamp is closed, the stop cock is positioned in the "closed to patient" setting (Figure 17.2t), and thoracic radiographs are taken to check tube placement. Once the proper tube placement is documented, three additional friction sutures[1] are applied and anesthesia may be discontinued, assuming no other procedures requiring anesthesia are planned.

If a thoracic bandage is applied to protect the thoracostomy tube, it must be applied loosely enough to avoid compromising thoracic wall excursions and must be removed at least daily to examine the thoracostomy site. Therefore, a patch bandage over the thoracostomy skin incision may be more practical if a bandage is desired.

When placing a thoracostomy tube during thoracotomy, the tube is placed immediately prior to intercostal apposition (or sternal apposition with median sternotomies). The same

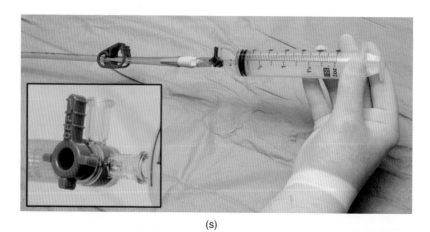

(s)

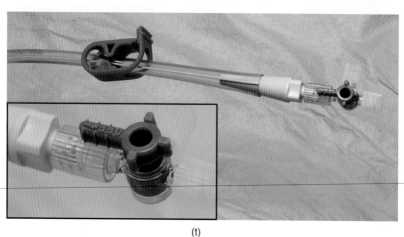

(t)

Figure 17.2 (*Continued*) (s) Adaptation of a thoracostomy tube for manual evacuation of intrathoracic air and fluid using a plastic tubing clamp, tubing adapter, three-way stopcock, and large syringe. Note that the clamp is open and the stopcock is open to the patient. (t) Position of thoracostomy tube clamp and three-way stopcock after air and fluid have been evacuated to achieve negative intrathoracic pressure. Note that the clamp is compressed, the stopcock is closed to the patient, and catheter caps cover the stopcock syringe adapters. Care is taken to make sure all junctions are tightened securely and leak-free to avoid introduction of air into the thoracic cavity.

stab incision and tunneling is performed as described above for percutaneous placement, but a trocar tube is unnecessary. Tubing may be pulled through the intercostal space with a Rochester-Carmalt forceps after incising the intercostal muscles or gently pushing the forceps through the intercostal muscles. Because of the exposure afforded by the surgical approach, blunt thrusting is not necessary. Once proper tube location is verified, a tube clamp is applied

and left open, and at least one friction suture is applied. When the thoracic cavity is closed in airtight fashion, air aspiration and final tube anchoring may progress as described above for percutaneous thoracostomy tube placement. A postoperative radiograph is typically unnecessary since proper placement is confirmed by direct visualization.

When placing a thoracostomy tube in conjunction with diaphragmatic hernia repair (or

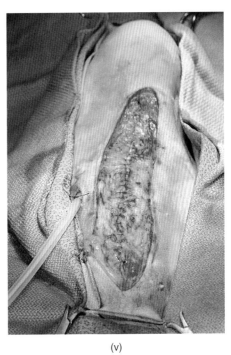

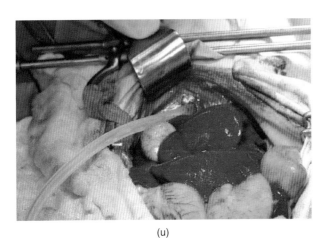

(u)   (v)

Figure 17.2 (*Continued*) (u) Thoracostomy tube placed during diaphragmatic herniorrhaphy. Note that the tube is placed through a stab incision in a healthy portion of the diaphragm before the rent in the diaphragm is closed. (v) Thoracostomy tube exiting the right abdominal wall after diaphragmatic herniorrhaphy. One friction suture is anchoring this tube during closure; three additional friction sutures will be added after or during skin closure.

whenever there is need for maintaining thoracic cavity negative pressure after an abdominal procedure), the tube enters the thoracic cavity through the diaphragm and exits the ventrolateral abdominal wall (Figures 17.2u and 17.2v). During diaphragmatic herniorrhaphy, the tube is placed through an uninjured portion of the diaphragm into the thoracic cavity before closure of the rent. Place a mattress or purse-string suture in the muscular portion of the diaphragm. Puncture the diaphragm in the center of the suture with a number 11 scalpel blade. The hole should be only large enough to accommodate the thoracic tube. Insert the tube through the stab incision and into the thorax. If not already done during hernia reduction, insert a hand through the rent and break down enough mediastinal tissue to make sure both sides of the pleural cavity communicate

and will be drained by the thoracic tube. Advance the tube toward the cranial aspect of the sternum, using a finger through the rent to ensure that the tube reaches the proper location. Tie the mattress (or purse-string) suture so that the diaphragm everts against the tube. Next, create an exit portal for the tube in the ventrolateral abdominal wall. Make a stab incision with a number 11 scalpel blade in the skin of the mid to cranial abdomen approximately 3–4 cm lateral to the midline incision, depending on the size of the patient. Place a Kelly hemostatic forceps into the stab incision and gently push it in a cranioventral direction to create a mound of tissue in the internal lateral abdominal wall caudal to the diaphragm. Incise this mound with the number 11 scalpel blade making a hole just large enough to accommodate the chest tube. Grasp the chest tube with the

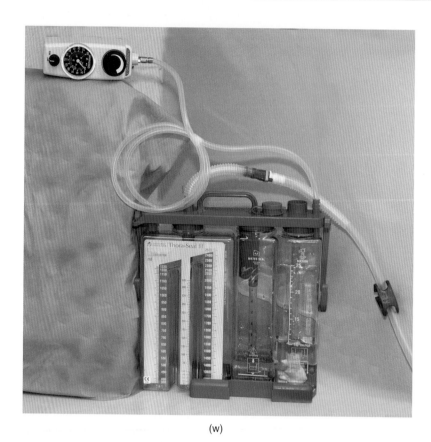

(w)

Figure 17.2 (*Continued*) (w) Continuous thoracic suction unit. This unit has a collection chamber (on the left in this photograph) that is attached by tubing to the patient's thoracostomy tube and a suction chamber (on the right in this photograph) that is attached by tubing to a regulator and continuous suction source. The suction chamber is filled to 10–12 cm of water to achieve that amount of negative intrathoracic pressure. The middle chamber is the water seal (also called an air trap). Filling the middle chamber with water to the indicated line will trap air and prevent air from moving into the collection chamber and toward the patient.

forceps and pull the tube through the abdominal wall. Verify proper tube placement, and anchor the tube to the skin and underlying abdominal fascia with a single friction suture. [Three additional friction sutures will be added later during final skin closure.]

Once a thoracostomy tube is in place, ongoing pneumothorax and pleural effusions are best managed by interfacing thoracostomy tubes with continuous suction thoracic drainage systems (Figure 17.2w). Intermittent manual aspiration of the thoracostomy tube is an alternative if continuous suction is not prac-

tical, but does not allow consistent lung expansion as air or fluid accumulates between aspirations.

Complications due to thoracostomy tubes are uncommon. Some complications to keep in mind include lung injury, tube malfunctions, tube site infection, and inadvertent pneumothorax from either loose or faulty connections or from damage of the tube by the animal.

Thoracostomy tube management includes efforts to prevent iatrogenic introduction of air. Continuous suction units (Figure 17.2w) have a safety mechanism, the water seal, that prevents atmospheric air from entering the patient, if there is a disconnection from the suction source. However, a hole in the thoracostomy tube or in the tubing between the patient and the continuous suction unit, or a loose connection between the thoracostomy tube and the tubing connecting it to the suction unit, will permit introduction of atmospheric air into the patient's pleural space. Fortunately, the water seal provides a means of monitoring for this situation. The water seal should not routinely bubble. Bubbling in the water seal indicates that the suction unit is pulling in air. That air is either atmospheric air being pulled into the tubing or air produced by ongoing pneumothorax. In the latter case, air bubbling indicates successful management of pneumothorax until the abnormality causing the pneumothorax is corrected and the bubbling stops. Bubbling due to a leak in the system between the patient and the suction unit must be ruled out by inspection of the tubing and connections because, if iatrogenic introduction of air into the pleural space is occurring, the patient's life could be in jeopardy in a matter of seconds. Tubes that are not attached to continuous suction units are monitored by periodic manual aspiration with a syringe. Care must be taken to avoid excessive suction pressure which could injure the lungs. Iatrogenic introduction of air is avoided by proper knowledge and use of connectors, tubing clamps, and three-way stopcocks.

Thoracostomy tubes must also be monitored to prevent premature dislodgement. Naive reliance on friction sutures that anchor the tube may result in premature removal. Likewise, bandages may provide a false sense of security because as a loose bandage slips it may actually pull the thoracostomy tube with it. Physical restraint (such as an Elizabethan collar) and sometimes chemical restraint (tranquilization) will be necessary to prevent premature dislodgement in active patients. If the animal's activity creates doubts as to the ability to prevent premature dislodgement, assess the true need for the tube, and remove the tube if it is not serving a useful and necessary purpose. Controlled removal

is less likely to create complications than the traumatic removal associated with the animal dislodging the tube.

Tube removal can be uncomfortable; therefore, analgesia is warranted. An injectable opiod or nonsteroidal anti-inflammatory drug given while preparing for tube removal is helpful, but local anesthesia is the main method of ensuring pain-free tube removal. Instill local anesthetic (e.g., a 9:1 solution of 2% lidocaine:sodium bicarbonate) in the subcutaneous tissues and musculature, including the intercostal space, surrounding the tube. The local block will not totally eliminate discomfort because the tube will traverse sensitive pleural surfaces on the way out. Interpleural bupivacaine can be used to obviate the intrathoracic component of the discomfort, but the initial burning sensation may be uncomfortable. Since sodium bicarbonate cannot be added to bupviacaine without resulting in a cloudy solution, a 9:1 solution of 2% lidocaine:sodium bicarbonate may be used interpleurally instead. In the latter case, care must be taken to avoid lidocaine overdose because lidocaine is also used for the subcutaneous and intercostal analgesia for tube removal. The skin around the tube is cleansed with chlorhexidine scrub, the friction sutures are cut, the tube is clamped, and gentle traction is applied to effect removal. It is important that the tube does not tear lung tissue on the way out. Lung damage could occur if excessive suction was applied to the tube immediately prior to removal. Therefore, inject 4–5 mL of air into the tube immediately prior to removal to ensure that no lung tissue has been sucked into the tube. Air injection should not be necessary as long as no suction is applied to the tube after instillation of interpleural bupivacaine.

Deciding when to remove a thoracostomy tube is not always straightforward. In cases of pneumothorax, thoracostomy tubes can usually be removed once negative pressure has been achieved for a 24-hour period, depending on the cause of the pneumothorax. For patients with pleural effusion, it has commonly been accepted in the past that thoracostomy tubes should be removed when the production of pleural fluid drops below 2 mL/kg/day; however, this targeted amount was challenged by a study in which both cats and dogs had chest tubes removed at volumes of 3–10 mL/kg/day without clinical consequence.[3] Rather than relying on strict daily pleural fluid volume assessment, the timing of thoracostomy tube removal is best based on volume trends, clinical signs and patient status, and gross and cytologic characteristics of the pleural fluid.

TRACHEOSTOMY TUBES

Temporary tracheostomy tube placement is performed to bypass upper airway obstructions caused by conditions, such as laryngeal paralysis, laryngeal collapse, laryngeal trauma, laryngeal masses, proximal tracheal obstruction, and brachycephalic upper airway syndrome. Tracheostomy tubes are commercially available, or they can be fashioned from an endotracheal tube. One specific commercially available tube (Shiley® Low Pressure Cuffed Tracheostomy Tube, Covidien Animal Health and Dental Division, Mansfield, MA) is a plastic tube that has a cuffed or uncuffed outer tube and an inner cannula which can be removed to facilitate cleaning the inner lumen (Figures 17.3a and 17.3b). Some tube sizes are too small to contain a cuff and inner cannula, so small dogs and cats will not benefit from these accessories. Commercially available tubes are usually supplied with an obturator (Figure 17.3a). The obturator is used only during placement to keep from dragging blood and secretions into the lumen. The obturator is removed as soon as the tracheostomy tube is in the tracheal lumen.

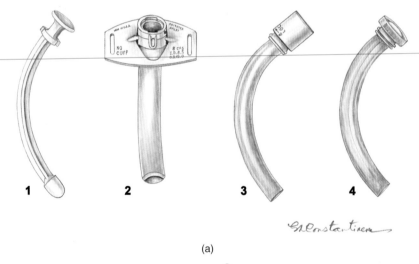

(a)

Figure 17.3 (a) Uncuffed tracheostomy tube (Shiley® Cuffless Tracheostomy Tube, Covidien Animal Health and Dental Division, Mansfield, MA). The components are: (1) obturator, which is inserted into the tracheostomy tube immediately before placement to keep secretions out of the tube during insertion and removed as soon as the tube is in the trachea; (2) tracheostomy tube, which is secured with umbilical tapes attached to eyelets in the flange of the swivel neck plate and tied behind the neck; (3) inner cannula, which is placed in the tracheostomy tube and replaced at regular intervals, and (4) closed-end cannula, which can be used to temporarily occlude the tracheostomy tube to test for the patient's ability to breathe around the tube.

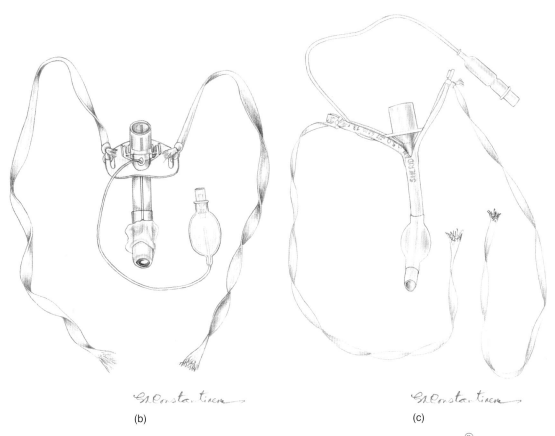

(b)   (c)

Figure 17.3 (*Continued*) (b) Commercially available cuffed tracheostomy tube (Shiley® Low Pressure Cuffed Tracheostomy Tube, Covidien Animal Health and Dental Division, Mansfield, MA) with inner cannula locked in place and umbilical tapes tied to eyelets in the flange. [Note: The cuff would only be inflated when positive-pressure ventilation is necessary. The deflated cuff increases the surface area on which secretions can accumulate, thereby complicating tracheostomy hygiene when cuffed tubes are used beyond the need for ventilation.] (c) Tracheostomy tube fashioned from a standard endotracheal tube. [Note: The inflation channel can be preserved if the cuff is needed. Preserving the inflation channel results in a curve to the tube that is rotated about 90° to the desired curve.]

If the animal requires manual or mechanical ventilation, a cuffed tube is necessary. Otherwise, an uncuffed tube is preferred. The cuff may be problematic in management of airway obstruction in awake patients because secretions may accumulate around the deflated cuff. The tube should not be larger than half the diameter of the trachea; however, multiple sizes should be available during placement. Commercially available tubes have been designed for use in humans and have a drastic curve approximately equal to 90°. This curvature may predispose the canine or feline patient to airway obstruction due to the straight anatomy of their tracheas.

A homemade tracheostomy tube can be constructed using an endotracheal tube (Figure 17.3c). Choose an endotracheal tube that is approximately one size smaller than what would ordinarily be used for orotracheal intubation. Remove the tube adapter and cut along both sides (180° apart) of the adapter end of the endotracheal tube to a level about half the length of the tube. If an inflatable cuff is needed, the cuts can be carefully made to preserve the inflation channel. Reattach the adapter at the apices of the cuts. Umbilical tape or intravenous tubing can be attached to both newly created wings and used to secure the tube around the patient's neck. This type of tracheostomy tube is often preferred by some clinicians because the shape of the tube conforms to the straight anatomy of the canine and feline trachea. One disadvantage of the homemade tracheostomy tube is that when the inflation channel is preserved the natural curve of the tube is about 90° rotated; however, no problems with this deviation have been reported.

Equipment needed for tracheostomy tube placement includes an endotracheal tube for orotracheal intubation, standard anesthetic supplies, clippers, prepping scrub and solution, barrier drape, sterile surgical gloves, sterile gauze, surgical instruments, suture material, and umbilical tape. The minimally suggested surgical instruments, which may be packaged together in a tracheostomy pack, are two towel forceps, a scalpel handle to accommodate a number 10 or number 15 scalpel blade, thumb forceps (Adson-Brown or DeBakey tissue forceps), Metzenbaum scissors, needle holders, two mosquito hemostatic forceps, and suture scissors. Self-retaining retractors, such as a Gelpi perineal retractor (preferably two) or a Weitlaner retractor, are quite helpful. Suction capability and an oxygen source should be readily available.

When placing a tracheostomy tube, ensure that the patient is under general anesthesia and is breathing supplemental oxygen through an endotracheal tube. The emergent "slash" tracheostomy should be a rare occurrence; usually, there is time to capture the airway with an endotracheal tube and prepare the patient for a controlled surgical approach. Patients in respiratory distress should be preoxygenated for approximately 5–10 minutes prior to beginning the procedure. Clip and aseptically prepare the ventral neck from the chin to the manubrium sterni with wide lateral margins. Make a ventral midline cervical skin incision just caudal to the larynx for a distance of approximately 4 cm, depending on the size of the patient (Figure 17.3d). Apply a self-retaining retractor to hold open the skin edges and clear just enough subcutaneous tissue to identify the midline division of the sternohyoideus muscles (Figure 17.3e). Separate the sternohyoideus muscles on the midline and reposition the self-retaining retractors on the sternohyoideus muscles to expose the trachea (Figure 17.3f). Incise the annular ligament between the second and third tracheal rings (Figure 17.3g). This tracheal location is chosen because it is the preferred stomal site for permanent tracheostomy should such be required. Place stay sutures around the second and third tracheal rings, knot the sutures and tag them with hemostats (Figure 17.3h). Traction on these sutures can be placed in opposite directions to open the tracheal incision to facilitate placement of the tracheostomy tube as the endotracheal tube is removed. [During the postoperative course, the stay sutures can be used for manipulation during reinsertion of a tube that has been inadvertently dislodged or requires changing.] The tracheostomy tube is inserted with the obturator in place (Figure 17.3i), but the obturator is quickly removed (Figure 17.3j) and replaced with an inner cannula, if available, as soon as the tracheostomy tube is positioned in the trachea. Secure the tracheostomy tube by attaching umbilical tape to each flange eyelet and tying the tapes behind the neck (Figures 17.3k and 17.3l).

A dressing/bandage is optional and only used to maintain cleanliness and absorb drainage of serosanguinous fluid from the incision. The authors prefer to leave the neck and incision uncovered for easy observation of swelling, bleeding, accumulated secretions, and tube position, and for prompt intervention if needed. If a bandage is desired, wait to apply it until the animal is awake and standing or in ventral recumbence. A bandage applied to a

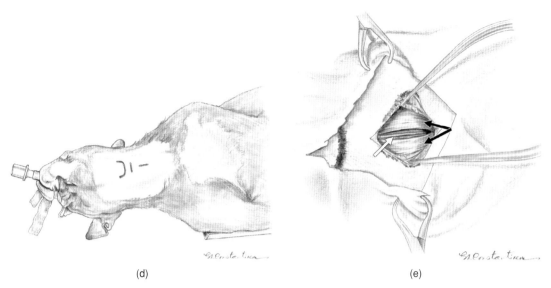

(d)   (e)

Figure 17.3   (*Continued*) (d) Positioning and preparation for tracheostomy tube placement. The dog is in dorsal recumbence with the thoracic limbs pulled caudally. An endotracheal tube is in place and should be attached to anesthetic tubing. The curved mark on the skin represents the caudal aspect of the thyroid cartilage, the straight mark immediately caudal to the curved mark represents the cricoid cartilage, and the midline straight mark indicates the proposed skin incision. Note that the surgical field is widely clipped and prepared. The endotracheal tube would be attached to an oxygen source and, most likely, inhalant anesthetic. The endotracheal tube cuff would be deflated for removal as the tracheostomy tube is inserted. (e) Surgical approach to the trachea for tracheostomy tube placement. Cranial is to the left. The skin incision is made immediately caudal to the cricoid cartilage over approximately the first through fourth tracheal rings. The skin edges are retracted with a Gelpi perineal retractor to facilitate identification of the sternohyoideus muscles (black arrows) and their midline division. The thyroidea caudalis vein (white arrow) located on the midline on the dorsal aspect of the sternohyoideus muscles is avoided to minimize hemorrhage.

recumbent extended neck is likely to change position when the patient recovers and becomes more active, causing patient discomfort or interfering with tube positioning. A neck bandage must be changed at least once daily to observe for tube site complications. Simply peeking under the bandage is not sufficient.

Immediately postoperatively, supplemental oxygen is continued while the animal recovers. Administer oxygen during recovery through a small tube (8 French) placed into the lumen of the tracheostomy tube. The oxygen flow rate should be nearly half of what is required with intranasal oxygen administration because oxygen is delivered directly into the trachea, making the trachea an oxygen-rich reservoir. Upon recovery from anesthesia the need for supplemental oxygen is based on the individual patient's needs.

Tracheostomy tube hygiene is extremely important because of the risk of iatrogenic respiratory infection and the possibility of acute fatal obstruction due to accumulated respiratory tract secretions. Immediately after surgical placement and for the first several hours, tracheostomy tubes require constant vigilance and hourly removal of intraluminal secretions. Around-the-clock observation and care are

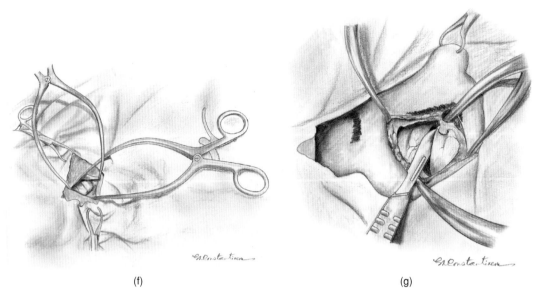

(f) (g)

Figure 17.3 (*Continued*) (f) Isolating the trachea prior to tracheotomy for tracheostomy tube placement. Cranial is to the left. The thyroidea caudalis vein is retracted laterally with one of the sternohyoideus muscles. The Gelpi perineal retractor is repositioned to retract the sternohyoideus muscles, and the loose fascia covering the ventral surface of the trachea is incised with Metzenbaum scissors. A second Gelpi perineal retractor is placed for craniocaudal retraction of skin and loose fascia exposing the tracheal rings. (g) Incising the annular ligament for tracheostomy tube placement. Cranial is to the left. The annular ligament between the second and third tracheal rings is isolated and incised. After the initial annular incision, the scalpel blade is turned upward to extend the incision, taking care to not damage the underlying endotracheal tube or its cuff. The tracheotomy is limited to 50% or less of the tracheal circumference.

mandatory. Preferably, the tube in place is one with an inner cannula that can be temporarily removed for cleaning and sanitizing and then replaced. Small tracheostomy tubes do not have inner cannulae; therefore, clean (ideally, sterile) soft suction catheters are inserted to clear the tubular lumens of secretions.

Strict adherence to asepsis cannot be overemphasized in tracheostomy tube maintenance. Unfortunately, it is rarely practical to use sterilized equipment at each tube cleaning session, but sanitization is possible. Use a 0.05% chlorhexidine solution to soak (and clean) tracheostomy tube components and suctioning accessories, but be sure to rinse with sterile saline any component that may come in contact with, or drip onto, respiratory tract tissues. Wear examination gloves when providing tracheostomy tube care, and remember to periodically cleanse the peristomal skin with warm 0.05% chlorhexidine solution. Scrub solutions are avoided to prevent contact of soap with respiratory epithelium.

Humidification of the airway is important to decrease the viscosity of respiratory secretions and facilitate their removal. Humidification is achieved by instillation of 2–3 mL of sterile isotonic saline solution into the trachea at the end of each tube cleaning session. If humidification is not sufficient to prevent respiratory tract desiccation and development of viscous secretions, aerosol therapy can be performed.

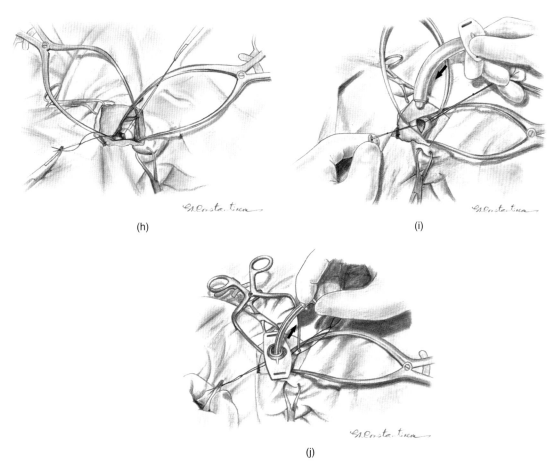

(h)   (i)

(j)

Figure 17.3   (*Continued*) (h) Placing tracheal stay sutures immediately before tracheostomy tube placement. Cranial is to the left. The suture needle is placed around the second tracheal ring, the ring just cranial to the tracheotomy, the suture is knotted such that a long loop is retained, and the free ends of the stay suture are tagged temporarily with a mosquito hemostatic forceps. A second identical stay suture is placed around the third tracheal ring, the ring just caudal to the tracheotomy. (i) Preparing to insert a tracheostomy tube. Cranial is to the left. The cranial and caudal stay sutures are retracted to pull open the tracheotomy. The endotracheal tube cuff will now be deflated and the endotracheal tube removed as the tracheostomy tube is inserted. The obturator is inserted into the tracheostomy tube immediately before placing the tube into the trachea. The purpose of the obturator is to keep blood and other secretions from being scraped into the tracheostomy tube lumen during placement. (j) Insertion of a tracheostomy tube. Cranial is to the left. The obturator is removed as soon as the tracheostomy tube is in place. After removing the obturator, the inner cannula (if applicable) is placed into the tracheostomy tube. The hemostatic forceps are removed from the stay sutures and the stay sutures are left in place.

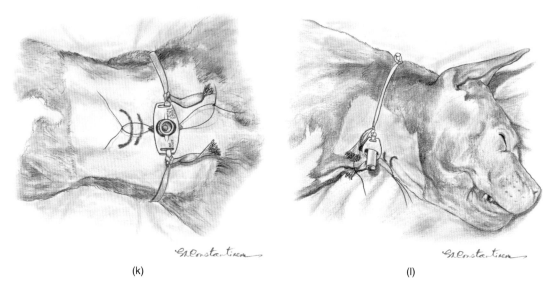

(k)   (l)

Figure 17.3 (*Continued*) (k) Completed tracheostomy tube placement (ventral view). Cranial is to the left. Umbilical tapes are tied to the eyelets in the tracheostomy tube flange. The knotted stay sutures are left in place. The stay sutures are used to facilitate replacement of the tracheostomy tube in the case of inadvertent or planned removal. Note the relationship of the tracheostomy tube to the thyroid cartilage (curved mark) and cricoid cartilage (straight mark). (l) Completed tracheostomy tube placement (lateral view). The umbilical tapes are tied on the back of the neck.

Potential complications of tracheostomy tubes include continued irritation of the tracheal lumen by the tube and accumulation of mucus, both which may result in gagging and coughing. Tracheal obstruction can occur due to mucus accumulation or due to occlusion of the tube opening as it lies against the tracheal mucosa. Tube dislodgement can also occur should the umbilical tape ties become loose. Local subcutaneous emphysema can sometimes occur as air leaks around the tube into the tissues. Long-term complications can include tracheal stenosis or stricture.

When it is determined that the tracheostomy tube is no longer needed, umbilical tapes are cut, the tube is extracted, and the resultant open wound is allowed to heal by second intention. The patient may continue to breathe through the stoma for several days until sufficient wound contraction occurs.

CYSTOSTOMY TUBES

Indications for cystostomy tube placement include urinary diversion in the face of urinary tract trauma or urinary tract obstruction (foreign body, cystic calculi, neoplasia, etc.), or to rest a surgically repaired urethra. It may also be advisable to place a cystostomy tube if urinary bladder atony is present to avoid over-distension. A Foley catheter (Figure 17.4a) or a Stamey Malecot catheter (Cook Medical Inc., Bloomington, IN; Figures 17.4b and 17.4c) may be used as a cystostomy tube. The Foley catheter is preferred because urine leakage into the peritoneal cavity has been noted with percutaneously placed Stamey Malecot catheters. These two catheters are better suited for temporary rather than long-term urinary diversion due to their length and likelihood of inadvertent premature removal. A long version of

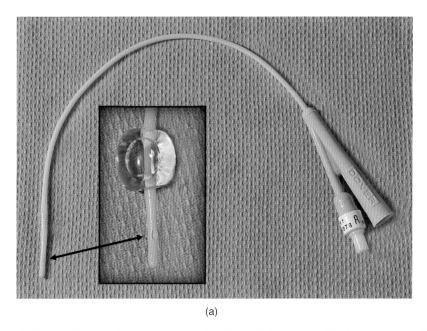

(a)

Figure 17.4   (a) Silicone Foley catheter. An 8 French catheter is illustrated. The insert shows inflation of the bulb. The arrow points to tube fenestrations.

Foley catheter is available for urethral catheterization of male dogs (Smiths Medical, Waukesha, WI; Figure 17.4d). This Foley catheter is not suitable as a cystostomy tube because it is excessively long. A low profile gastrostomy tube (Cook Medical Inc., Bloomington, IN; Figure 17.4e) may be used as a long-term cystostomy tube to decrease the chances that the tube will be damaged or removed by the patient. Planned removal is more difficult with this device compared to Foley and Stamey Malecot catheters. The following description of cystostomy tube placement technique employs a standard silicone Foley catheter.

Prior to placing a cystostomy tube, clip and aseptically prepare the ventral abdomen from the xyphoid cartilage to the distal pubis with wide lateral margins. The standard approach is a ventral midline celiotomy. If a full abdominal exploration is not necessary, make a ventral midline incision approximately 5 cm long just cranial to the brim of the pubis in female dogs and all cats and a 5 cm long parapreputial incision just cranial to the pubis in male dogs. Enter the abdomen through a standard linea alba incision. Locate the urinary bladder and place a stay suture in its apex (Figure 17.4f). Perform a test inflation of the Foley catheter bulb to make sure it is not defective (Figure 17.4g). Then, introduce the catheter into the peritoneal cavity through the abdominal wall to one side of the linea alba. Make a tiny stab incision in the internal abdominal wall with a number 11 scalpel blade just big enough to accommodate the tube (typically an 8 French Foley catheter) approximately 4 cm lateral to the linea alba, depending on the size of the patient (Figures 17.4h and 17.4i). Insert a mosquito hemostatic forceps into the stab and push outward to create a mound of tissue as visualized on the skin (Figures 17.4j and 17.4k). Using the number 11 scalpel blade, incise the mound of skin and underlying tissue over the tip of the mosquito forceps until the tip of the forceps is

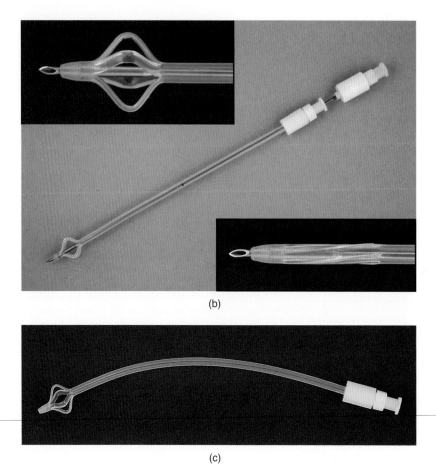

(b)

(c)

Figure 17.4 (*Continued*) (b) Stamey Malecot catheter. A polyethylene catheter is illustrated. The inserts demonstrate how the needle obturator straightens the flanged portion of the catheter for penetration into the abdomen and into the urinary bladder. (c) Stamey Malecot catheter without the needle obturator. The flanged portion of the catheter is designed to keep the catheter in the urinary bladder. [Note: Urine leakage around this catheter has been reported with percutaneous placement.

exposed (Figures 17.4l and 17.4m). Again, this stab should be just big enough to accommodate the catheter. Gently grasp the tip of the Foley catheter with the mosquito hemostatic forceps and pull the catheter into the abdomen (Figures 17.4n through 17.4p). Place a purse-string suture directly at the proposed catheter site using absorbable suture material (Figure 17.4q). Puncture the urinary bladder in the center of the purse-string using a number 11 scalpel blade

(Figure 17.4r). Suction any urine that is present inside the lumen of the urinary bladder. Ensure that the hole is just large enough to accommodate the tube. It is acceptable for the hole to be snug around the tube. If the hole is too large, it will be difficult to maintain a leak-proof seal once the purse-string suture is tied. Place the tube into the urinary bladder (Figure 17.4s). Advance the tube into the lumen of the urinary bladder well past the level of the deflated

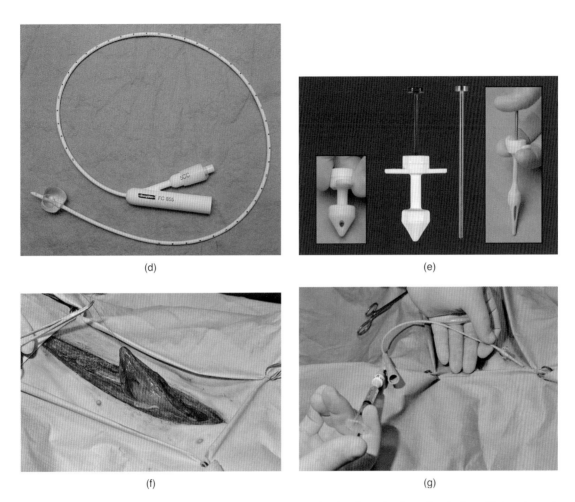

(d)   (e)

(f)   (g)

Figure 17.4   (*Continued*) (d) Silicone Foley catheter for urethral catheterization of male dogs. This catheter is not suitable for cystostomy tube placement because of its excessive length. (e) Silicone low profile gastrostomy tube. This tube has two side holes (see insets) in the triangulated tip. The tip is elongated with a plastic or metal obturator to facilitate insertion through the abdominal wall and into the stomach (or into the bladder if used for a cystostomy tube). In this photograph, a plastic obturator is inserted into the tube. A metal obturator is pictured next to the low profile gastrostomy tube. The right insert demonstrates using the metal obturator to elongate the tube. Pushing the obturator with a thumb while holding the tube flanges with the first and second fingers in syringe-like fashion elongates the tip. (f) Isolation of urinary bladder for cystostomy tube placement. A stay suture of 3–0 poliglecaprone 25 is placed in the apex of the urinary bladder and tagged with a mosquito hemostatic forceps. The suture is placed using a wide bite that penetrates the full thickness of the urinary bladder wall in order to ensure engagement of the submucosa. (g) Performing test inflation of a Foley catheter prior to use as a cystostomy tube. The preferred inflation medium is sterile water. The bulb is deflated before insertion.

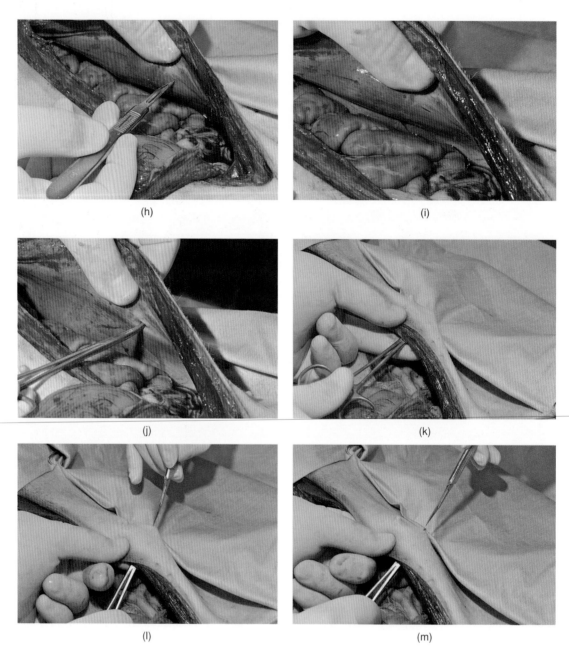

(h)

(i)

(j)

(k)

(l)

(m)

Figure 17.4 (*Continued*) (h) Preparing to make a stab incision in the left abdominal wall with a number 11 scalpel blade. (i) Tiny stab incision in the left abdominal wall just large enough to accommodate the tips of a mosquito hemostatic forceps. (j) Inserting tips of mosquito hemostatic forceps into left abdominal wall stab incision. (k) Advancing tips of mosquito hemostatic forceps laterally through the left abdominal wall stab incision until a mound of skin is visible over the forceps tips. (l) Preparing to make a stab incision in the skin of the left abdominal wall over the mosquito hemostatic forceps tips with a number 11 scalpel blade. (m) Incising the left abdominal wall with a number 11 scalpel blade just enough to permit protrusion of the mosquito hemostatic forceps tips.

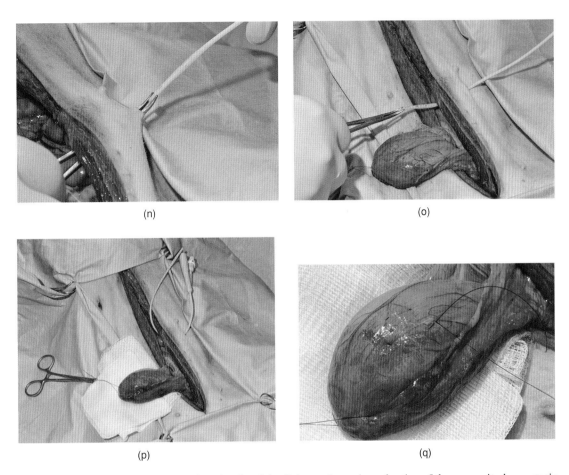

(n)   (o)

(p)   (q)

Figure 17.4 (*Continued*) (n) Grasping the tip of the Foley catheter into the tips of the mosquito hemostatic forceps in preparation for pulling the catheter into the abdomen. (o) Pulling the Foley catheter into the abdomen. (p) Foley catheter introduced into the abdomen and urinary bladder exteriorized in preparation for cystostomy. (q) Purse-string suture (3–0 poliglecaprone 25) in the left dorsolateral portion of the urinary bladder encircling the proposed site of cystostomy. Suture bites for the purse-string suture must engage the submucosa, and it is acceptable to place these bites full-thickness through the urinary bladder wall to ensure submucosal engagement.

balloon (Figure 17.4t). Tie the purse-string suture snugly (Figure 17.4u) and cut the strands (Figure 17.4v). If the purse-string is tied too tightly, ischemia and necrosis of the stoma may develop. Preplace two to four absorbable sutures from the urinary bladder (near the catheter entrance) to the body wall (Figure 17.4w). At this point, the balloon should be inflated with sterile water (Figure 17.4w). Then,

tie the preplaced sutures to tack the urinary bladder to the abdominal wall (Figure 17.4x). Gently pull the catheter until the purse-string suture inhibits its extraction and use four friction sutures[1] to secure the tube to the skin and underlying fascia (Figure 17.4y).

If a low-profile gastrostomy tube is being placed to serve as a cystostomy tube, the incision in the abdominal wall will need to be large

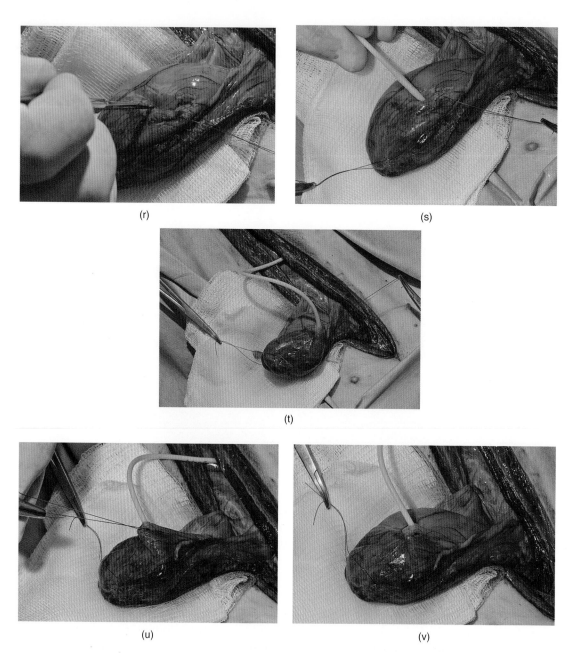

(r)

(s)

(t)

(u)

(v)

Figure 17.4 (*Continued*) (r) Making a stab incision in the urinary bladder for placement of a cystostomy tube. The stab is made in the center of the preplaced purse-string suture using a number 11 scalpel blade. The sharp edge of the blade is oriented toward the purse-string strands to avoid inadvertent severing of the suture within the bladder tissue. (s) Inserting a Foley catheter into a stab incision in the center of a preplaced purse-string suture in the urinary bladder. (t) Advancing the Foley catheter into the urinary bladder before the purse-string suture is tied. (u) Tied purse-string suture after the Foley catheter is advanced deeply into the urinary bladder. (v) Finished purse-string suture with strands cut. Next, the urinary bladder will be anchored to the body wall.

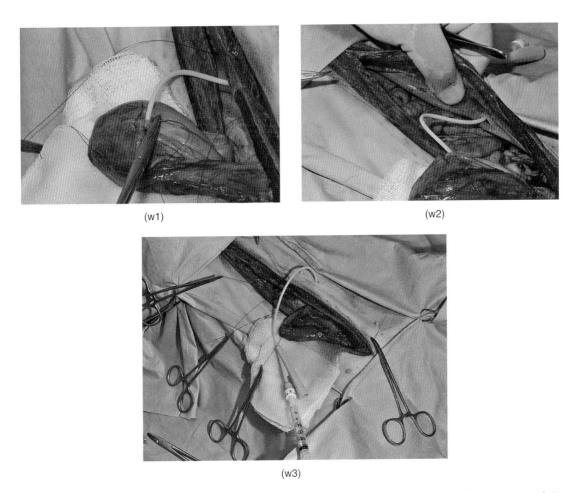

(w1)   (w2)

(w3)

Figure 17.4 (*Continued*) (w) Preplacing sutures from the abdominal wall to the urinary bladder to result in a cystopexy when tied. All sutures are placed full-thickness into the urinary bladder taking care not to hit the tube with suture bites. (1) The first suture is placed dorsal to the tube in the body wall and dorsal to the tube in the urinary bladder. (2) The first suture is tagged with mosquito hemostatic forceps and one to three similar sutures are additionally preplaced around the tube. (3) Four tacking sutures have been preplaced from the abdominal wall to the urinary bladder and the Foley bulb is inflated with sterile water.

in order to accommodate the size of the tube's tip. This tube comes with an obturator (Figure 17.4e) that can be used to stretch the catheter into a more slender tube that will allow both the abdominal wall and urinary bladder incisions to be as small as possible. Once the tube is through the abdominal wall and into the urinary bladder, remove the stylet to deploy the catheter into its intended shape. Tighten the purse-string suture and preplaced tacking sutures as directed above. One or two interrupted sutures may be required in the abdominal wall and skin incisions to ensure a snug fit. If that is the case, the abdominal sutures must be placed before the tacking sutures are tied.

The method of cystostomy tube removal depends on whether a Foley catheter or low-profile gastrostomy tube is used. For the Foley

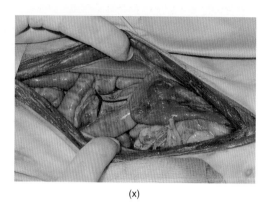

(x)

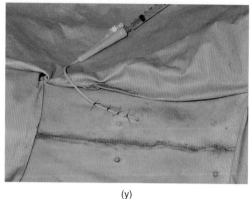

(y)

Figure 17.4 (*Continued*) (x) Cystopexy completed. Four preplaced sutures from the abdominal wall to the urinary bladder around a Foley catheter have been tied and the stay suture in the apex of the urinary bladder has been removed. (y) Four friction sutures anchoring a cystostomy tube. The first friction suture (closest to the tube exit) is placed while the abdomen is still open and with mild traction on the catheter so that the Foley bulb is against the urinary bladder wall. The remaining friction sutures are placed after abdominal closure. Note the syringe with saline attached to the catheter. After each friction suture is tied, saline is injected and aspirated to make sure that no friction suture occludes the lumen of the catheter.

catheter, first remove the friction sutures. Then, empty the bulb by attaching a syringe to the inflation valve port and aspirating. Emptying the bulb will not be possible if the friction sutures are occluding the inflation channel; therefore, it is best to remove the friction sutures completely from the Foley catheter. After emptying the bulb, the catheter should be easily extracted. Low profile gastrostomy tubes are rarely removed unless the reason for which they were used as a cystostomy tube has resolved. To remove a low profile gastrostomy tube, insert the obturator to stretch the tube into a skinnier shape while extracting. Moderate force will be necessary to remove the low profile gastrostomy tube. Local infiltration of surrounding tissues with a 9:1 solution of 2% lidocaine:sodium bicarbonate will help control patient discomfort during removal. Local anesthetic is also used for removal of a Foley catheter cystostomy tube, although there should be minimal pain with Foley catheter removal.

The most significant complication of cystostomy tubes is inadvertent dislodgement of the tube. If dislodgement occurs before the urinary bladder stoma has adhered to the abdominal wall, uroabdomen may occur resulting in urine peritonitis. If dislodgement occurs after the urinary bladder stoma has adhered to the abdominal wall, urine scalding on the peristomal skin may occur or cystitis could develop from locally introduced bacteria. Another minor complication is transient hematuria; however, this is generally self-limiting and should clear within a few days after surgery.

ESOPHAGOSTOMY TUBES

Esophagostomy tubes can be used for nutritional support as long as the animal is not vomiting and does not have esophageal dysfunction. Some clinicians prefer esophagostomy tubes over gastrostomy tubes because of potentially more serious complications with gastrostomy tubes, such as peritonitis. Dogs and cats generally tolerate esophagostomy tubes and they can eat voluntarily with the tube in place when appetite returns. Due to the large bore nature

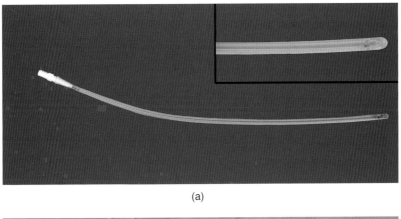

(a)

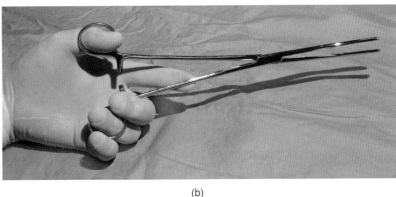

(b)

Figure 17.5   (a) Commercially available silicone esophagostomy tube (Feline Esophagostomy Tube – Silicone, Smiths Medical, Waukesha, WI). (b) 12-inch curved Rochester-Péan forceps for use as an esophagostomy tube placement forceps.

of esophagostomy tubes (14 French or larger), blenderized diets may be used, in contrast to liquid diets required for nasoesophageal/nasogastric feeding. Silicone esophagostomy tubes are commercially available (Feline Esophagostomy Tube—Silicone, Smiths Medical, Waukesha, WI; Figure 17.5a), but esophagostomy tubes can be made from most types of tubing by fashioning side holes in the tip (Figure 17.2c). Some general guidelines for size of esophagostomy tube are 14 French for animals less than 10 kg and 19 French or larger for animals greater than 10 kg. The esophagostomy tube placement technique described here employs a red rubber tube, whereas silicone tubes are preferred.

Prior to placing an esophagostomy tube, place the patient in right lateral recumbence. Clip and aseptically prepare an area on the left lateral neck extending from the ramus of the mandible to the caudal cervical area and from the wing of the atlas to the trachea. Premeasure the length of the tube from the seventh intercostal space to the proposed exit point of the feeding tube in the mid portion of the neck. Using a long Rochester-Péan (Figure 17.5b) or similar forceps, introduce the forceps with tips closed into the oral cavity and esophagus caudal

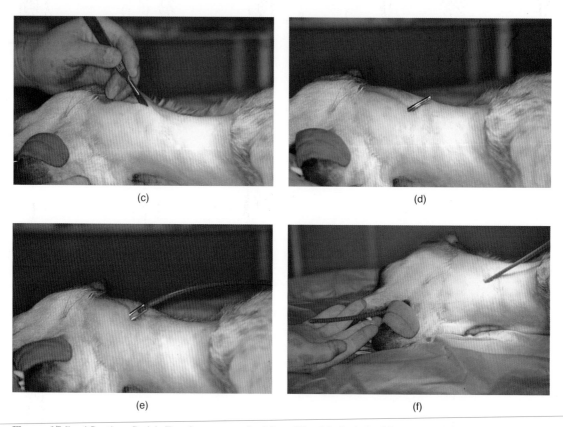

Figure 17.5 (*Continued*) (c) Esophagostomy incision. The blade is incising over tips of the esophagostomy placement forceps, making an incision just large enough to accommodate the chosen tube. (d) Esophagostomy placement forceps emerging through the skin from the esophagus. (e) Grasping the tip of the esophagostomy tube in the tips of the esophagostomy placement forceps. Note that a red rubber tube is being used, but silicone tubing is preferred. (f) Esophagostomy tube pulled into the esophagus and out the oral cavity.

to the hyoid apparatus so that the incision over the forceps tip will be in the mid portion of the neck. Make a small skin incision over the tips of the forceps using a number 10 scalpel blade (or number 15 blade for cats and small dogs) just large enough to accommodate the tube (Figure 17.5c) and deepen this incision to the esophagus until the forceps tips emerge (Figure 17.5d). Grasp the tip of the tube with the forceps (Figure 17.5e) and pull the tube into and out of the oral cavity (Figure 17.5f). Using the forceps, redirect the distal end of the feeding tube back into the mouth (Figures 17.5g

and 17.5h). Advance the tube into the esophagus until a "pop" is palpated, indicating that the tube has straightened into the distal esophagus. When the tube is directed down the esophagus the external portion of the tube shifts from a caudal-to-cranial orientation (Figure 17.5g) to a cranial-to-caudal orientation (Figure 17.5i). The tube should be slid cranially and caudally to ensure that it is straight and not kinked in the pharynx. At this point, a lateral thoracic radiograph should be taken to confirm proper placement of the tube. Once proper placement is confirmed, the tube is anchored with a

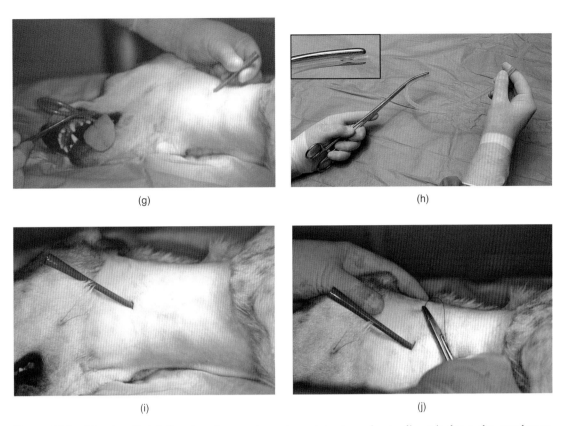

Figure 17.5 (*Continued*) (g) Turning the esophagostomy tube in order to direct it down the esophagus. Note that the tube is grasped by the esophagostomy placement forceps in the curved portion of the forceps. In this photo, the tube is positioned along the outer portion of the forceps' curve. (h) Positioning of an esophagostomy tube along the inner portion of an esophagostomy placement forceps curve as would be done to advance the tube down the esophagus. Grasping along the inner portion of the forceps' curve will make release of the forceps easier and less likely to inadvertently pull the tube back out the oral cavity. (i) External position of the esophagostomy tube when the tube is effectively directed caudally down the esophagus. The tube in this position should easily slide cranially and caudally within the esophagus without changing direction if proper placement has been achieved. (j) Deep passage of a suture needle to engage the periosteum of the wing of the altas and surrounding fascia in preparation for the first friction suture to anchor the esophagostomy tube. [Make sure that a large needle is chosen to achieve this objective and be careful to not lose the needle under the skin.]

friction suture[1] (1–0 or larger, depending on the size of the tube) that engages the fascia and periosteum of the wing of the atlas. The suture needle is passed deeply to hit the wing of the atlas before turning upward and exiting the skin (Figure 17.5j). Tug on the suture strands to ensure adequate fascia and periosteal engagement (Figure 17.5k) before tying the knot. Tie a square knot gently against the skin (Figure 17.5l), place the tube onto the square knot, and then tie a surgeon's knot so that the suture slightly indents the tube to complete

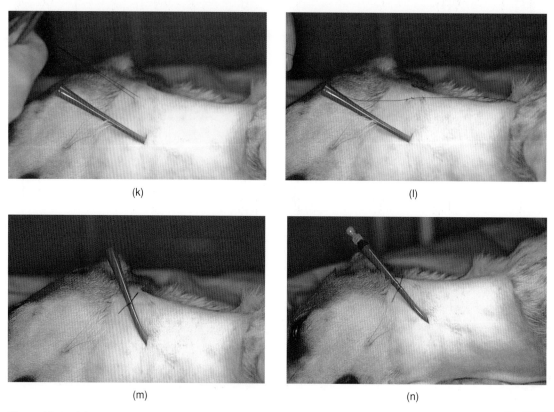

(k)

(l)

(m)

(n)

Figure 17.5 *(Continued)* (k) Tugging on suture strands to verify that the planned friction suture has engaged the periosteum of the wing of the atlas and surrounding fascia. (l) Square knot tied in the suture engaging the periosteum of the wing of the atlas and surrounding fascia. This knot is tied as if placing a skin incision suture. Then, the tube is placed against the knot and a surgeon's knot is applied to sandwich the tube between the square knot and surgeon's knot, thus completing the friction suture. (m) Completed friction suture anchoring the esophagostomy tube to the periosteum of the wing of the atlas and surrounding fascia. Additional friction sutures may be placed to assist anchoring the tube to skin and underlying fascia. (n) Completed esophagostomy tube placement with tubing adapter and cap in place. When the dog is in dorsal recumbence or standing and the ear is hanging downward, the esophagostomy tube should lie naturally behind the ear.

the friction suture (Figure 17.5m). Additional friction sutures may be placed to secure the tube to the skin and underlying cervical fascia. Flush the tube and cap it (Figure 17.5n). Flush the tube with approximately 5 mL of saline (preferred) or water prior to and after each feeding. Immediately prior to removing an esophagostomy tube, flush the tube with saline or water to ensure that residual food is flushed into the esophageal lumen so that no food residue is dragged through and deposited in the subcutaneous tissues around the stoma site. The stoma is allowed to heal by second intention. Complications of esophagostomy tubes can include stomal infections, aspiration of water or food with possible secondary aspiration pneumonia, esophagitis due to reflux of gastric acid and regurgitation, and inadvertent tracheal placement. Other complications of esophageal tubes may include occlusion or inadvertent removal by the patient.

GASTROSTOMY TUBES

Gastrostomy tubes can be used for nutritional support for animals that are not vomiting and are particularly useful when esophageal function is in question. Gastrostomy tubes may be placed with an endoscope (percutaneous endoscopic gastrostomy) or with the aid of specially designed instrumentation (percutaneous nonendoscopic gastrostomy). These minimally invasive methods of gastrostomy tube placement are preferred over surgical placement; however, if a celiotomy is being performed for other reasons and the patient requires a gastric tube, it is more efficient to place the tube surgically than to close the celiotomy and apply one of the nonsurgical techniques. Surgical placement is described below.

Gastrostomy tubes should have a diameter large enough to accommodate feeding of gruels, meaning that they must be 14 French or larger. Most commonly, 20 French tubes are used for cats and small dogs (up to 10 kg)

and 24 French for dogs greater than 10 kg. Although a large Foley catheter could be used for gastrostomy, the bulb may eventually burst in the presence of gastric acid, posing a threat for premature dislodgement or leakage of gastric contents around the tube. Therefore, a Pezzer mushroom tip catheter (Peg Feeding Tube, Smiths Medical, Waukesha, WI; Figure 17.6a) is preferred, and silicone is preferred over latex. Large (20 mm for 16 French tubes and 25 mm for 20 French tubes) and small (15 mm for 16 French tubes and 20 mm for 20 French tubes) mushroom tip diameters are available (Smiths Medical, Waukesha, WI); the small mushroom is preferred for ease of removal when the tube is no longer needed.

During celiotomy the gastrostomy tube may be placed in the gastric fundus to exit through the left body wall, as is done with minimally invasive techniques. However, intraoperative placement affords the option of placing the tube in the pyloric antrum to exit through the right body wall. The latter choice is a good idea in dogs that are predisposed to gastric dilatation-volvulus, because right-sided gastrostomy tube placement results in a prophylactic gastropexy. Right-sided gastrostomy tube placement in a large breed dog is described here.

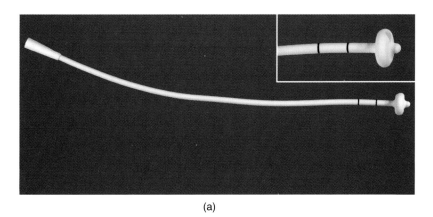

(a)

Figure 17.6   (a) Silicone Pezzar mushroom-tipped gastrostomy tube (Peg Feeding Tube, Smiths Medical, Waukesha, WI). Inset is a closeup view of mushroom tip of the tube.

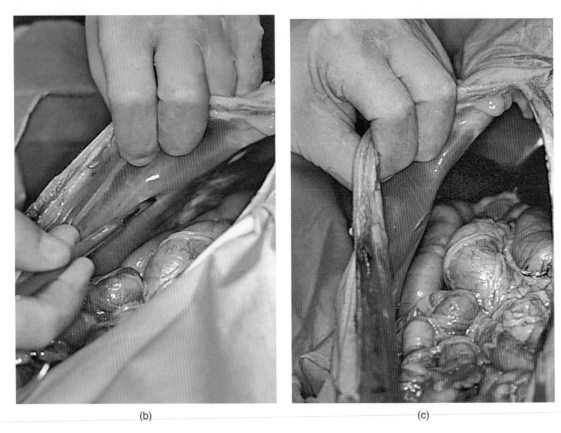

(b)   (c)

Figure 17.6   (*Continued*) (b) Scalpel pointing to the proposed incision site in the right body wall caudal to the last rib for surgical gastrostomy tube placement. (c) Incision in the right body wall for surgical gastrostomy tube placement. This incision will need to be deepened and lengthened to accommodate the Pezzar tube mushroom tip. (d) Elongation of a Pezzar tube mushroom tip using Rochester-Carmalt forceps as would be done to pass the tube through the abdominal wall. Care must be taken to not tear the tip of the tube with the forceps. (e) Advancing a Rochester-Carmalt forceps through the right body wall incision until the tip can be palpated under a mound of skin. (f) Incising the skin over a Rochester-Carmalt forceps that has been passed through the right abdominal wall musculature. This skin incision must be large enough to accommodate the mushroom tip of the Pezzar tube.

Upon completion of the surgical procedures for which the celiotomy was performed, create an exit stoma for the tube in the right lateral abdominal wall immediately caudal to the last rib. Using a number 10 scalpel blade, make an incision in the abdominal musculature approximately 6 cm lateral to the linea alba incision (Figures 17.6b and 17.6c). This incision must be large enough to accommodate the Pezzar tube mushroom. [Note: The mushroom may be slightly elongated, but not entirely (Figure 17.6d); therefore, the incision in the abdominal musculature must be larger than the tube diameter.] Place a Rochester-Carmalt forceps through the abdominal wall incision and advance through the subcutaneous tissue until the skin is reached. Advance the forceps to create a conical elevation of skin (Figure 17.6e). Make

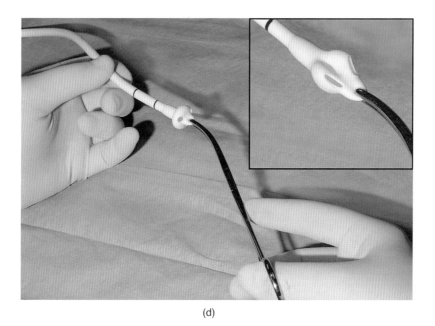

(d)

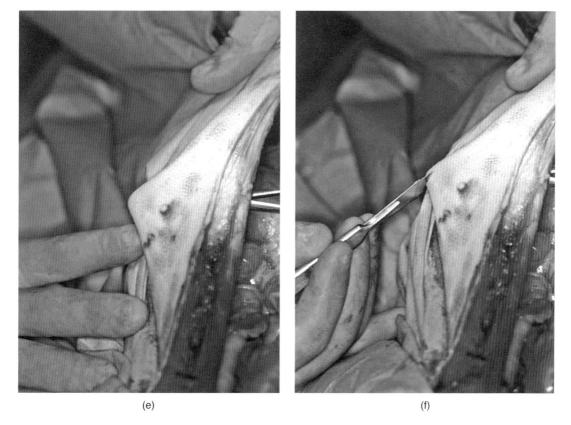

(e)

(f)

Figure 17.6   (*Continued*)

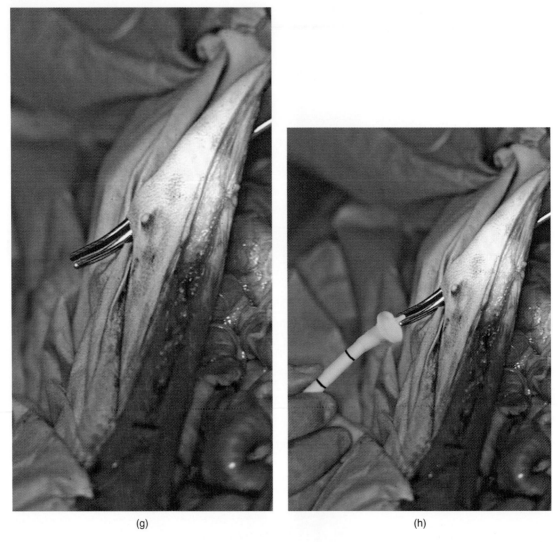

(g)   (h)

Figure 17.6 (*Continued*) (g) Tips of a Rochester-Carmalt forceps emerging through the skin to grasp the gastostomy tube tip. (h) Grasping the tip of a gastrostomy tube with Rochester-Carmalt forceps to pull the tube into the peritoneal cavity.

an incision over the tips of the forceps until the forceps protrudes through the hole (Figures 17.6f and 17.6g). Increase the size of the skin incision to accommodate the Pezzar mushroom. Grasp the tip of the feeding tube with the forceps (Figure 17.6h) and pull the feeding tube through the hole and into the abdomen

(Figure 17.6i). Place a purse-string suture in the stomach at the proposed tube site (pyloric antrum immediately to the right of the incisura angularis) using 2–0 or 3–0 absorbable suture material. A short-lasting suture material, such as poliglecaprone 25, is preferred for the purse-string suture because the diminishing tensile

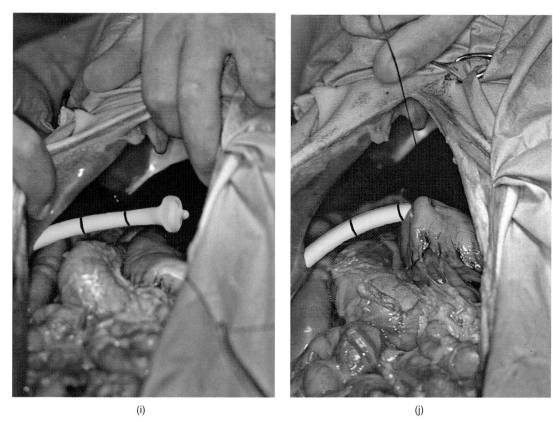

(i)   (j)

Figure 17.6 (*Continued*) (i) Gastrostomy tube within the peritoneal cavity from the right abdominal wall. (j) Gastrostomy tube coursing from the right abdominal wall into the stomach. The tip of the tube is in the stomach and the purse-string suture around the gastrostomy has been tied.

strength will be advantageous at the time of tube removal. Stab into the stomach in the area surrounded by the purse-string suture using a number 11 scalpel blade. Extend this incision so that it is just large enough to accommodate the mushroom, being careful not to cut the purse-string suture. Insert the tube into the gastrostomy incision and tie the purse-string suture so that the stomach is snugly against the tube and the mushroom is deep in the stomach lumen (Figure 17.6j). Preplace two to four sutures from the stomach to the body wall using 1–0 monofilament suture (Figure 17.6k). Absorbable suture is acceptable, but the prin-

cipal author prefers polypropylene. Take full-thickness bites in the stomach to ensure engagement of the submucosa, taking care not to incorporate the tube or its mushroom in the process. Also, make sure that there is enough distance between these preplaced sutures so that the mushroom will not be impeded by them when the tube is removed. When preplacing four sutures, place the dorsal suture first, followed by the cranial and caudal sutures, and lastly the ventral suture. Pull the gastrostomy tube to draw the mushroom against the purse-string suture and the stomach against the abdominal wall (Figure 17.6l). Tie the preplaced

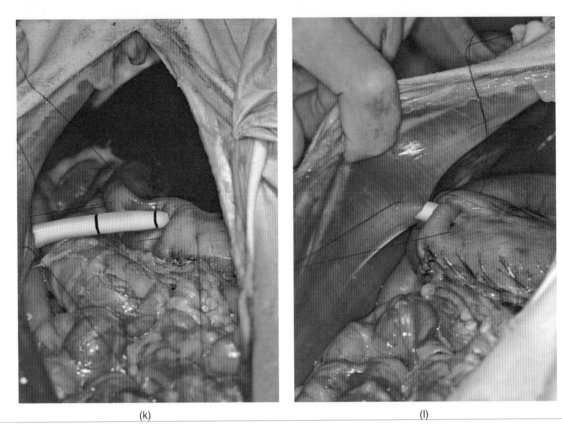

(k)   (l)

Figure 17.6 (*Continued*) (k) Two sutures (one cranial to the tube and one caudal to the tube) to anchor the stomach to the right abdominal wall have been preplaced around the gastrostomy, taking care to not touch the tube or its tip during suture bites. If four tacking sutures are used (recommended), the dorsal suture is preplaced first, followed by the cranial and caudal sutures, and the ventral suture is preplaced last. (l) Pulling the gastrostomy tube to bring the stomach in apposition with the right body wall.

sutures (dorsal, then cranial and caudal, and lastly ventral) to complete the pexy of the stomach to the body wall (Figures 17.6m and 17.6n). Place a friction suture[1] externally to secure the tube to the skin and underlying fascia, and later add three additional friction sutures after the abdomen is closed.

When removing a gastrostomy tube, inject the tube with 10–15 mL of water or saline to ensure that residual food is flushed into the gastric lumen and not dragged through the subcutaneous tissues of the abdominal wall. Inject

local anesthetic (9 parts lidocaine mixed with 1 part sodium bicarbonate) into the subcutaneous tissue and muscle surrounding the tube. After allowing the local anesthetic to take effect, pull snugly on the tube with one hand while the other hand presses against the body wall at the tube exit site. Continue to pull until the mushroom collapses and the tube comes out.

Potential complications of gastrostomy tubes include stomal infections, inadvertent complete or partial removal, tube occlusion, and peritonitis. An Elizabethan collar is essential for as long

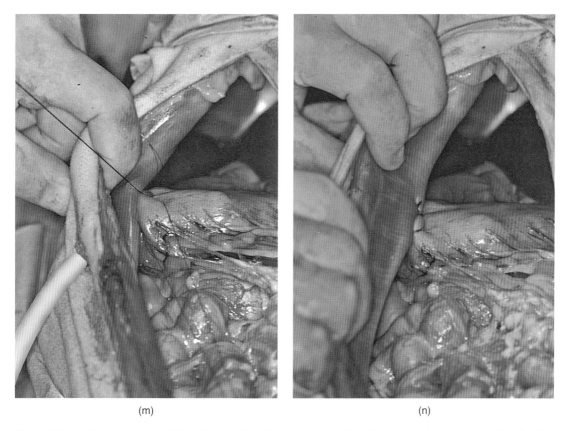

(m) (n)

Figure 17.6 (*Continued*) (m) Tying the preplaced stomach-to-body wall sutures. (n) Completed anchoring of the stomach to the right body wall.

as the gastrostomy tube is present in order to avoid chewing the tube or inadvertently pulling it out of the abdomen.

JEJUNOSTOMY TUBES

Jejunostomy tubes are indicated for nutritional support in patients that are vomiting and may be placed preemptively during celiotomy whenever postoperative vomiting is a realistic possibility. Feeding into jejunostomy tubes is limited to liquid diets because of the small diameter of the tube (10 French or smaller). Red rubber (SOVEREIGN Feeding Tube and

Urethral Catheter, Covidien Animal Health & Dental Division, Mansfield, MA; Figure 17.1a), polyurethane (Argyle Indwell Polyurethane Feeding Tube, Covidien Animal Health & Dental Division, Mansfield, MA), polyvinyl chloride (Argyle Polyvinyl Chloride Feeding Tube with Sentinel Line, Covidien Animal Health & Dental Division, Mansfield, MA; Figure 17.7a), and silicone (Nasal Oxygen/Feeding Tube-Silicone, Smiths Medical, Waukesha, WI) tubes (usually 5, 8, or 10 French) may be used. Silicone (Figure 17.7b) is preferred because of minimal tissue reactivity compared to other tube biomaterials. If not damaged, silicone tubes can be cleaned, steam sterilized, and used again. Minimally invasive nasojejunostomy tubes can be placed, but

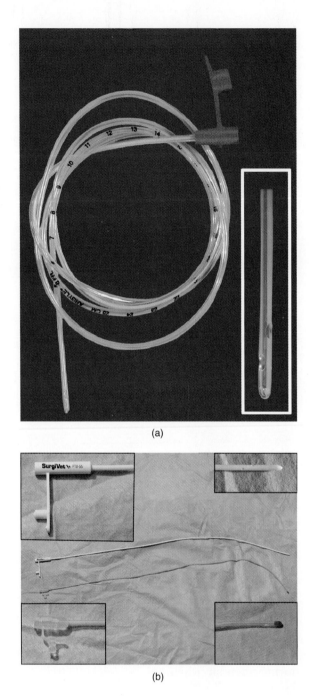

(a)

(b)

Figure 17.7   (a) Polyvinyl chloride feeding tube (Argyle Polyvinyl Chloride Feeding Tube with Sentinel Line, Covidien Animal Health & Dental Division, Mansfield, MA). The green cap indicates that the tube is made of polyvinyl chloride. A blue cap would indicate that the tube is made of polyurethane. (b) Silicone nasogastric tube (Nasal Oxygen/Feeding Tube-Silicone, Smiths Medical, Waukesha, WI) for use as a jejunostomy tube. Manufacture of the white tube was discontinued in 2009. The clear tube substitute is less stiff, more stretchable, and a little more collapsible than the white tube.

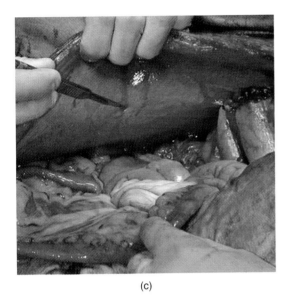

(c)

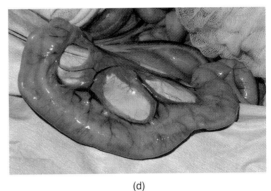

(d)

Figure 17.7 *(Continued)* (c) Location for jejunostomy tube entry in the middle portion of the right abdominal wall. [Cranial is to the right; view is from the perspective of an assistant to a right-handed surgeon.] Note the location of the incisional gastropexy cranial to the proposed jejunostomy tube entry site. The number 11 scalpel blade points to the proposed tube exit site. (d) Isolated loop of jejunum for placement of a jejunostomy tube. [Cranial is to the left; view is from a right-handed surgeon's perspective.]

surgical jejunostomy is currently more commonly performed and is described here.

Upon completion of the surgical procedures for which the celiotomy was performed, identify the site in the abdominal wall where the tube will exit. The exit stoma for the tube should be located in the right lateral abdominal wall in the mid abdomen caudal to where a gastropexy would typically be performed (Figure 17.7c). Whereas a left abdominal wall stoma would be acceptable, the authors find the right abdominal wall more practical for a right-handed surgeon and more anatomically appropriate for the segment of small intestine that will accommodate the tube. Isolate the loop of intestine into which the jejunostomy tube will be placed (Figure 17.7d) and place a stay suture to maintain orientation (Figure 17.7e). The tube should enter the jejunum as cranially as is practical. It is acceptable for the tube to span an enterotomy or anastomosis site, but avoid having the tip of the tube come

to rest at such sites. The tube is introduced into the abdomen before placing it in the jejunum (Figure 17.7f). A tiny stab incision is made with a number 11 scalpel blade in the transversus abdominis muscle in the caudal aspect of the incision and approximately 4 cm from the midline incision. A mosquito hemostatic forceps is introduced into the stab and force applied in a craniolateral direction until the tip can be palpated just lateral to the nipples of the mammary chain. A tiny stab incision is made over the tip of the forceps, taking care not to make the incision any larger than that necessary to permit exposure of the forceps' tip. Then, the tip of the jenunostomy tube is grasped with the forceps and the tube is pulled into the abdomen. After it is in the abdomen, the tube is placed into the jejunum (Figure 17.7g). A purse-string suture (or horizontal mattress suture, as preferred by the principal author) is placed in the antimesenteric border of the previously isolated cranial segment of

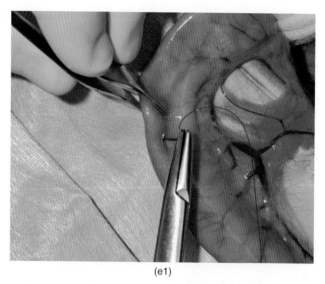

(e1)

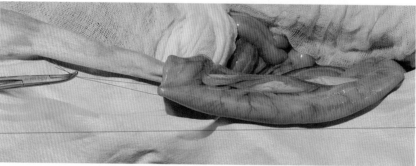

(e2)

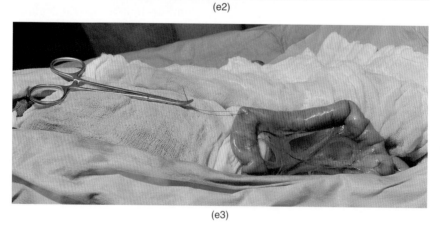

(e3)

Figure 17.7   (*Continued*) (e) Placing a 3–0 poliglecaprone 25 stay suture just cranial to the proposed jejunostomy site. [Cranial is to the left; view is from a right-handed surgeon's perspective.] (1) A full-thickness bite of intestine is made. (2) The stay suture is tagged with mosquito hemostatic forceps. (3) The jejunal loop is moved to the animal's left and the stay suture maintains orientation while the tube is introduced into the abdomen.

jejunum using 3–0 absorbable monofilament suture material (such as poliglecaprone 25 or glycomer 631). A tiny stab incision just large enough to accommodate the tube is made with a number 11 blade in the center of the horizontal mattress suture, and the jejunostomy tube is introduced into the stab and advanced caudally for a generous distance (one long intestinal loop, the length supplied by at least three vascular arcades). The mattress suture is tied and the jejunum is secured to the body wall using 3–0 monofilament suture (poliglecaprone 25 or glycomer 631) in an interlocking box pattern (Figures 17.7h and 17.7i).

The interlocking box pattern is chosen instead of simple interrupted sutures that tack the jejunum to the body wall because the interlocking boxes keep fluid around the tube in the intestine. Fluid could potentially leak around the tube into the subcutaneous tissues, but intestinal fluid should not be able to leak into the peritoneal cavity. There is no need to wait for adhesions to seal the area around the tube for safe tube removal as is the case with simple tacking sutures. With the interlocking box technique the tube may be safely removed at any time,[4]

and there should be little concern for peritonitis if the tube is prematurely removed by the patient. Prior to the development of the interlocking box suture pattern jejunostomy tubes were left in place for 5–7 days to wait for the adhesive seal regardless of whether or not the feeding tube was being used.

The feeding tube is placed into the intestine as described above before the interlocking box sutures are placed. Then, the box sutures are placed in the following order. The first box is started by passing caudocranially in the abdominal wall ventral (superficial) to the jejunostomy site. The suture is then passed transversely across the jejunum (full-thickness bite) ventrodorsally just cranial to the jejunostomy. The third pass is from cranial to caudal in the abdominal wall dorsal (deep) to the jejunostomy, and the final pass is from dorsal to ventral transversely in the intestine caudal to the jejunostomy. The suture strands are left long and tagged with hemostats. The second box is started by passing ventrodorsally in the abdominal wall cranial to the jejunostomy. The second suture is passed craniocaudally in the intestine dorsal (deep) to the jejunostomy. The third

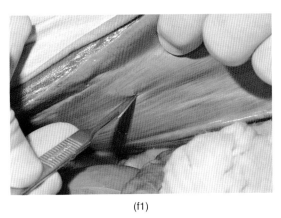

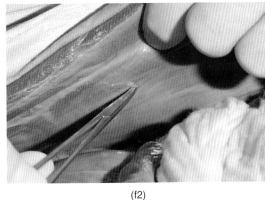

(f1)

(f2)

Figure 17.7 (*Continued*) (f) Pulling the jejunostomy tube into the abdomen. [Cranial is to the right; view is from an assistant surgeon's perspective, assuming that the surgeon is right handed.] (1) A tiny puncture is made in the transversus abdominis muscle with a number 11 scalpel blade 2–3 cm from the linea alba incision, depending on the size of the patient. (2) A mosquito hemostatic forceps is introduced into the tiny puncture in the transversus abdominis muscle.

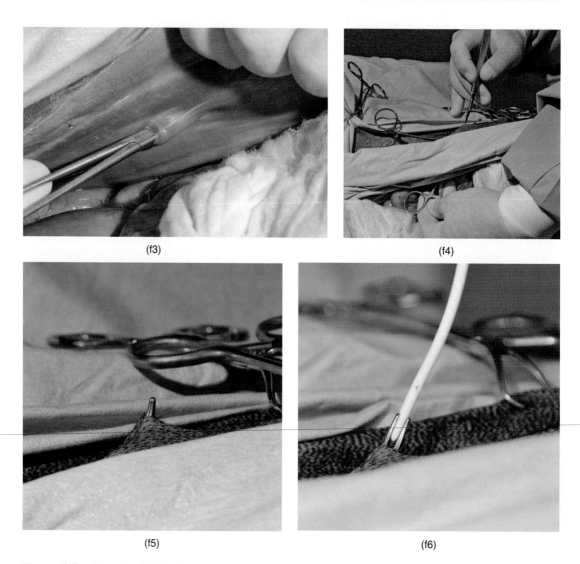

(f3)   (f4)

(f5)   (f6)

Figure 17.7   (*Continued*) (3) The forceps is advanced in a craniolateral direction until the tip can be felt under the skin just lateral to the nipple line. (4) A number 11 scalpel blade is used to make a tiny incision over the forceps' tips just large enough to permit the tips to exit the skin immediately lateral to the nipple line. (5) The forceps' tips exit the skin with the jaws closed. (6) The forceps' tips are opened to grab the tip of the tube.

suture is passed dorsoventrally in the body wall caudal to the jejunostomy, and the final pass is from caudal to cranial in the intestine ventral (superficial) to the jejunostomy. The cranial suture strands are pulled together as are the previously placed caudal strands. The caudal strands are tied to secure the first box and the cranial strands are tied to secure the second box. Externally, the jejunostomy tube is anchored to skin and underling fascia with four interrupted friction sutures placed 1 cm apart (Figure 17.7j).[1] Size 2–0 nylon or polypropylene is preferred for

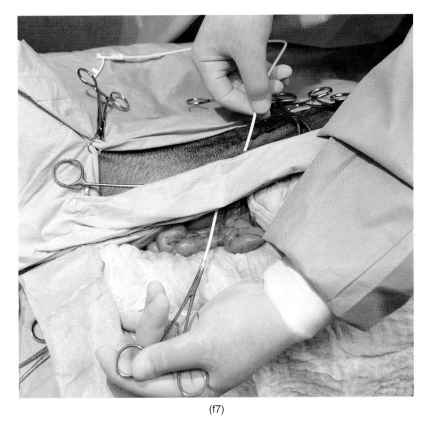

(f7)

Figure 17.7   (*Continued*) (7) The tube is pulled into the abdominal cavity.

anchoring 8 French and 10 French tubes; size 3–0 is used for 5 French tubes.

When removing a jejunostomy tube, inject the tube with approximately 10 mL of water or saline to ensure that residual food is flushed into the intestinal lumen and not dragged through the subcutaneous tissues of the abdominal wall. Cut the friction sutures and gently extract the tube. Although jejunostomy tube removal is well tolerated by dogs and cats, infiltration with local anesthetic around the exit stoma skin and body wall will lessen tube removal discomfort. Periodically, cleanse the stoma as needed to remove secretions. Secretions from the stoma are usually mild and typically resolve in 3–5 days.

Complications of jejunostomy tubes include local cellulitis, inadvertent complete or partial removal of the tube, tube occlusion, stomal infection, and peritonitis. Self-limiting local cellulitis is the most common complication.

WOUND DRAINS

Drains are generally made of latex, silcone, or other pliable material, and are mostly tubular in shape. Some of the varieties, particularly, Penrose drains (Penrose Drain, Cardinal Health, McGaw Park, IL; Figures 17.8a and 17.8b), are easily collapsible. Drain use is indicated when normally apposed tissue has been separated

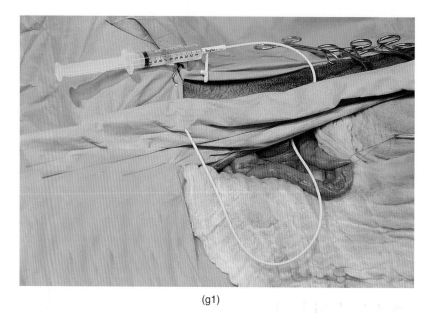

(g1)

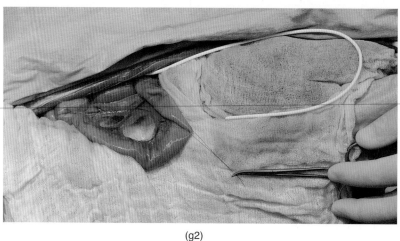

(g2)

Figure 17.7   (*Continued*) (g) Placing the jejunostomy tube into the intestine. [Cranial is to the right; view is from an assistant surgeon's perspective, assuming that the surgeon is right handed.] (1) A saline-filled syringe is attached to the jejunostomy tube to later dilate the intestine with saline to aid advancement of the tube caudally in the intestinal lumen. The stay suture marks the cranial direction of the intestine. (2) The tube is positioned in the cranial aspect of the field while the purse-string suture (actually a horizontal mattress suture) is placed.

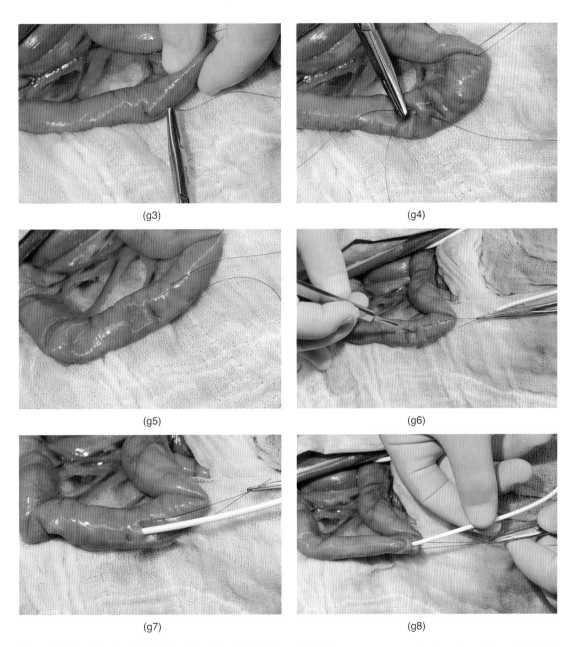

(g3)

(g4)

(g5)

(g6)

(g7)

(g8)

Figure 17.7 (*Continued*) (3) The first bite (full thickness) of the mattress suture is placed craniocaudally. (4) The second bite (full thickness) of the mattress suture is placed caudocranially. (5) The properly executed mattress suture resembles a "smiley face." (6) A number 11 blade is used to make a hole in the center of the mattress suture (a "nose" in the "smiley face"). The blade is held upside down with the sharp edge toward the "eyes" of the "smiley face" to avoid cutting the suture as could occur if the blade penetrated too close to the "mouth" of the "smiley face." Note that the cranial stay suture has been removed and the tube is in position to be threaded into the hole that will be made in the intestine. (7) The hole in the intestine should be just large enough to accommodate the tube. (8) The tube is threaded caudally in the jejunum while gentle counter tension is applied to the tagged ends of the mattress suture.

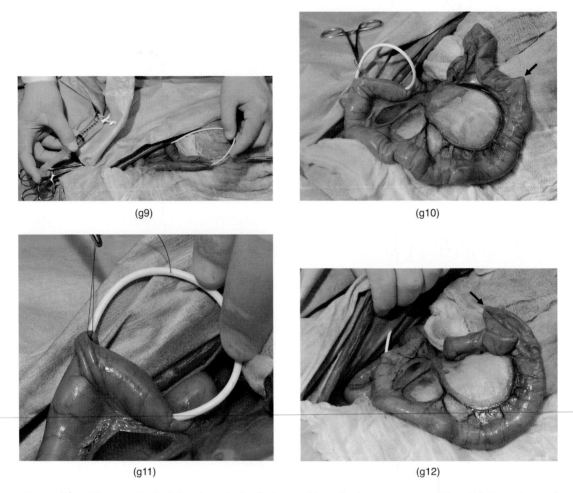

(g9) (g10)

(g11) (g12)

Figure 17.7 (*Continued*) (9) Saline is periodically injected into the intestine to provide mild distention and lubrication for ease of tube passage. (10) The tube is advanced for a generous distance (the amount of intestine supplied by about three vascular arcades). The arrow indicates the position of the tube's tip. (11) The horizontal mattress suture is tied to prevent leakage around the tube during remaining manipulations. The tube can still slide through the hole in the intestine so care must be taken to make sure the tube does not back out during the remainder of the procedure. (12) The strands of the mattress suture have been cut and the jejunum aligned with the body wall in preparation for jejunopexy. The arrow points to the tip of the tube within the jejunum.

and a pocket of dead space is created that cannot be sufficiently closed. When this pocket is created, blood vessels and lymphatics are destroyed, which may lead to accumulation of fluid inside the newly created pocket. If the character of the fluid is that of frank blood (clotted or unclotted), it is termed a hematoma. If the character of the fluid is that of serosanguinous fluid, it is termed a seroma. Regardless of the fluid characteristics, its presence provides a rich culture medium for bacteria to multiply, a barrier for new blood vessels to form in the

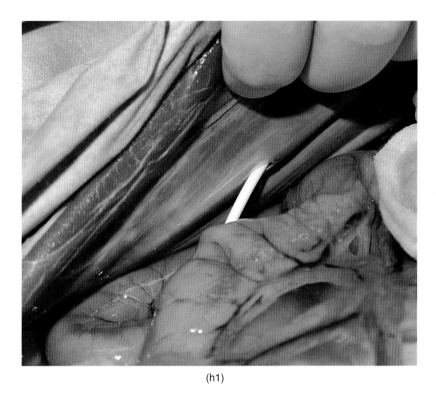

(h1)

Figure 17.7 (*Continued*) (h) Anchoring the jejunum to the body wall using the interlocking box suture pattern. [Cranial is to the right; view is from an assistant surgeon's perspective, assuming that the surgeon is right handed.] (1) The jejunostomy site is brought close to the tube exit site on the body wall leaving a short segment of tube visible for orientation.

apposing tissue, and, in general, leads to a delay in wound healing. However, drains should only be placed when clearly indicated, because the inappropriate use of a drain can be detrimental to the animal and lead to wound dehiscence, infection, abscess formation, or even death. The surgeon should carefully consider the likelihood of a seroma, the viability of the tissue, the ability to appropriately close the wound, and the ability to restrict the movement of the wound area and the patient after surgery. Drains can also be placed in the peritoneal cavity to remove bile, urine, or other aberrant fluids.

Drains are classified as either passive or active. Passive drains rely on gravity and capillary action to drain fluid from a wound. The most common passive drain used in veterinary medicine is the flattened, cylindrical latex or silicone tube called the Penrose drain (Figure 17.8a); however, stiffer tubular drains can also act as passive drains. Since passive drains rely on gravity, they must be placed such that the distal end of the drain exits from the wound in the most dependent site (Figure 17.8b). A Penrose drain should never be fenestrated for two reasons: (1) fenestrations may increase the chances that the drain will break upon attempted removal and (2) fenestration will decrease the surface area of the drain thereby limiting capillary action, which is necessary for the Penrose drain to work in the first place. Noncollapsible, tubular passive drains can be fenestrated because, in addition to fluid running along the outside of the drain via capillary action, there is a pressure

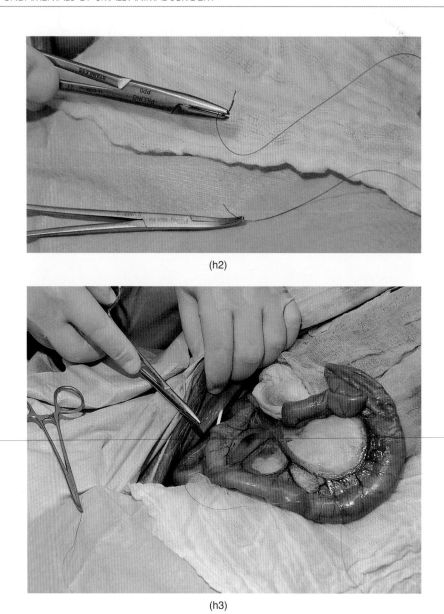

(h2)

(h3)

Figure 17.7 (*Continued*) (2) Synthetic absorbable suture (3–0 poliglecaprone 25) is used for the interlocking box suture. Note that the end is tagged with a mosquito hemostat to prevent inadvertently pulling the suture through during one of the passages. During passage all suture bites must avoid hitting the tube. (3) For the first box, the tagged suture end is left in the caudal aspect of the surgical field and the first suture bite will be from caudal to cranial in the body wall.

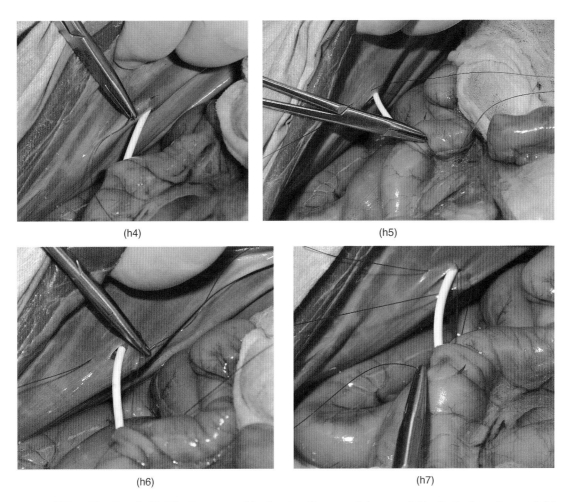

(h4)

(h5)

(h6)

(h7)

Figure 17.7   (*Continued*) (4) The first suture bite is taken from caudal to cranial in the body wall superficial to the tube. (5) The second bite of the first box is placed full thickness transversely across the intestine from superficial to deep cranial to the tube such that the passage is orientated at a right angle to the first body wall suture. (6) The third bite of the first box is passed from cranial to caudal in the body wall deep to the tube. This passage is perpendicular to the intestinal suture passage and parallel to the original body wall suture passage. (7) The fourth and final suture passage for the first box is made full thickness transversely across the intestine from deep to superficial caudal to the tube.

difference between the wound pocket and the inner lumen of the tube which will encourage luminal drainage. Passive drains should be covered by a bandage after placement. Bandaging affords protection from ascending bacterial infections, protection of surrounding skin from wound fluid scalding as well as a method for semiquantification of exudative volume from the drain. Bandages must be changed daily or more frequently should strike through occur. Frequency of bandage changing can be decreased once drainage volume has decreased.

Active drains, also known as closed suction drains, are more efficient than passive drains

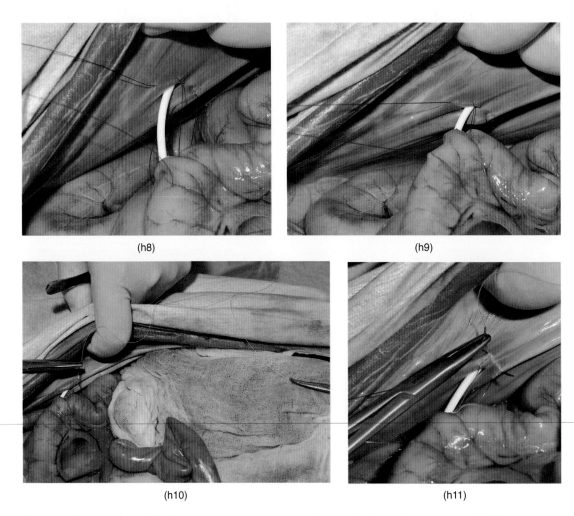

(h8) (h9)

(h10) (h11)

Figure 17.7 (*Continued*) (8) The four suture passages of the first box have been completed. (9) The suture strands have been tagged with a hemostatic forceps (not shown) so that mild tension on the strands can provide orientation while the second box is developed. A small segment of tube is left visible for orientation during development of the second box. (10) The strand of suture for the second box is tagged with a mosquito hemostatic forceps and that forceps is placed in the cranial aspect of the surgical field to maintain orientation. [Note that 3–0 fluorescent polypropylene is being used for demonstration purposes to more easily discern the two boxes, but synthetic absorbable suture would be used in clinical cases.] (11) The first pass of the second box is placed in the body wall cranial to the tube from superficial to deep, essentially connecting the dots from the two body wall bites from first box passages.

in removing fluid from a wound or a body cavity. Active drains also decrease the likelihood of drain-related infection compared to passive drains. These drains are termed "active" because they actively remove fluid from the wound by application of external suction. In applying suction, not only is wound fluid removed from the local area, but also the wound layers are drawn closer in apposition, which in effect decreases dead space, decreases the likelihood of

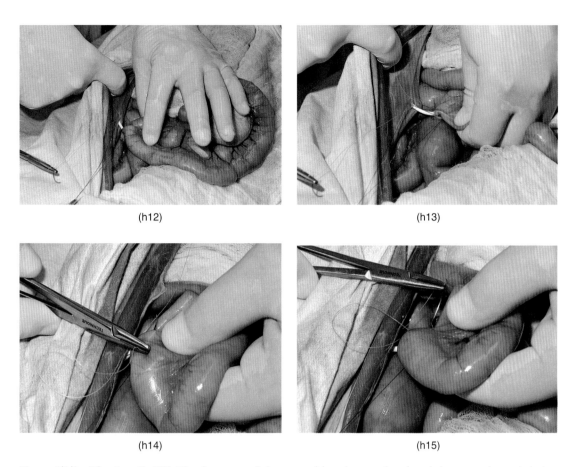

(h12)

(h13)

(h14)

(h15)

Figure 17.7 (*Continued*) (12) The first pass of the second box is completed and the second pass is being planned. The second pass of the second box is the most difficult suture pass because it goes craniocaudally in the intestine deep to the tube. To achieve this passage, the surgeon is positioning the nondominant hand to rotate the down side of the intestine upward. (13) The intestine has been rotated so that the intestine deep to the tube is now accessible for an easy pass by the right-handed surgeon. (14) With the intestine rotated, the deep pass appears to be going caudocranially. The true cranial to caudal passage will be evident when the intestine is rotated back to its normal position. (15) The needle is grasped at the point before rotating the intestine back to its normal location.

seroma formation, and facilitates early adhesion of skin to the underlying wound bed. The most commonly used active drain in veterinary practice is what is known as a Jackson-Pratt closed suction drain (Jackson-Pratt Silicone Flat Drain and Jackson-Pratt Reservoir, Cardinal Health, McGaw Park, IL; Figure 17.8c). This drain is composed of a flat or round, flexible, fenes-

trated section molded to a silastic tube that is attached to a flexible bulb ("grenade"). Activation of the grenade by depression of this bulb establishes negative pressure in the wound cavity.

A homemade closed suction drain, for small wounds, can be constructed using a butterfly catheter and a vacutainer blood collection tube (Figure 17.8d). Cut off the luer lock portion

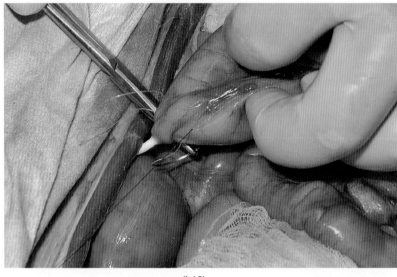

(h16)

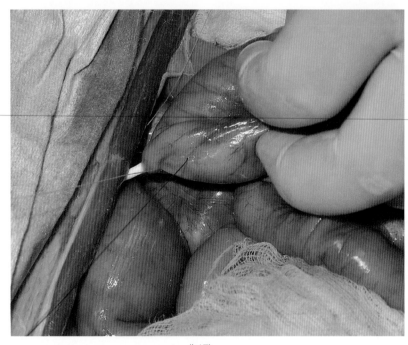

(h17)

Figure 17.7 (*Continued*) (16) As the intestine is rotated back to normal position, the needle is passed craniocaudally so that it will be in proper orientation for the third suture passage of the second box. (17) With the intestine back in normal orientation and the second pass suture running craniocaudally, the third pass may be performed.

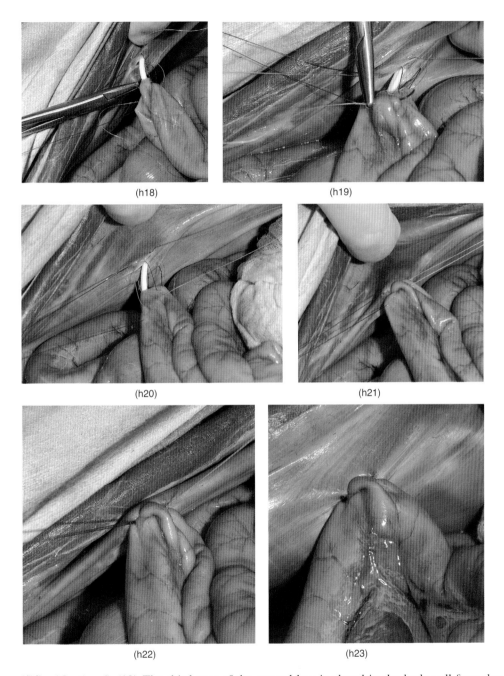

(h18)

(h19)

(h20)

(h21)

(h22)

(h23)

Figure 17.7   (*Continued*) (18) The third pass of the second box is placed in the body wall from deep to superficial caudal to the tube essentially connecting the dots created there by first box body wall suture passes. (19) The fourth and final pass of the second box is made full thickness in the intestine superficial to the tube caudocranially. (20) Both boxes of the interlocking box are completed. (21) When the strands of both boxes are pulled, the intestine abuts the body wall and the tube is no longer visible. (22) The strands of each box are tied. Either box may be tied first. (23) Cutting the free strands after tying the knots completes the interlocking box jejunopexy.

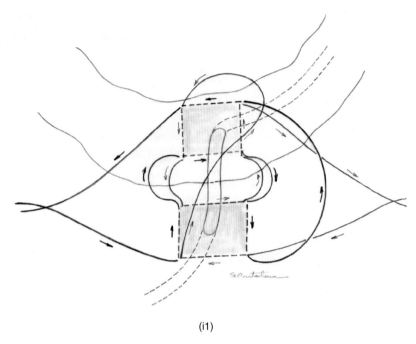

(i1)

Figure 17.7 (*Continued*) (i) Artistic summary of the interlocking box jejunopexy. [These drawings are oriented from the perspective of a right-handed surgeon; therefore, they will appear upside down compared to Figure 17.7h.] (1) The red suture represents the first box with suture passes in the following order: (a) caudal to cranial in the body wall superficial to the tube, (b) superficial to deep in the intestine cranial to the tube, (c) cranial to caudal in the body wall deep to the tube, and (d) deep to superficial in the intestine caudal to the tube. The black suture represents the second box with suture passes in the following order: (a) superficial to deep in the body wall cranial to the tube, (b) cranial to caudal in the intestine deep to the tube, (c) deep to superficial in the body wall caudal to the tube, and (d) caudal to cranial in the intestine superficial to the tube.

of the butterfly catheter and create small fenestrations 1–2 cm from the end of the catheter. These fenestrations should not be larger than 25% of the circumference of the catheter. The end of the drain is then inserted into the wound through a separate stab incision. After the wound is closed, the butterfly needle portion of the catheter is inserted into a vacutainer blood collection tube. Secure the drain to the skin and underlying fascia with four friction sutures. Monitor the collection tube frequently and change to a new collection tube before complete filling so as to always maintain negative pressure. Vacuum blood collection tube

drains are not very efficient because they require frequent changing of the collection tubes when there is significant drainage.

Another alternative for a closed suction drain is to use fenestrated tubing attached to a 35–60 mL syringe. Gently pull back on the syringe. Once negative pressure is obtained, place an 18-gauge hypodermic needle through the syringe plunger at the level of the syringe wings to maintain negative pressure (Figure 17.8e). Always completely occlude the tube prior to emptying or changing to a new receptacle such that air is not drawn into the wound pocket. The sharp needle that maintains the plunger in an

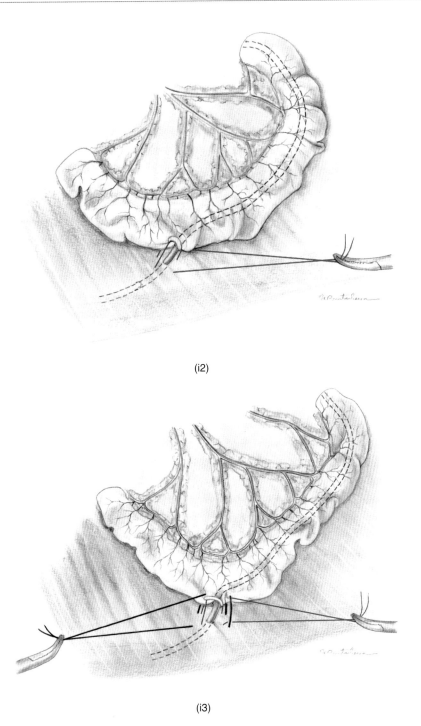

(i2)

(i3)

Figure 17.7 (*Continued*) (2) The first box is completed and the (red) suture strands tagged with the forceps in the caudal aspect of the surgical field. (3) Both boxes are completed with the black suture strands tagged with forceps in the cranial aspect of the surgical field.

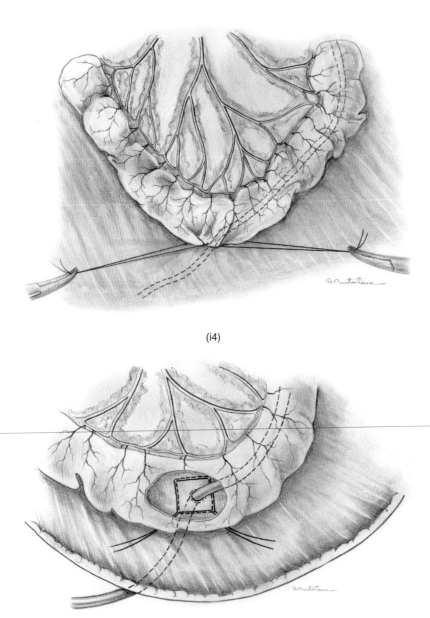

(i4)

(i5)

Figure 17.7   (*Continued*) (4) When the strands of both boxes are pulled, the tube is no longer visible. (5) The holes in the body wall and jejunum are juxtaposed and sandwiched between the jejunum and body wall within the interlocking boxes. Therefore, any fluid around the tube will stay in the intestine or could potentially leak into the subcutaneous tissues, but intestinal fluid should not be able to leak into the peritoneal cavity. The suture strands are retained in this drawing for orientation purposes, but would be knotted and cut at this point.

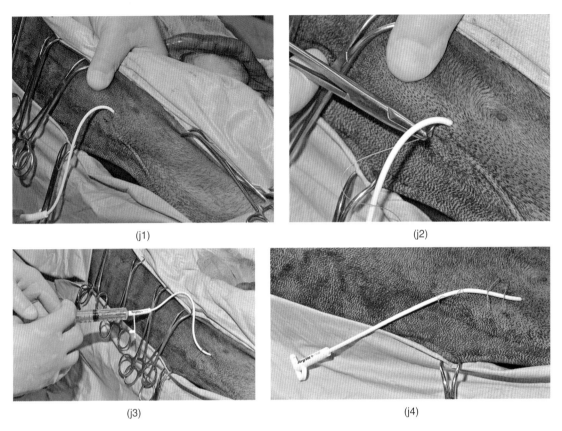

(j1)　　　　　　　　　　　　　　　　(j2)

(j3)　　　　　　　　　　　　　　　　(j4)

Figure 17.7 (*Continued*) (j) Anchoring the jejunostomy tube to the skin and underlying fascia with four friction sutures. (1) The first friction suture is placed as soon as the interlocking box jejunopexy is complete so that inadvertent tube withdrawal does not occur during remaining surgical manipulations. The surgeon's nondominant hand is stabilizing the body wall at the jejunsotomy site from within the peritoneal cavity to serve as a reference point for placement of the first friction suture and ensure that the friction suture penetrates underlying fascia without entering the abdomen. (2) The first friction suture is placed immediately cranial and slightly lateral to the tube exit site. (3) Saline is injected into the tube after each friction suture is placed to make sure that the lumen of the tube is not obstructed by the suture. (4) Three additional friction sutures are placed after the abdominal incision is closed.

aspirating position poses injury risk to the patient and care givers; therefore, this type of suction drain is not recommended.

When placing a passive drain, clip and aseptically prepare a wide area around the wound. The portion of the drain that will be placed inside the wound should be measured and recorded. The length of the drain when removed should be compared to the length of the drain when it was installed to ensure removal of the entire drain. Place the drain inside the wound in a vertical alignment. The proximal end of the drain is then advanced away from the wound opening and then sutured to the skin in a nondependent area by passing a simple interrupted transcutaneous nonabsorbable suture. Next, a new stab incision is created at the dependent aspect of the wound, away from

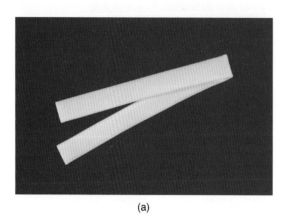

(a)

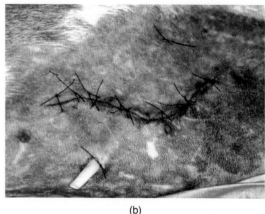

(b)

Figure 17.8 (a) Collapsible latex drain (Penrose Drain, Cardinal Health, McGaw Park, IL). (b) Latex Penrose drain in place on the left side of a dog. [Cranial is to the left and ventral is to the bottom of the photograph.] A curved laceration just dorsal to the nipple line spanning the junction of the thorax and abdomen has been sutured. Prior to closure a Penrose drain was placed because of a pocket of dead space under the wound and dorsal to it. Note that the exit hole for the Penrose drain is ventral to the wound so that gravity flow will be facilitated when the dog is standing or in sternal recumbence. There is no drain exposed dorsally. Instead, a single nylon suture through the skin anchors the drain in the subcutaneous space to help prevent the drain from sliding out. A second anchoring suture is seen where the drain exits. The second anchoring suture is placed to help prevent retraction of the drain into the wound. Both anchoring sutures must be removed in order to remove the Penrose drain.

the primary wound opening. This stab incision will act as an exit portal for the distal end of the drain and should be large enough for the drain to exit and for fluid to discharge. A drain should never exit through the primary incision because there is an increased risk of incision dehiscence. If the wound pocket is especially deep and there is adequate subcutaneous closure, it is acceptable for the drain to lie beneath the suture line. Once the drain is passed through the exit portal, the distal end of the drain should be tacked to the portal edge with a simple interrupted nonabsorbable suture (Figure 17.8b).

When placing an active drain, many of the rules mentioned above still apply. There are only a few differences when placing active drains. First, the exit portal should be just large enough to accommodate the drain tube. This will ensure a leak proof seal such that the drain can maintain suction within the wound. Second, the proximal portion of the drain does not

have to be sutured to the skin. Third, because the drain works under suction, the exit portal does not need to be placed in a dependent location. Four friction sutures[1] should be used to secure the drain to the skin and underlying fascia.

Jackson-Pratt drains are particularly helpful in deep wounds. The drain may be pulled through the wound with hemostatic forceps via a small stab incision in the skin, or the drain may be passed from within outward using a sharp metal trocar (Figures 17.8f through 17.8k). Once the drain is placed (Figure 17.8j), the wound is closed. After wound closure the drain is anchored to skin and underlying fascia with four friction sutures, a reservoir is attached, and suction is activated (Figure 17.8k).

Active drains may also be used to remove fluid from the abdominal cavity. Indications for abdominal drainage include septic abdomen, uroabdomen, and bile peritonitis. Once the

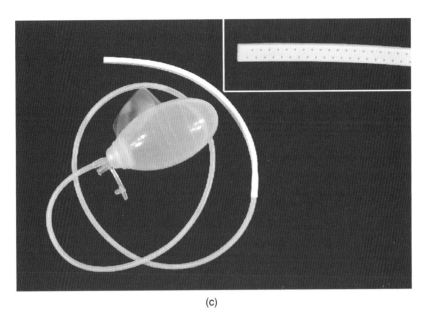

(c)

Figure 17.8 (*Continued*) (c) Jackson-Pratt closed suction drain (Jackson-Pratt Silicone Flat Drain and Jackson-Pratt Reservoir, Cardinal Health, McGaw Park, IL). Inset is a close up of the tip of the drain showing fenestrations. The tubular nonfenestrated portion of the drain is attached to the reservoir. The drain reservoir is squeezed and the air exit is plugged to initiate and maintain suction.

primary condition has been surgically addressed, a drain is placed prior to abdominal closure. Create an exit stoma for the tube in the right or left lateral abdominal wall. Using a number 11 scalpel blade, make a stab incision in the skin approximately 5–6 cm lateral to the midline incision. Place a hemostatic forceps through the stab incision and advance through the subcutaneous tissue until the peritoneum is reached. Visualize the tips of the Kelly hemostat as a conical elevation protruding from the peritoneum. Lightly incise a small hole over the tips such that the tips protrude through the hole. Grasp the proximal end of the drain tube with the hemostatic forceps and gently pull the tube through the hole and out through the skin. Alternatively, a sharp metal trocar fixed to the end of the drain tube (Figure 17.8f) may be pushed from the inside of the abdomen out through the skin, negating the need to incise an exit portal.

Four friction sutures should be used to secure the drain tube to the skin and underlying fascia.

There are no set duration guidelines that govern when to remove surgical drains. However, most passive drains must remain in place for at least 5 days for maximal benefit, and most active drains can be removed within 3–5 days. Generally, drains are maintained for 3–5 days and rarely as long as 10 days. A rule of thumb for drain removal is that drains should be removed once the volume of drainage trends downward or the character of the discharge changes to a serous or serosanguinous appearance. The drain itself will elicit a small amount of transudation just from being in the tissue, so it is unlikely that there will ever be complete cessation of fluid discharge. If the discharge does stop flowing, suspect an outflow occlusion. Rule out kinking of the drain tube, blood or tissue clot in the lumen of the drain, and tissue

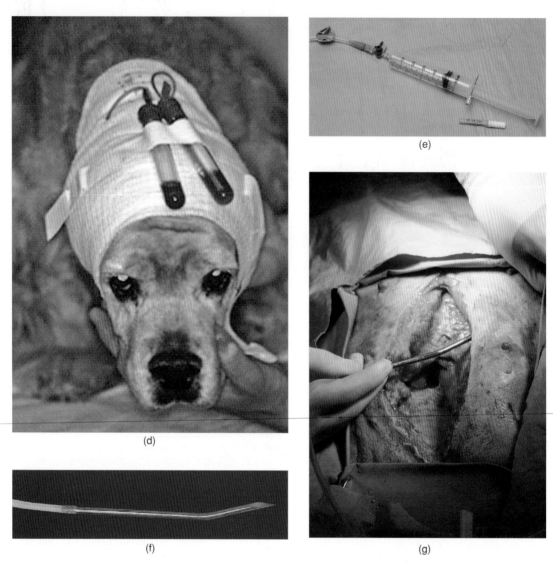

Figure 17.8 (*Continued*) (d) Active drains using modified butterfly catheters attached to vacutainer blood collection tubes. In this case, the drains are placed in the subcutaneous tissue under the ears. This was once a method to provide drainage after total ear canal ablation, but drains are no longer used for that procedure. (e) Active drain using a syringe to provide suction. An 18-gauge hypodermic needle is driven through the syringe plunger and rests on the wings of the syringe barrel to provide suction. A clamp or stopcock is necessary to prevent introduction of air in the wound when the syringe is being emptied. Both clamp and stopcock are pictured here. The clamp and stopcock must remain open during suctioning and closed when emptying the syringe. (f) Sharp metal trocar fixed to the nonfenestrated end of a Jackson-Pratt drain tube. (g) Jackson-Pratt drain placement at the time of secondary wound closure subsequent to incisional drainage of a surgical wound abscess. The surgeon is using a sharp metal trocar to make the exit portal such that the drain is pulled from within outward.

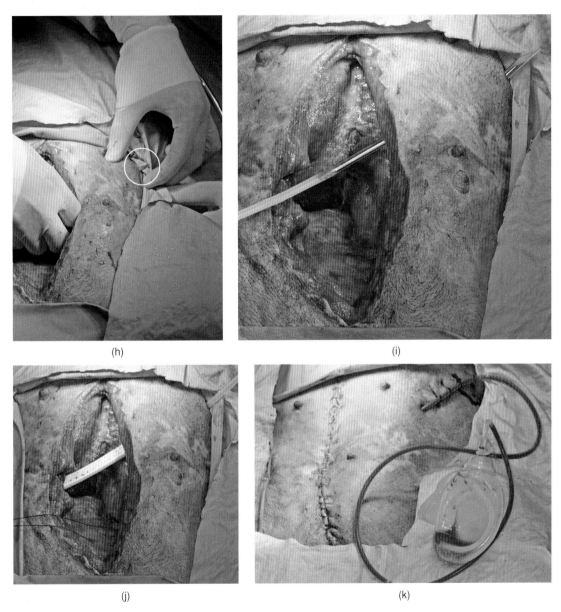

(h)

(i)

(j)

(k)

Figure 17.8 (*Continued*) (h) Exit of a drain trocar distant from the wound edge. The circle shows the tip of the trocar coming through the skin. (i) Using a drain trocar to pull a Jackson-Pratt drain into the wound toward the exit hole. Note the metal trocar has been passed through the abdominal skin. (j) Jackson-Pratt drain in a deep wound prior to wound closure. Note the fenestrated portion of the drain is entirely in the wound and the tubular nonfenestrated portion exits the skin. It is important to have a tight seal around the tube at the exit with no fenestrations showing so that negative pressure can be maintained within the wound. (k) Completely placed Jackson-Pratt drain. Note the reservoir holding constant suction drawing red tinged fluid coming from the wound. Also note that the tube is anchored to the skin and underlying fascia with four friction sutures.

blocking the fenestrations of the drain (i.e., omentum in an abdominal drain). If the cause of the obstruction cannot be corrected, the malfunctioning drain should be removed. Cytology of the wound fluid may be helpful in determining if it is safe to remove a drain. A decrease in the number of bacteria and the appearance of healthy neutrophils may be good indicators that the drain may be removed. Remove a wound drain after local anesthetic infiltration by cutting the friction sutures and extracting manually.

REFERENCES

1. Song EK, Mann FA, Wagner-Mann CC. Comparison of different tube materials and use of Chinese finger trap or four friction suture technique for securing gastrostomy, jejunostomy, and thoracostomy tubes in dogs. *Vet Surg* 2008;37:212–221.
2. Yoon H, Mann FA, Lee S, Branson KR. Comparison of the amounts of air leakage into the thoracic cavity associated with four thoracostomy tube placement techniques in canine cadavers. *Am J Vet Res* 2009;70:1161–1167.
3. Marques AI, Tattersall J, Shaw DJ, Welsh E. Retrospective analysis of the relationship between time of thoracostomy drain removal and discharge time. *J Small Anim Pract* 2009;50:162–166.
4. Daye RM, Huber ML, Henderson RA. Interlocking box jejunostomy: a new technique for enteral feeding. *J Am Anim Hosp Assoc* 1999;35:129–134.

ADDITIONAL RESOURCES

Additional information about tubes and drains in small animal surgery can be found in the following textbooks:

1. Hackett TB, Mazzaferro EM. *Veterinary Emergency and Critical Care Procedures.* Ames, Iowa: Blackwell Publishing Professional, 2006.
2. Silverstein DC, Hopper K. *Small Animal Critical Care Medicine.* St. Louis, Missouri: Saunders Elsevier, 2009.
3. Slatter D, ed. *Textbook of Small Animal Surgery,* 3rd ed. Philadelphia, Pennsylvania: Saunders, 2003.
4. Fossum TW, ed. *Small Animal Surgery,* 3rd ed. St. Louis, Missouri: Mosby Elsevier, 2007.

Chapter 18

CANINE OVARIOHYSTERECTOMY

Fred Anthony Mann

Ovariohysterectomy is one of the most common surgical procedures performed by small animal veterinarians. While the basics of the surgical procedure to remove the ovaries and uterus must be performed each time to be successful, there are many variants of certain portions of the surgical procedure that are based on individual preferences. This chapter covers canine ovariohysterectomy in a meticulous step-by-step fashion in a manner used by the principal author to teach veterinary students.

Liberally clip the ventral abdomen from the mid-thorax to the vulva. The surgical preparation should include a wide clip that extends from cranial to the xiphoid cartilage to caudal to the brim of the pelvis and lateral to the symmetrical folds of the flank and mammae to at least the level of the ventral border of the ribs (see also Chapter 10). A long and wide clip and aseptic surgical preparation are necessary to be prepared to extend the incision in case of an unforeseen event, such as a dropped ovarian pedicle.

Empty the dog's urinary bladder by manual expression prior to surgery, typically after clipping and prior to the first surgical scrub application. Emptying the urinary bladder is important to help avoid inadvertent cystotomy when the scalpel enters the abdominal cavity. Palpate the urinary bladder and gently squeeze to express as much urine as possible. Urinary bladder expression is more easily achieved with the dog in lateral recumbence. Apply pressure on both sides forcing the urine caudally to the trigone. Continue to increase pressure until the urethral sphincter relaxes and urine starts to flow. Maintain pressure on the sides of the urinary bladder until it is empty. Be careful to avoid excessive pressure that will traumatize the urinary bladder and result in hematuria. If expression would require excessive pressure, it is better to wait and aspirate the urine intraoperatively with a syringe and hypodermic needle than risk iatrogenic injury.

After urinary bladder expression, a rough surgical scrub is performed and the dog is moved to the operating table. The dog is placed in dorsal recumbence with the limbs extended and loosely secured to the operating table (Figures 18.1–18.4), and a sterile surgical preparation is performed (see also Chapter 10).

Fundamentals of Small Animal Surgery, 1st edition.
By Fred Anthony Mann, Gheorghe M. Constantinescu and Hun-Young Yoon.
© 2011 Blackwell Publishing Ltd.

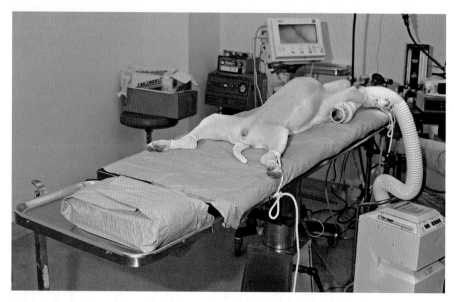

Figure 18.1   Dorsally recumbent positioning for canine ovariohysterectomy viewed from the left caudal aspect of the patient: Limbs are extended and tied loosely to the operating table. [Caution: Tying limbs too tightly can cause a tourniquet effect and resultant ischemic injury.] The instrument table (Mayo stand) is positioned at the caudal edge of the operating table so that a continuous sterile field can eventually be developed from the surgical site to the instruments after the instrument pack has been opened. [The device with the large corrugated tubing is a warming device that will be turned on once surgical drapes are applied.]

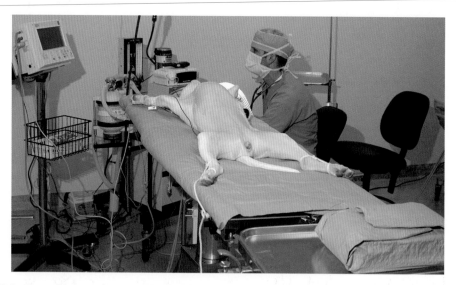

Figure 18.2   Dorsally recumbent positioning for canine ovariohysterectomy viewed from the caudal aspect of the patient. Note the positioning of anesthetist and monitoring devices at the cranial aspect of the patient and the instrument table (Mayo stand) at the caudal edge of the operating table.

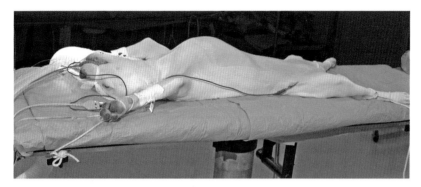

Figure 18.3 Dorsally recumbent positioning for canine ovariohysterectomy viewed from the right lateral aspect of the patient, the side of the table at which a right-handed surgeon will work.

After the sterile preparation is complete, the surgical instrument pack is placed on the Mayo instrument stand (or other instrument table) positioned at the caudal edge of the operating table (Figures 18.1 and 18.2). A nonsterile assistant opens the outer wrap of the surgical instrument pack (Figure 18.5). The gowned and gloved surgeon opens the inner wrap of the instrument pack such that the wrap overlaps the edge of the operating table and covers the dog's paws (Figures 18.6–18.8). The surgeon uses drapes from a separate pack (Figure 18.7) to apply four quarter drapes (Figures 18.9–18.14). The surgical field is quadrant draped to allow a midline incision extending from the xiphoid cartilage to the brim

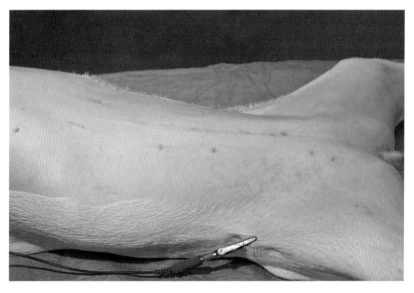

Figure 18.4 Dorsally recumbent positioning for canine ovariohysterectomy viewed from the right lateral aspect of the patient, closeup view of the ovariohysterectomy surgical site. [The alligator clip outside the surgical field is one of the electrocardiographic monitoring leads.]

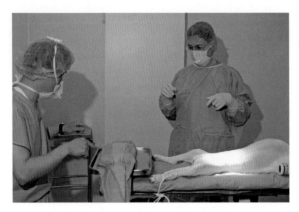

Figure 18.5   Opening the outer wrap of the sterile instrument pack by a nonsterile assistant. [Note the position of the instrument table such that the outer wrap will cover the patient's distal pelvic limbs when opened.]

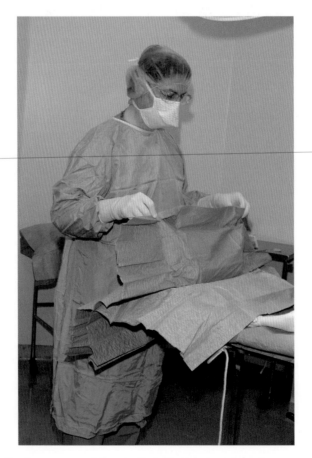

Figure 18.6   Opening the inner wrap of the sterile instrument pack by the gowned and gloved surgeon. Care is taken to protect the hands from contamination as the wrap is allowed to fall.

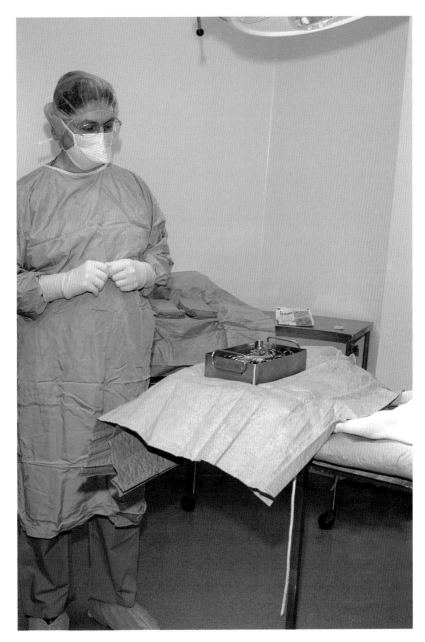

Figure 18.7   Opened sterile instrument pack. Note the opened sterile drape pack in the background.

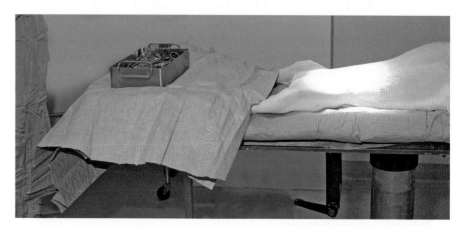

Figure 18.8   Opened sterile instrument pack and patient as viewed from the dog's left side. Note that the wraps have covered the distal pelvic limbs of the dog. The next step is to apply four quarter drapes.

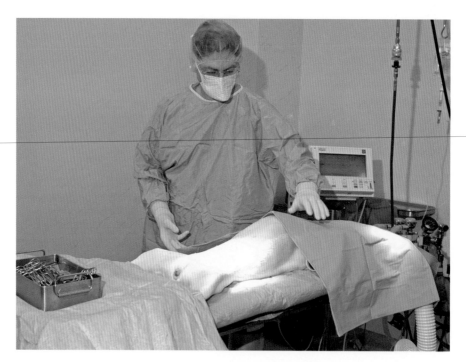

Figure 18.9   Application of the first quarter drape over the cranial aspect of the dog with the edge at the level of the xiphoid cartilage. Care is taken to simply drop the drape so as to avoid contaminating gloved hands in the process. If the drape is placed too far caudally, it can be pulled cranially by grasping the area of drape just below the left hand of the surgeon in this picture. If the drape is placed too far cranially, there is no correction except to apply a new drape in the appropriate position. In such a case, a nonsterile assistant should discard the inappropriately applied drape before the new drape is applied. Alternately, the inappropriate drape may remain and a new sterile drape can be placed over it.

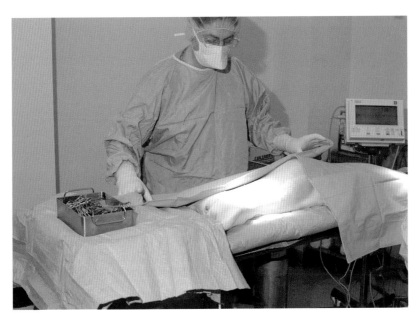

Figure 18.10 Application of the second quarter drape on the right side of the dog. Notice how the surgeon holds the drape corners and releases them to protect the fingers from inadvertent contamination during drape application. If the drape is placed too far medially, it can be pulled laterally by grasping the drape just lateral to the surgical field. If the drape is placed too far laterally, there is no correction except to apply a new drape in the appropriate position.

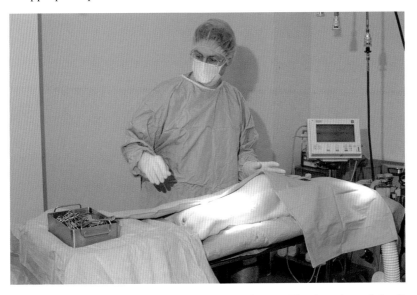

Figure 18.11 Attachment of the first and second quarter drapes. The junction of the first two drapes (near the surgeon's left hand in this picture) will be attached to each other and the underlying skin with towel forceps. A conveniently packed instrument pack will have towel clamps on top since they are the first instruments to be used.

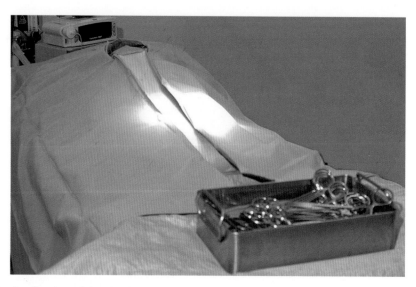

Figure 18.12 Application of the third quarter drape on the dog's left side. An assistant surgeon may apply this drape, or the surgeon may move to this side of the table temporarily to do so. If the drape is placed too far medially, it can be pulled laterally by grasping the drape just lateral to the exposed skin. [Note: Fingers should not touch the dog's skin in this process.] If the drape is placed too far laterally, there is no correction except to apply a new drape in the appropriate position. Towel clamps are used to secure the first and third drapes to each other and the underlying skin before placing the final (caudal) quarter drape.

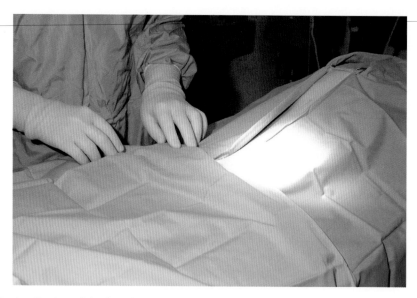

Figure 18.13 Application of the fourth quarter drape at the caudal aspect of the dog. If the drape is placed too far cranially, it can be pulled caudally by grasping the drape just caudolateral to the exposed skin. [Note: Fingers should not touch the dog's skin in this process.] If the drape is placed too far caudally, there is no correction except to apply a new drape in the appropriate position.

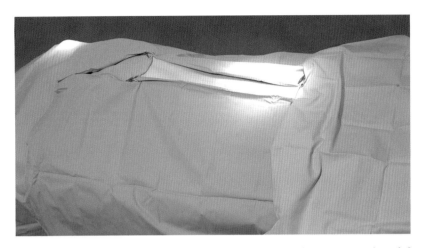

Figure 18.14 Completed quarter drapes with a towel forceps at each corner, as viewed from the dog's right side (right-handed surgeon's perspective). The dog's head is to the left in this photograph. Note that the instrument pack is covered by the caudal drape. The caudal drape will be aseptically lifted to grasp the instrument tray and place in on top of the quarter drape. The same maneuver will be necessary when the full drape is applied to cover the quarter drapes.

of the pelvis. The edge of each lateral drape should be approximately 2 cm from the proposed skin incision (just medial to the nipples). There are two common methods of quarter drape placement with regard to order of placement. With the first method, the cranial and caudal drapes are applied first. The cranial drape should be at the base of the xiphoid cartilage. The caudal drape should be at the cranial brim of the pelvis. The lateral drapes are applied next and secured with towel forceps to themselves and to the skin at the intersecting corners. With the second method, the quarter drapes are placed in the following order: (1) caudal, (2) lateral, (3) cranial, and (4) lateral, towel clamping at each intersecting corner along the way.

Before applying the full drape, it is helpful to identify the landmarks for the ovariohysterectomy skin incision (Figures 18.15 and 18.16). The surgeon's nondominant hand is placed with the thumb on the cranial aspect of the pubis and the fifth finger on the umbilicus. The midpoint between the fifth finger and thumb is identified with the index fin-

ger, which indicates the caudal extent of the skin incision for dogs. Incise from just caudal to the umbilicus to the point identified by the index finger. In cats, the index finger indicates the middle of the skin incision. In other words, make the skin incision in cats more caudally to better exteriorize the uterine body.

After applying the full drape (Figures 18.17 and 18.18), the incision landmarks are estimated before fenestrating the full drape (Figure 18.19). The full drape is fenestrated by cutting in the form of an "I" with flaps oriented laterally (Figures 18.20–18.22). The flaps of the full drape are rolled under (but exterior to the quarter drapes) and secured with two towel forceps (Figure 18.23).

Perform a sponge count prior to making the skin incision and have the anesthetist record the number of sponges. Count any additional sponges received during the procedure and have the anesthetist add them to the original count. Organize the surgical instruments on the instrument table prior to making the skin incision.

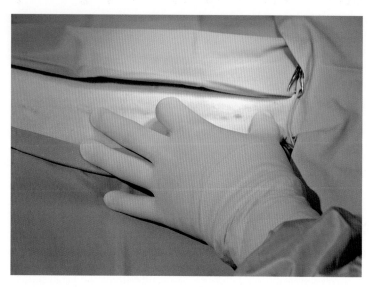

Figure 18.15 Ascertaining the location of the ovariohysterectomy skin incision prior to application of the full drape, as viewed from the right-handed surgeon's perspective. The third finger of the left hand points to the umbilical scar and the thumb palpates the cranial brim of the pubis. The index finger finds the midpoint of the line between the umbilicus and pubis. This midpoint approximates the caudal aspect of the ovariohysterectomy incision in dogs, the cranial start of the incision being the caudal edge of the umbilical scar. [In cats, the index finger point marks the mid portion of the ovariohysterectomy incision.]

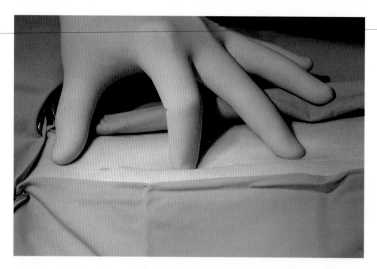

Figure 18.16 Ascertaining the location of the ovariohysterectomy skin incision prior to application of the full drape, as viewed from the dog's left side. The dog's head is to the right. The third finger of the left hand points to the umbilical scar and the thumb palpates the cranial brim of the pubis. The index finger finds the midpoint of the line between the umbilicus and pubis. This midpoint approximates the caudal aspect of the ovariohysterectomy incision in dogs, the cranial start of the incision being the caudal edge of the umbilical scar. [In cats, the index finger midpoint marks the mid portion of the ovariohysterectomy incision.]

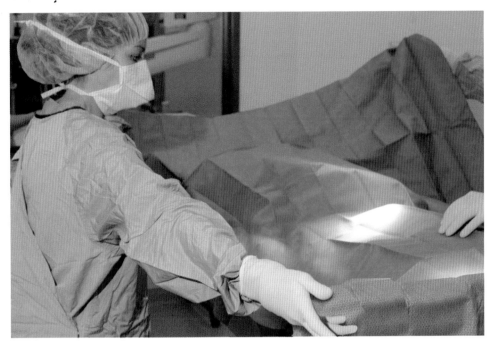

Figure 18.17   Application of a full drape to cover the quarter drapes. The dog's head (covered by drape) is to the right in this photograph. Large full drapes are more easily applied with the aid of a sterile surgical assistant. Smaller drapes than what is demonstrated here are typically used for canine and feline ovariohysterectomies performed by solo surgeons.

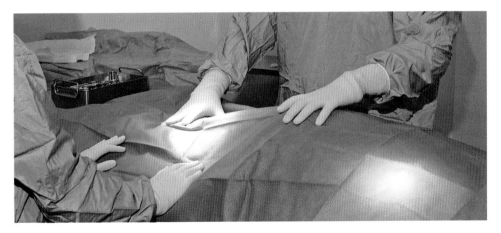

Figure 18.18   Completed application of a full drape to cover the quarter drapes. The dog's head (covered by drape) is to the right in this photograph. Note that the instrument pack (left of picture) has been placed on top of the full drape and that there is a continuous sterile field from the instrument stand to the surgical site.

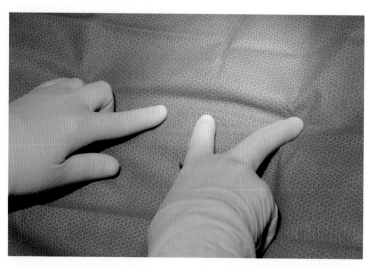

Figure 18.19   Ascertaining the site for fenestration of the full paper drape. The dog's head is to the left in this photograph. The third finger of the surgeon's right hand is palpating the cranial brim of the pubis and the other fingers are estimating the previously determined skin incision, the flexed left third finger at the level of the cranial aspect of the incision and the right index finger at the caudal aspect of the incision. The fenestration will be made such that the edges are approximately 2 cm from the skin incision laterally, cranially, and caudally.

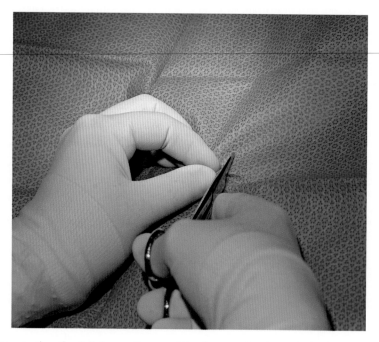

Figure 18.20   Fenestrating the full drape, first cut. The fenestration is made in the form of an "I" with the top and bottom of the "I" in the cranial and caudal aspects of the drape. In this picture, the caudal (bottom of the "I") cut is being made. The cut should be approximately 4 cm.

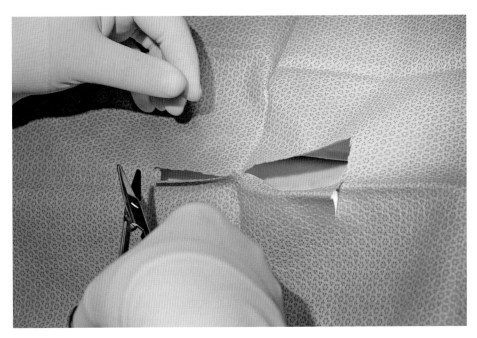

Figure 18.21 Nearly completed full drape fenestration. An I-shaped fenestration is being completed by cutting the top of the "I" at the cranial aspect of the fenestration.

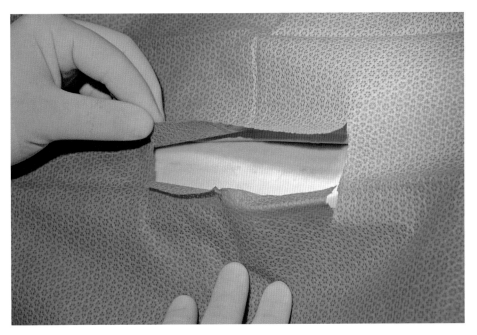

Figure 18.22 Completed fenestration of the full drape. An I-shaped incision has been made in the drape creating approximately 2 cm lateral flaps which will be rolled under and secured with towel clamps.

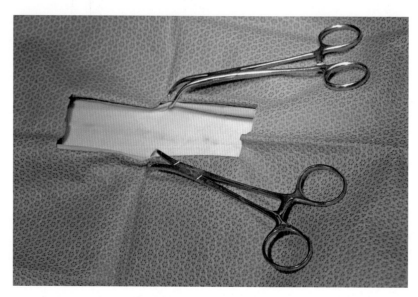

Figure 18.23 Completed draping for canine ovariohysterectomy. The lateral edges of the fenestration are rolled under, placed on top of the quarter drapes, and secured with towel forceps in the central portion of the fenestration. The towel forceps clamp through both drapes and skin laterally and through only skin medially, with the rings of the forceps resting caudally.

Verify the location of the skin incision (Figures 18.24–18.26) and incise the skin from cranial to caudal (Figures 18.27–18.30). The index finger and thumb of the nondominant hand are used to tense the skin and apply lateral pressure as the skin is incised. Apply enough pressure to incise the full thickness of the skin. Continue the incision caudally with one continuous motion.

Hemostasis using gauze pressure (Figure 18.31), mosquito hemostatic forceps, and/or electrocoagulation should be achieved prior to incising the next level. Use sponges with a slow (paused) dabbing motion rather than a wiping motion. Wiping may remove blood clots that are sealing smaller vessels and causes unnecessary tissue trauma. Wiping also "paints" the field red, making it difficult to differentiate tissue planes and identify anatomical landmarks.

Find the midline and incise the subcutaneous tissue, using Metzenbaum scissors to expose the linea alba (Figures 18.32–18.39). Incise the subcutaneous fat from both sides of the linea alba using a push cut (Figures 18.35 and 18.36) and avoid undermining of the subcutaneous tissue. Undermining creates dead space, which will predispose to seroma formation postoperatively. The subcutaneous fat attaches to the linea alba bilaterally; therefore, a push cut is necessary on both the left and right sides of the linea alba. The linea alba is very thin in cats and in the caudal part of the abdomen in dogs, making its identification more difficult.

Lift the linea alba with thumb forceps in the cranial aspect of the incision and carefully stab the abdominal wall into the peritoneal cavity with a scalpel held such that the sharp edge of the blade points upward (Figures 18.40–18.42). The blade of the scalpel faces upward so that when it penetrates the peritoneal cavity, the risk of damaging abdominal contents is reduced. The stab incision should be made at the cranial aspect of the incision near the umbilicus, if possible, because the fat in the falciform ligament at this location offers additional protection against iatrogenic injury.

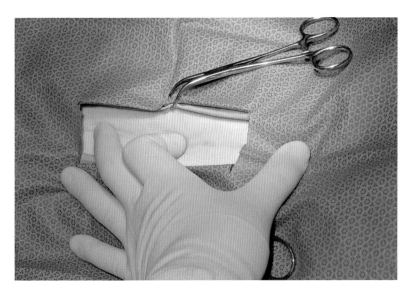

Figure 18.24 Final identification of the proposed ovariohysterectomy skin incision, as viewed from the right-handed surgeon's perspective. The third finger of the left hand points to the umbilical scar and the thumb palpates the cranial brim of the pubis. The index finger finds the midpoint of the line between the umbilicus and pubis. This midpoint approximates the caudal aspect of the ovariohysterectomy incision in dogs, the cranial start of the incision being the caudal edge of the umbilical scar. [In cats, the index finger point marks the mid portion of the ovariohysterectomy incision.]

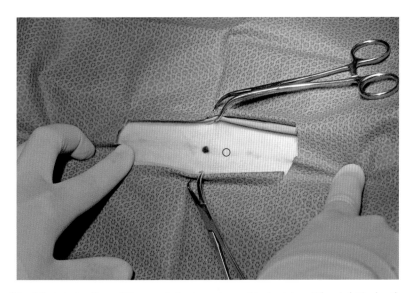

Figure 18.25 Final determination of the ovariohysterectomy skin incision. The right index finger is pointing to the cranial brim of the pubis and the left index finger is pointing to the umbilical scar. For illustrative purposes, a sterile black marker has been used to demonstrate the midpoint of the line between the two index fingers. [Note: The midpoint was originally estimated too far cranially; therefore, the actual caudal extent of the incision is marked with the colored circle.]

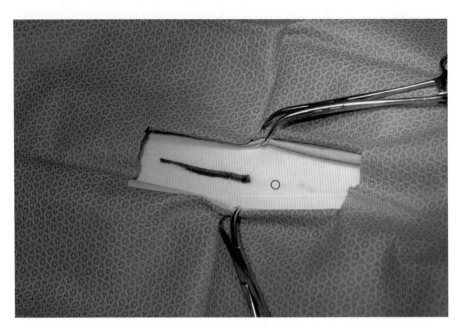

Figure 18.26 The canine ovarioyhsterectomy skin incision outline. For illustrative purposes, a sterile black marker has been used to draw the proposed incision. [The caudal extent of this incision was underestimated by approximately 2 cm; therefore, the skin incision was continued for that distance past the caudal end of the black ink.]

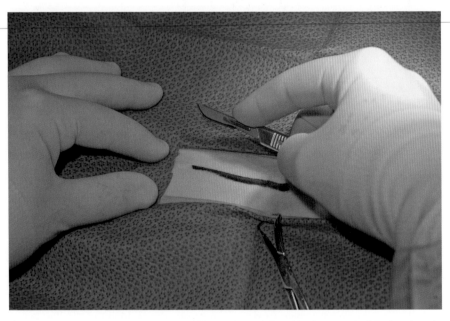

Figure 18.27 The canine ovariohysterectomy skin incision. The skin is tensed with the thumb and index finger of the nondominant hand while the dominant hand uses a scalpel.

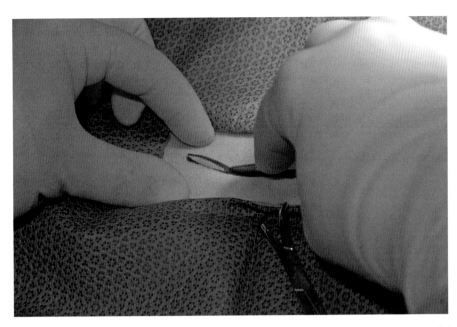

Figure 18.28 Making the canine ovariohysterectomy skin incision. The skin is incised from cranial to caudal. Ideally, the full thickness of the skin is incised in one cranial-to-caudal motion.

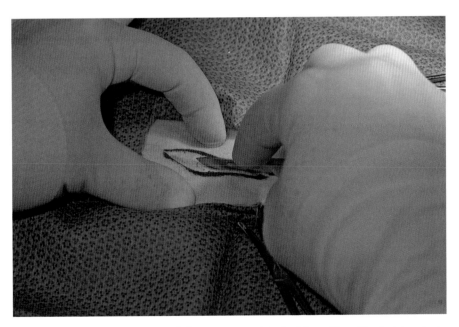

Figure 18.29 Deepening the canine ovariohysterectomy skin incision. The skin incision is deepened by tensing the skin laterally with the thumb and index finger of the nondominant hand while gentle pressure is applied to the scalpel as it is moved from cranial to caudal. Care is taken to stay on midline and avoid filleting of subcutaneous tissues.

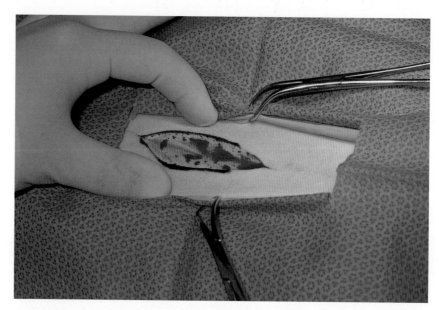

Figure 18.30 Completed canine ovariohysterectomy skin incision. The skin edges should be easily spread apart before incising the subcutaneous tissues to expose the linea alba.

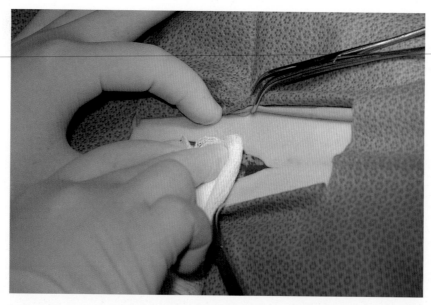

Figure 18.31 Skin incision hemorrhage control. Direct pressure with a gauze sponge is usually sufficient to control ovariohysterectomy skin incision hemorrhage before progressing to subcutaneous tissue incision. Gauze is applied directly with pressure for a few seconds and then removed. Rapid blotting and wiping are traumatic to tissues, fail to efficiently control bleeding, and serve to paint the field red, making it difficult to differentiate tissue layers.

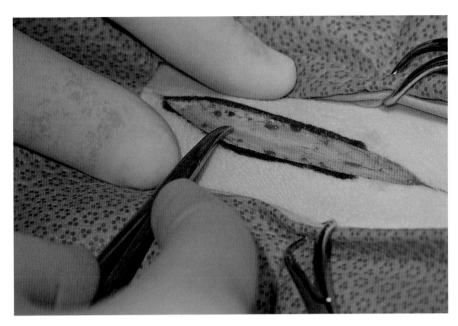

Figure 18.32   Subcutaneous tissue incision: identifying the midline. In very thin dogs and cats, the linea alba might be visible through the subcutaneous fat. In other cases, the midline can be found by observing the subtle trough effect when the skin edges are gently spread. The hemostatic forceps in this picture is pointing to the trough effect indicating the midline.

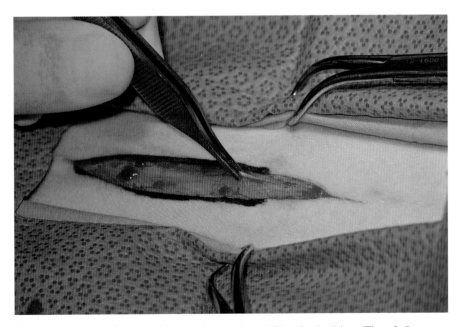

Figure 18.33   Subcutaneous tissue incision: isolating the midline for incision. Thumb forceps are used to elevate the subcutaneous fat at the midline in preparation for incision with Metzenbaum scissors.

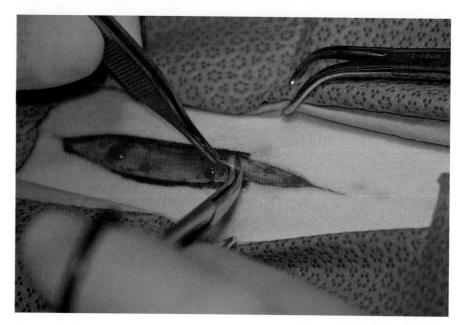

Figure 18.34 Subcutaneous tissue incision: beginning the incision. While thumb forceps elevates the subcutaneous fat at the midline, Metzenbaum scissors are used to snip a fenestration that is deep enough to contact the external rectus sheath at the linea alba in the caudal aspect of the incision.

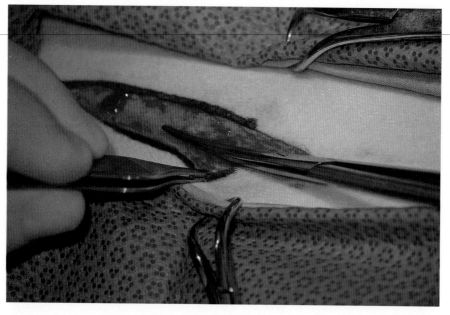

Figure 18.35 Subcutaneous tissue incision: continuing the incision. One blade of the Metzenbaum scissors is placed in the fenestration and against the external rectus sheath trapping the full thickness of the subcutaneous fat between the scissor blades.

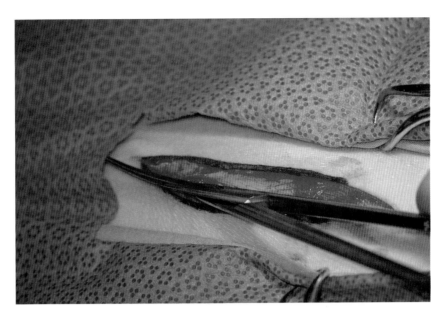

Figure 18.36 Subcutaneous tissue incision: extending the incision. With one blade of the Metzenbaum scissors against the external rectus sheath and subcutaneous fat between the scissor blades, the blades are partially closed and the scissors are pushed cranially to incise the subcutaneous tissue. This maneuver cuts the subcutaneous fat off one side of the linea alba. A second fenestration and push cut are then performed to remove the subcutaneous attachment from the other side of the linea alba.

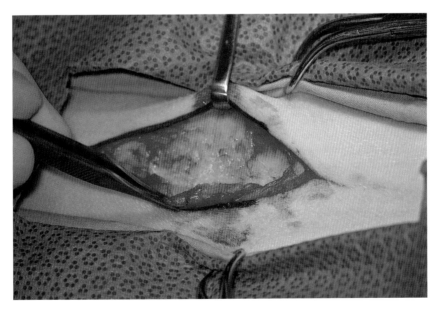

Figure 18.37 Subcutaneous tissue incision: completion of subcutaneous incision from the right side of the linea alba.

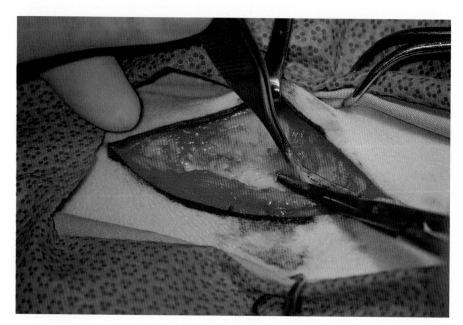

Figure 18.38 Subcutaneous tissue incision: fenestration of subcutaneous tissue on the left side of the linea alba. A push cut is then performed to remove the subcutaneous attachment from the left side of the linea alba.

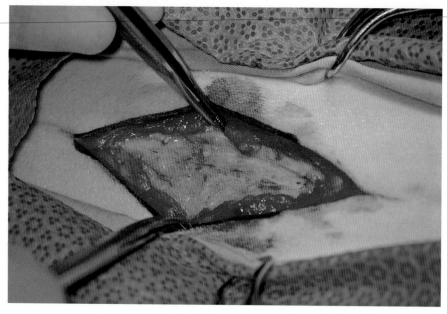

Figure 18.39 Completed subcutaneous incision. The subcutaneous fat has been incised from the linea alba bilaterally.

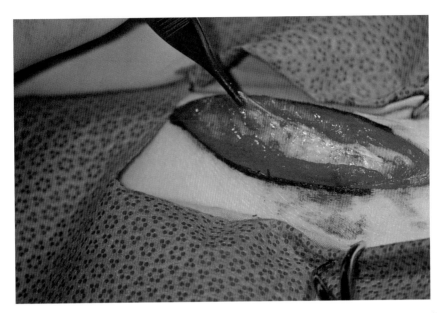

Figure 18.40 Entering the peritoneal cavity: lifting the linea alba with thumb forceps. The linea alba is grasped with thumb forceps in the cranial aspect of the incision and lifted outward so that abdominal contents will fall away from the site where the scalpel blade will puncture.

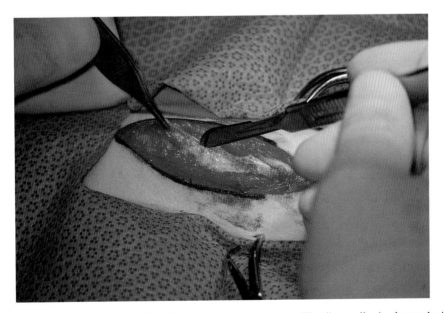

Figure 18.41 Entering the peritoneal cavity: stab incision location. The linea alba is elevated with thumb forceps in the cranial aspect of the incision so that a stab incision may be made as close to the umbilicus as possible. The scalpel is held in pencil grip fashion with the sharp edge of the blade positioned upward.

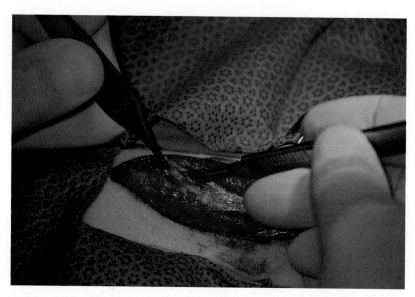

Figure 18.42   Entering the peritoneal cavity: stab incision. While the linea alba is elevated with thumb forceps, a scalpel held in pencil grip fashion with the sharp edge of the blade positioned upward is carefully stabbed through the linea alba. By making the stab in the cranial portion of the incision the internal organs should be somewhat protected by fat extending caudally from the falciform ligament. Nonetheless, care should be exercised to avoid inadvertently injuring an internal organ, which most commonly is the urinary bladder, especially if it had not been fully evacuated during surgical preparations.

Insert the thumb forceps into the stab incision to use as a groove director for the scalpel as the linea alba incision is made from cranial to caudal (Figures 18.43 and 18.44). The thumb forceps and scalpel blade should be moved in tandem so that the incision is completed with one continuous motion. The entire linea alba incision may be made in this fashion, or Mayo scissors can be used to extend the incision caudally (Figure 18.45) and cranially (Figure 18.46). Be sure to keep the tip of the scissors against the linea alba as they are inserted into the abdomen and lift outward while cutting. The linea alba is generally too tough to cut with a push-cutting motion. Once the opening is large enough to accommodate a finger, palpate for adhesions to the ventral midline cranially and caudally. Stop the linea alba incision at the cranial and caudal aspects of the skin incision. Extending the lineal incision beyond the limits of the skin incision will make closure of the linea alba difficult. Incision off of the midline will also make closure difficult. Paramedian incisions may require more time and effort to suture to ensure appropriate apposition.

Before searching for the ovaries and uterus, it is important for the surgeon to have a comfortable knowledge of the regional anatomy. Some structures will be visualized, but other important regional structures will be out of sight, yet easily damaged if their locations are not noted for their protection. For ovariohysterectomy, the surgeon must have an accurate and comfortable knowledge of the following anatomical structures and their locations: kidneys, ureters, suspensory ligament of the ovary, ovaries, mesovarium (the cranial part of the broad ligament), ovarian vascular pedicles, proper ovarian ligament, uterine horns, uterine body, uterine arteries, mesometrium (the caudal and larger part of the broad ligament),

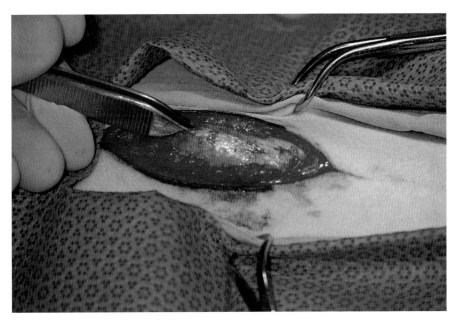

Figure 18.43   Extending the linea alba incision: groove director. After the stab incision is made, the thumb forceps is inserted to confirm that the peritoneal cavity has been entered and, with the tips directed caudally, is used to lift upward on the linea alba while a scalpel is used to incise from cranial to caudal.

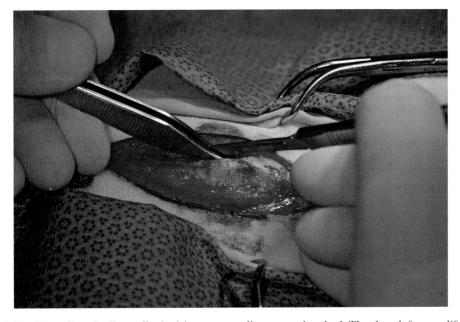

Figure 18.44   Extending the linea alba incision: groove director and scalpel. The thumb forceps lift upward and move in concert with the scalpel to extend the linea alba caudally.

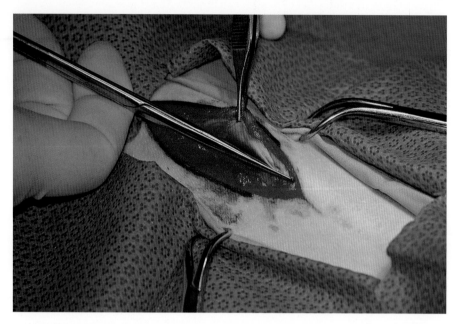

Figure 18.45   Extending the linea alba incision with Mayo scissors: caudal extension. Mayo scissors may be used instead of the scalpel and groove director technique. The scissor method is particularly helpful for directing off-midline incisions back to the midline.

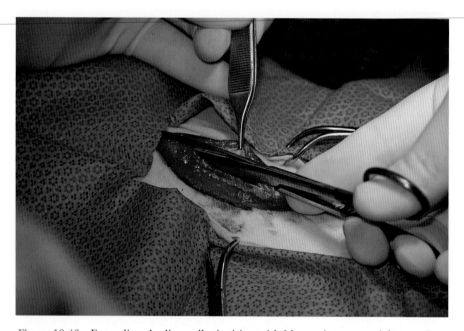

Figure 18.46   Extending the linea alba incision with Mayo scissors: cranial extension.

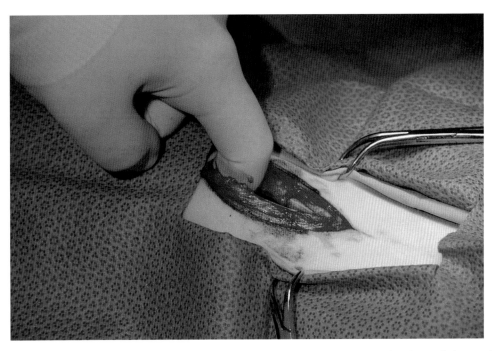

Figure 18.47   Completed linea alba incision for ovariohysterectomy. The left index finger is inserted into the cranial aspect of the linea alba incision to lift the abdominal wall outward in preparation for placement of an ovariohysterectomy hook.

round ligament of the uterus, and the inguinal canal. Complete understanding of abdominal anatomy is mandatory for any surgeon operating in the peritoneal cavity, but the above structures are a sample of important structures relative to routine ovariohysterectomy. When unplanned events occur, such as a dropped ovarian pedicle, more in depth understanding of abdominal anatomy is required to efficiently and effectively rectify the situation.

An ovariohysterectomy hook is used to locate the first ovary to be removed. The left ovary is situated more caudal than the right ovary and is more easily exteriorized; therefore, it is recommended to remove the left ovary first. To facilitate retrieval of the left ovary, insert the index finger of the nondominant hand into the cranial portion of the abdominal incision and lift upward (Figure 18.47). Hold the ovariohysterectomy hook with the hook facing upward (Figure 18.48). Insert the ovariohysterectomy hook into the mid to caudal portion of the incision (Figures 18.49 and 18.50). Keep the hook facing outward (laterally) against the body wall. When the hook reaches the deepest point, turn the hook medially and sweep the hook toward the midline and slowly withdraw it (Figures 18.51 and 18.52). If immediate resistance is felt, stop, release the tissue and try again. If intestine or omentum is exteriorized, replace the structure into the peritoneal cavity and try again. Initially, the uterus or the broad ligament may be exteriorized in the hook. Gently retract the broad ligament until the uterus is visualized. Then, gently exteriorize the remainder of the uterine horn and trace it to the ovary (Figures 18.53 and 18.54).

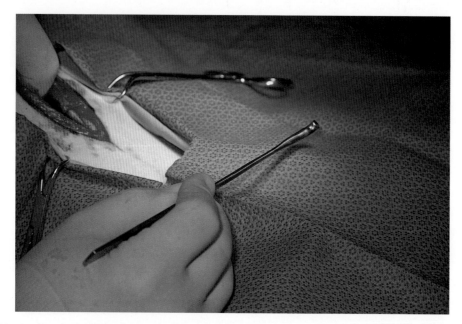

Figure 18.48   Snook ovariohysterectomy hook. The ovariohysterectomy hook is held with the inner surface of the hook pointing upward in preparation for placement into the left side of the peritoneal cavity.

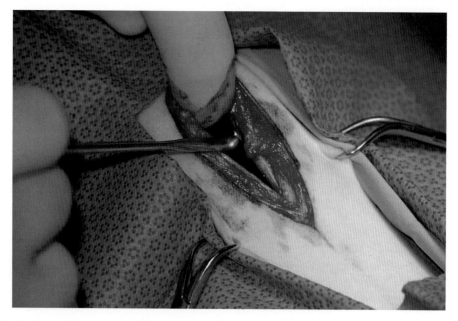

Figure 18.49   Introducing the ovariohysterectomy hook. With the left index finger lifting the abdominal wall outward, the ovariohysterectomy hook, with the inner surface of the hook pointing upward, is placed into the peritoneal cavity along the left abdominal wall.

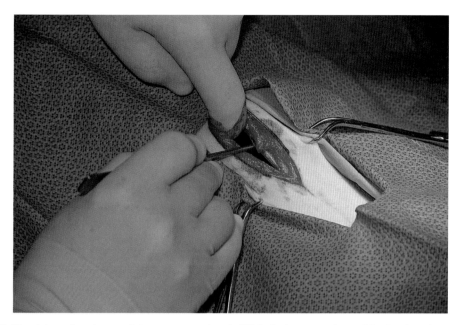

Figure 18.50 Advancing the ovariohysterectomy hook. With the inner surface of the hook pointing upward, the hook is advanced into the peritoneal cavity by rubbing it along the left abdominal wall until the hook hits the dorsal portion of the abdomen.

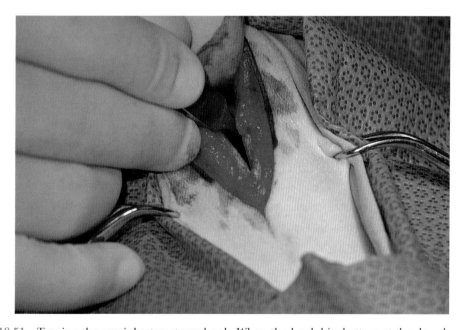

Figure 18.51 Turning the ovariohysterectomy hook. When the hook hits bottom at the dorsal portion of the peritoneal cavity, the hook is rotated so that the inner surface of the hook is directed medially.

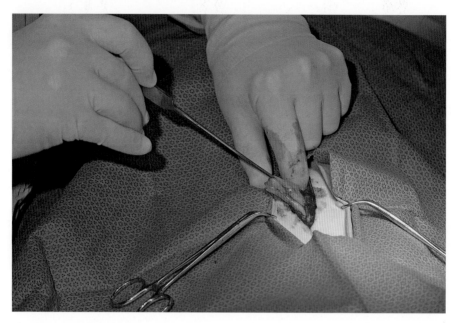

Figure 18.52   Extracting the ovariohysterectomy hook. The hook is pulled outward and toward the surgeon to exteriorize the left uterine horn.

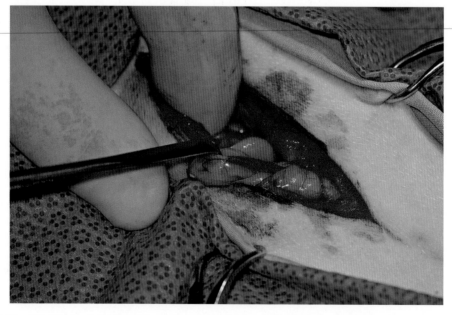

Figure 18.53   Finding the left ovary. Once the ovariohysterectomy hook is extracted as far as it will go without damaging its catch, the index finger and thumb of the surgeon's nondominant hand may be used to locate the ovary.

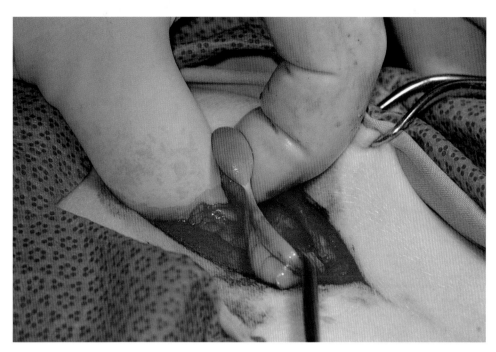

Figure 18.54 Exteriorizing the left ovary. With the ovariohysterectomy hook still attached to the left uterine horn, the ovary is exteriorized and the proper ligament is identified.

Identify the ovary and uterine horn before applying any hemostatic forceps. Place a mosquito hemostatic forceps on the proper ovarian ligament (Figure 18.55) to aid retraction of the ovary. Hold the mosquito forceps in the dominant hand so that the ovary is exteriorized in a direct outward (ventral) direction (Figure 18.56). The forceps is used to hold the ovarian pedicle in this position to prevent inadvertent caudal traction that could result in premature tearing of the ovarian pedicle. Use the nondominant hand (thumb and index finger) to strum and eventually tear the suspensory ligament from its attachment on the diaphragm in the region of the last rib (Figures 18.56–18.66). Slide the index finger of the nondominant hand down the lateral aspect of the suspensory ligament as far as possible (Figure 18.56). Apply increasing pressure in a caudomedial direction until the ligament breaks. Use the flat part of the index finger on the cranial surface of the ligament. Placing the index finger on the side of the ligament increases the chance of poking a hole in the mesovarium and possibly lacerating the ovarian vessels rather than rupturing the suspensory ligament. Alternatively, and preferred by the principal author whenever possible, the index finger may be inserted along with the thumb to grasp the suspensory ligament between the thumb and index finger as far down in the abdomen as possible (Figure 18.57). Then, a twisting motion is used to break the suspensory ligament (Figures 18.58–18.64). Sharp transection of the suspensory ligament is generally avoided since the blood vessels in the suspensory ligament will bleed more when this technique is used. When the suspensory ligament is adequately broken, the ovary and part of the ovarian pedicle should be readily exteriorized (Figures 18.65 and 18.66).

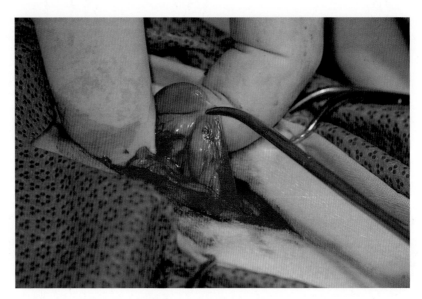

Figure 18.55 Clamping the proper ligament. A mosquito hemostat is applied to the proper ligament to maintain the ovary in an exteriorized position and to assist manipulations.

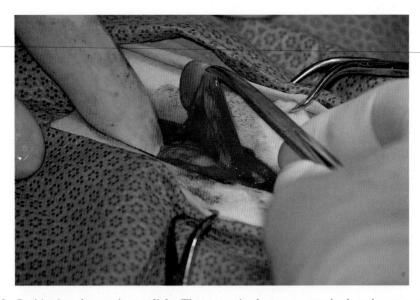

Figure 18.56 Positioning the ovarian pedicle. The mosquito hemostat attached to the proper ligament is held in the surgeon's dominant hand and manipulated to make sure that the ovarian pedicle is loose relative to the suspensory ligament and that the pedicle is directed outward instead of caudally. [Note: Pulling the ovarian pedicle caudally causes it to become parallel to and in close proximity with the suspensory ligament, increasing the chance of causing hemorrhage as the suspensory ligament is tensed and torn.]

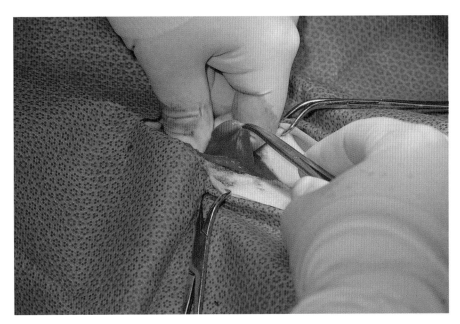

Figure 18.57 Stretching the suspensory ligament. The index finger and thumb of the nondominant hand are used to strum and stretch the suspensory ligament. Increased pressure is applied to the suspensory ligament in a caudomedial direction until the ligament breaks.

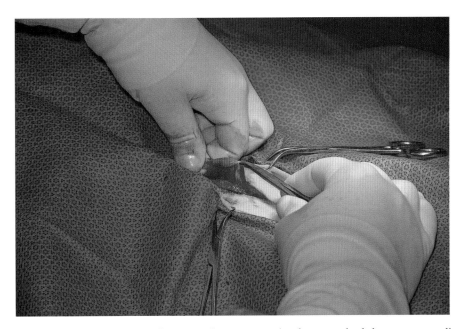

Figure 18.58 Tearing the suspensory ligament. Once strumming has stretched the suspensory ligament to somewhat exteriorize it, the ligament may be grasped between the thumb and index finger to apply force in a twisting action.

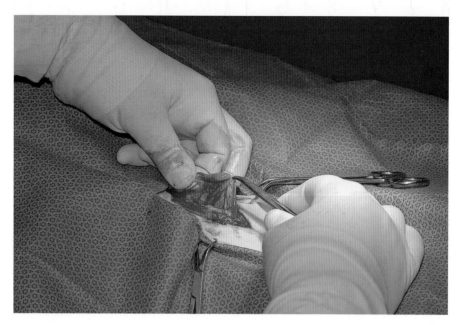

Figure 18.59   Incomplete tearing of the suspensory ligament. Partial tearing of the suspensory ligament may allow good exteriorization of the ovary and pedicle, but the remaining suspensory ligament will interfere with ligation.

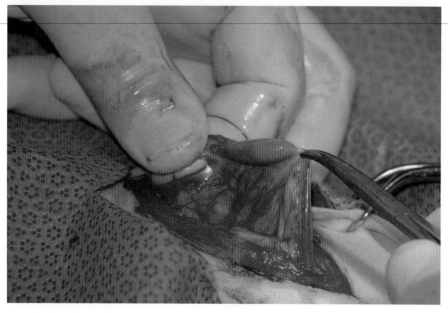

Figure 18.60   Incomplete tearing of the suspensory ligament (closeup view). A small band of the suspensory ligament remains between the thumb and index finger.

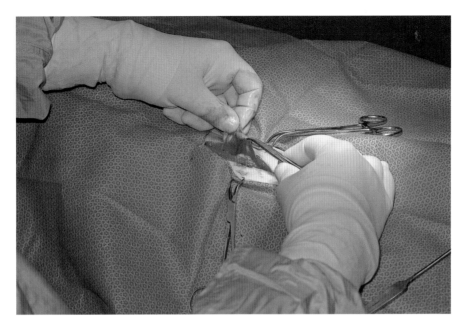

Figure 18.61 Remaining band of suspensory ligament. The remaining band of suspensory ligament cranial to the ovarian pedicle must be removed for optimal forceps placement and ligation.

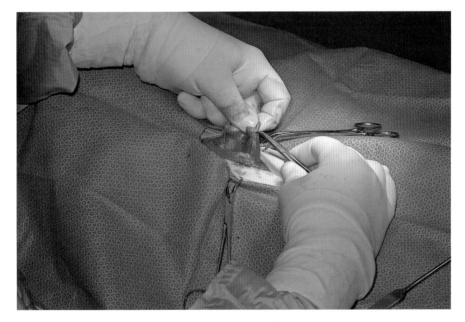

Figure 18.62 Detaching the remaining band of suspensory ligament. While steadying the ovarian pedicle with the mosquito forceps on the proper ligament and holding the suspensory ligament between the thumb and index finger, the middle finger can be used to tear the remaining band out of the abdomen.

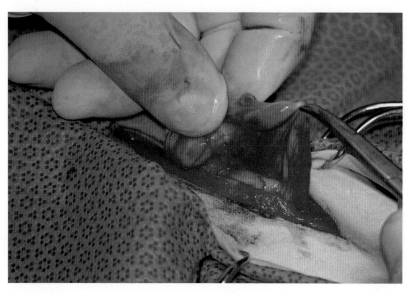

Figure 18.63   Detaching the remaining band of suspensory ligament (closeup view). The middle finger of the nondominant hand is used to help apply caudomedial pressure on the remaining band of suspensory ligament while the dominant hand and mosquito hemostat on the proper ligament steady the ovarian pedicle to prevent tearing of ovarian vessels in the process. [Note that the ovarian pedicle remains loose while the remaining suspensory ligament band is tight.]

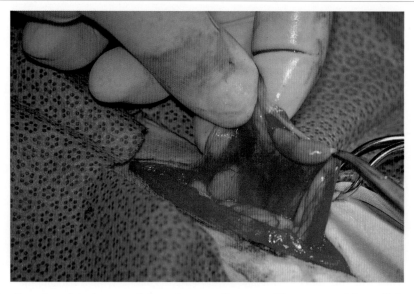

Figure 18.64   Complete detachment of the suspensory ligament. The ovary and its pedicle are optimally exteriorized.

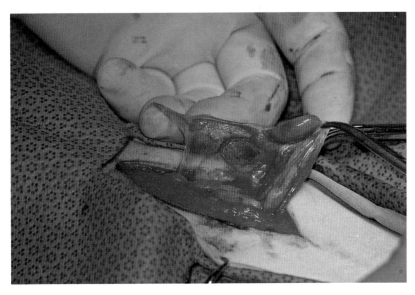

Figure 18.65 Verification of complete detachment of the suspensory ligament. The torn cranial aspect of the suspensory ligament should be exteriorized, as noted on the tip of the ring finger of this surgeon's left hand.

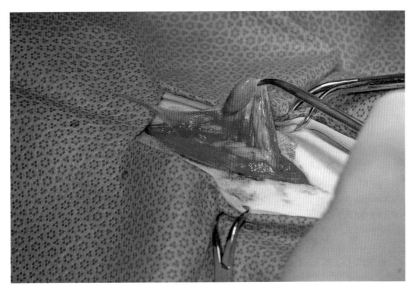

Figure 18.66 Preparation for ligating the left ovarian pedicle. The tip of the suspensory ligament noted lying on the drape in the cranial aspect of this picture will be pulled up toward the ovary when the forceps are applied so that the suspensory ligament is eventually excised along with the ovary.

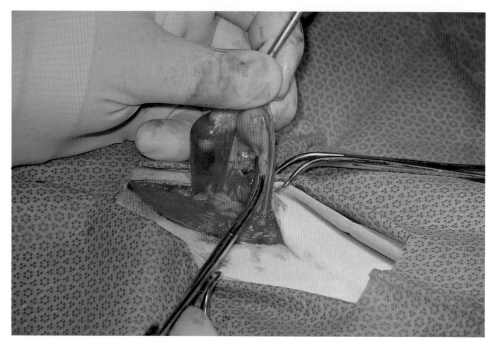

Figure 18.67   Isolating the left ovarian pedicle. Using a Rochester-Carmalt forceps, an avascular area of mesovarium adjacent to the ovarian vessels is identified for perforation to make a window as close to the ovarian vessels as possible.

Use a Rochester-Carmalt forceps intended for the ovarian pedicle to create a window in the broad ligament between the ovary and uterine horn (Figures 18.67–18.72). [Note: In cats and very small dogs, a mosquito or Kelly hemostatic forceps may be used in place of a Rochester-Carmalt forceps.] The ovarian pedicle typically contains a lot of fat in addition to the vessels (Figure 18.67). Look for a clear area in the broad ligament caudal to the pedicle and make a window with the tips of the forceps (Figures 18.67–18.69). Make sure all branches of the ovarian artery will be included. Open the Rochester-Carmalt forceps so that the window is spread open parallel to the vascular pedicle (Figures 18.70 and 18.71). Lift the suspensory ligament so that it will not be incorporated in clamping of the vascular pedicle but will be distal to the clamps as it is attached to the ovary (Figures 18.71 and 18.72).

Apply Rochester-Carmalt forceps to the ovarian pedicle using a three-clamp technique. The most proximal clamp should be placed first, taking care to leave enough room between that clamp and the ovary for a second clamp and also a cut between the second clamp and the ovary, and making sure that the entire ovary will be excised when the cut is made (Figure 18.73). Place the second clamp immediately distal to the first clamp so that a minimal amount of tissue (approximately 5 mm) can be seen between the two clamps (Figures 18.74–18.76). Always hold the ovary while applying these two clamps to be sure all ovarian tissue will be excised. Remove the mosquito forceps from the suspensory ligament and place a clamp across the uterine horn at this location (Figures 18.77 and 18.78). This third clamp is to control backflow bleeding when the ovarian pedicle is incised.

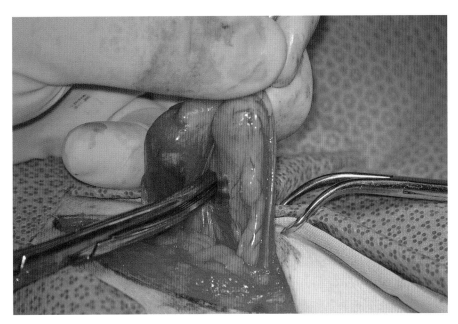

Figure 18.68   Perforating the left mesovarium. Rochester-Carmalt forceps are used to perforate the mesovarium and are orientated so that the jaws will open parallel to the ovarian pedicle.

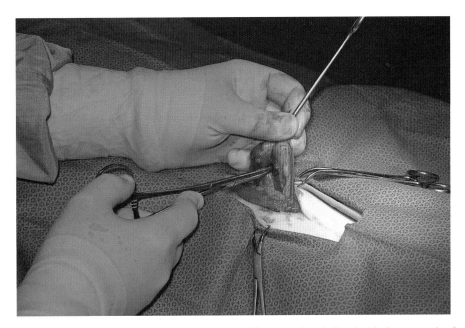

Figure 18.69   Preparing to make a mesovarium window. The ovary is stabilized with the mosquito forceps on the proper ligament and the Rochester-Carmalt forceps penetrating the mesovarium is positioned to open the jaws parallel to the ovarian pedicle.

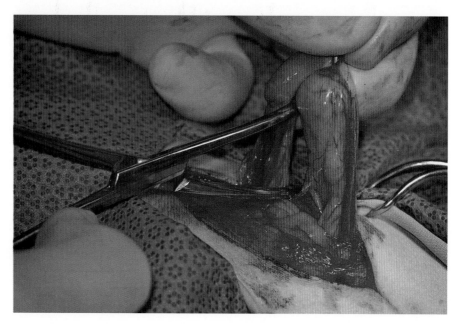

Figure 18.70 Making the mesovarium window next to the left ovarian pedicle. The Rochester-Carmalt forceps jaws are maximally spread parallel to the ovarian pedicle to create a large window.

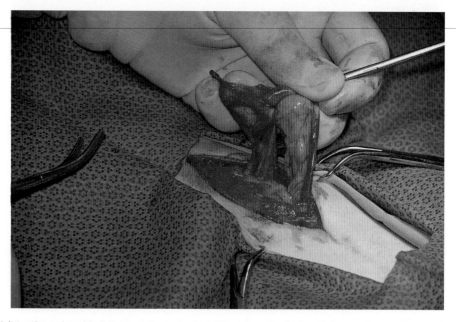

Figure 18.71 Completed left mesovarium window. Note the proximity of the window to the ovarian pedicle and the location of the suspensory ligament resting on the tip of the surgeon's left little finger.

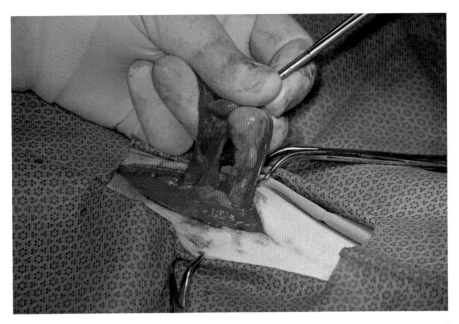

Figure 18.72   The left ovarian pedicle ready for forceps application. Note that the suspensory ligament is held out of the way so that it is not entrapped in the eventually applied forceps and ligatures.

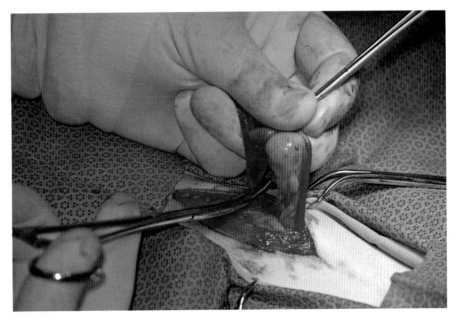

Figure 18.73   Application of the first hemostatic forceps on the left ovarian pedicle. The curved Rochester-Carmalt forceps is applied with the tips pointed upward and as far proximal as possible leaving a comfortable amount of room proximal to the forceps for ligature application.

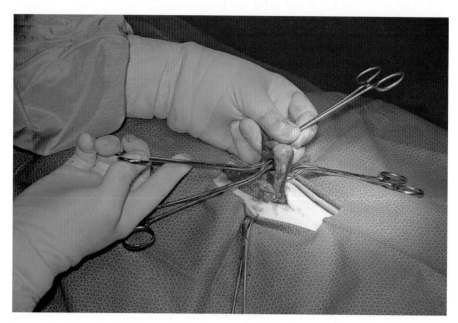

Figure 18.74   Application of the second hemostatic forceps on the left ovarian pedicle. The second curved Rochester-Carmalt forceps is applied parallel to the first forceps with the tips pointing upward.

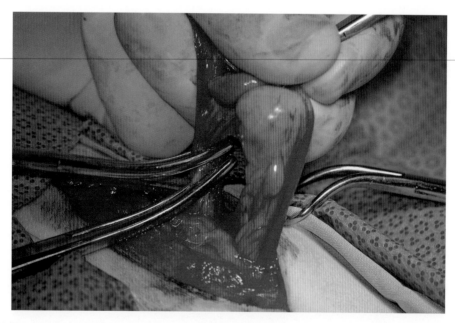

Figure 18.75   Application of the second hemostatic forceps on the left ovarian pedicle (closeup view). The tips of both Rochester-Carmalt forceps are parallel with only a small amount of tissue (4–5 mm) between them. Note that the tips protrude only a couple mm beyond the pedicle to allow easy manipulation of suture around them.

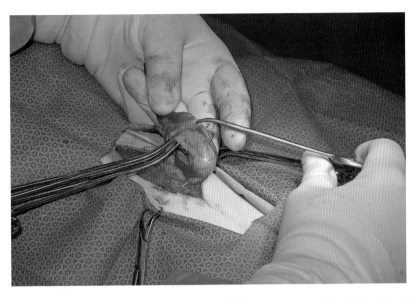

Figure 18.76 Preparation for placing a third hemostatic forceps to control backflow bleeding at the left ovarian pedicle. A third hemostatic forceps (not shown) may be placed immediately distal to the second forceps on the ovarian pedicle and a cut made between the second and third forceps. Alternately, the third forceps (not shown) may be applied across the mesometrium and uterus at the level of the proper ligament after removing the mosquito hemostatic forceps attached to that structure. Then, the incision may be made immediately distal to the second Rochester-Carmalt forceps.

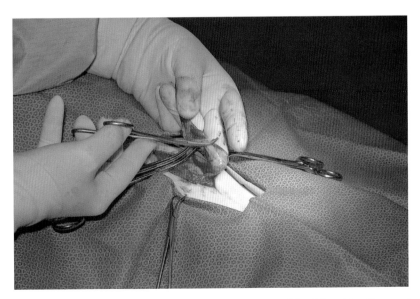

Figure 18.77 Application of the third hemostatic forceps to control backflow bleeding at the left ovarian pedicle. A Kelly hemostatic forceps is applied across the mesometrium and uterus at the level of the proper ligament where the mosquito hemostatic forceps was previously attached. Notice that the tips of the Kelly hemostatic forceps are oriented toward the ovary.

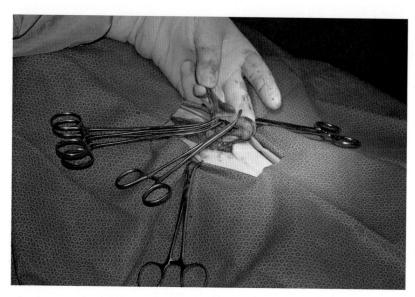

Figure 18.78   Completion of three forceps application prior to incising the left ovarian pedicle. Two parallel Rochester-Carmalt forceps are attached to the ovarian pedicle, and a Kelly hemostatic forceps across the mesometrium and uterus at the level of the proper ligament will control backflow bleeding. The suspensory ligament is being held between the surgeon's left thumb and ring finger to demonstrate that this structure is not incorporated within the forceps.

As soon as the clamps are applied, Metzenbaum scissors are used to incise the ovarian pedicle between the middle clamp and the ovary (Figures 18.79–18.83). Transecting the pedicle before placing ligatures makes manipulations easier, but if a forceps slips, the pedicle will retract into the peritoneal cavity. Leaving the ovary attached during ligature application actually creates a false sense of security because tissues can tear at any forceps even if the forceps does not slip. Transecting the ovarian pedicle first allows for less manipulation during ligature placement and, therefore, less chance of tearing tissue at the forceps.

Move the ovary caudally so that it and the entire left uterine horn rest in the caudal aspect of the surgical field while ligating the left ovarian pedicle (Figures 18.84–18.94). To fully exteriorize the uterine horn, manually remove the broad ligament and round ligament (Figures 18.85–18.94). Pull the round ligament entirely out of the abdomen (Figures 18.89 and 18.90).

Be careful to avoid the uterine arteries that run parallel to the uterine horns when tearing and pulling the broad and round ligaments.

There are multiple surgeon preferences for ligating ovarian pedicles. The principal author prefers a simple transfixation suture method as illustrated in this chapter (Figures 18.92–18.115). To begin transfixation of the left ovarian pedicle, gently push a closed mosquito hemostatic forceps through the pedicle just proximal to the proximal clamp (Figures 18.92–18.95). This manipulation pushes the vessels away from the mosquito forceps and is less likely to injure vessels than passing a suture needle through the pedicle. Some surgeons pass the suture end of the needle through the pedicle to avoid spearing vessels with the needle point. However, the hemostat method described here is even less likely to injure a vessel and also results in less dragging of suture through the pedicle tissue. Open the hemostat and grab the free

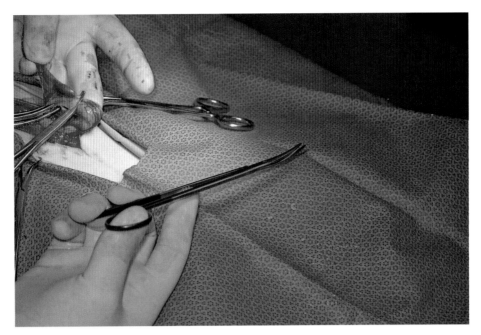

Figure 18.79   Preparation to incise the left ovarian pedicle with Metzenbaum scissors. The curve of the Metzenbaum scissors is oriented upward, similar to the orientation of the Rochester-Carmalt forceps.

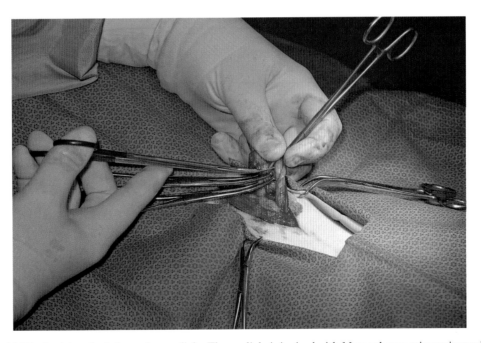

Figure 18.80   Incising the left ovarian pedicle. The pedicle is incised with Metzenbaum scissors immediately distal to the second Rochester-Carmalt forceps.

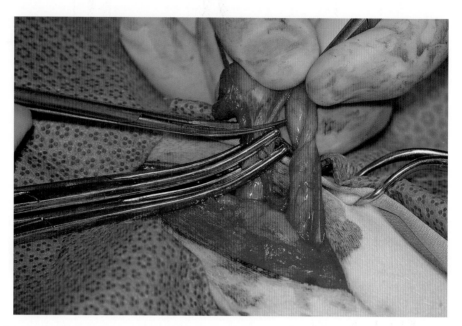

Figure 18.81   Incising the left ovarian pedicle (closeup view). Note how close the incision is made to the second Rochester-Carmalt. The pedicle is incised with Metzenbaum scissors so that only a couple mm of tissue will remain immediately distal to the second Rochester-Carmalt forceps.

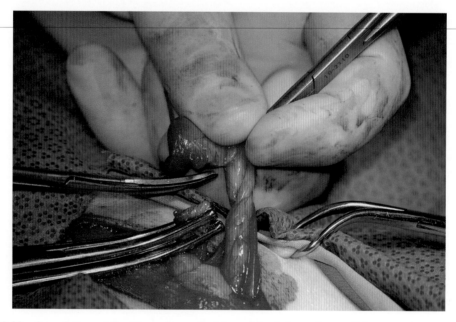

Figure 18.82   Completion of the Metzenbaum incision of the left ovarian pedicle. Note the parallel orientation of the scissor blades and Rochester-Carmalt forceps tips.

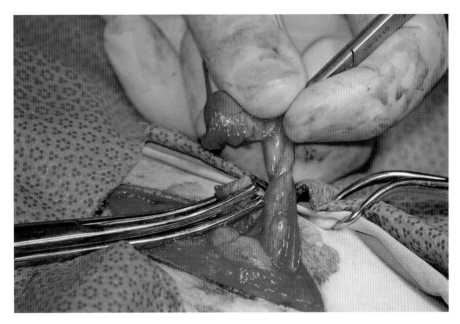

Figure 18.83 Completed left ovarian pedicle incision. The ovary, uterus, and backflow controlling forceps can now be moved caudally out of the way.

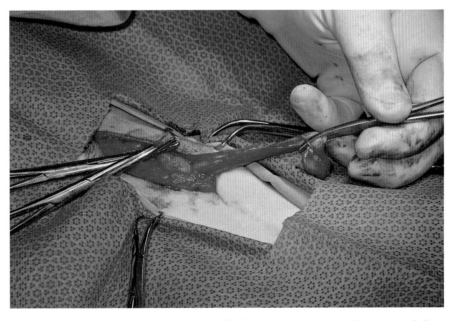

Figure 18.84 Moving the left ovary and uterus caudally. Directing the ovary and uterus caudally makes room for manipulating and ligating the ovarian pedicle.

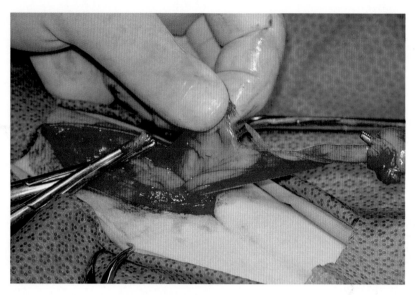

Figure 18.85 Removing the left broad ligament. The broad ligament is manually extracted from the peritoneal cavity to free the uterine horn and facilitate caudal displacement of the ovary and uterine horn. It is best to extract the broad ligament now to maximally get the uterine horn and ovary out of the way. Furthermore, this maneuver will be necessary later, if not done now, when it is time to ligate the uterine body.

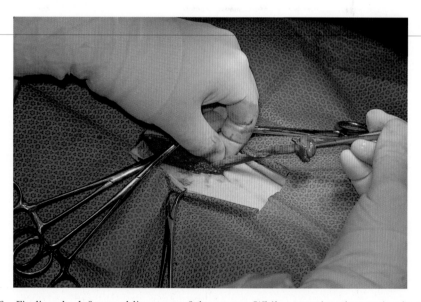

Figure 18.86 Finding the left round ligament of the uterus. While retracting the uterine horn and ovary caudally with the dominant hand, the surgeon uses the left hand to locate the round ligament. Removing the round ligament allows for maximal caudal exteriorization of the uterine horn, which will become handy later when the second uterine horn must be traced.

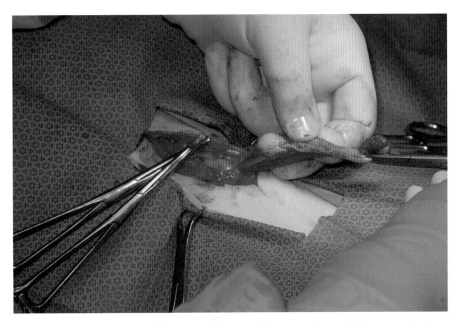

Figure 18.87   Isolating the left round ligament. The round ligament is carefully grasped as it runs parallel to the uterine horn on the edge of the broad ligament.

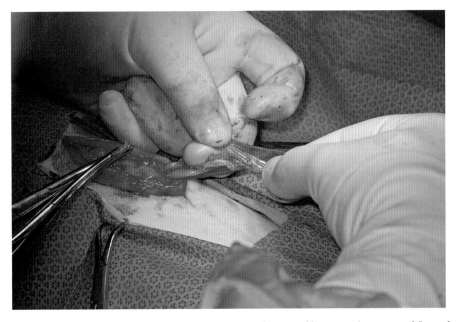

Figure 18.88   Preparing to extract the left round ligament. The round ligament is separated from the uterine horn to avoid damaging the uterine artery and vein during its extraction.

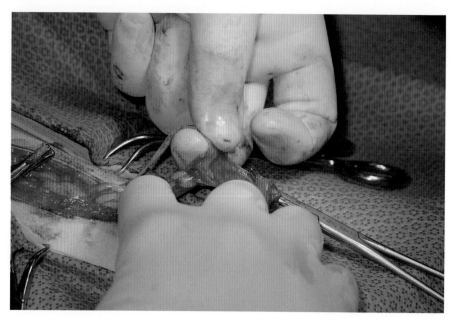

Figure 18.89   Visualizing the left round ligament. The round ligament is fully visualized before manually extracting it.

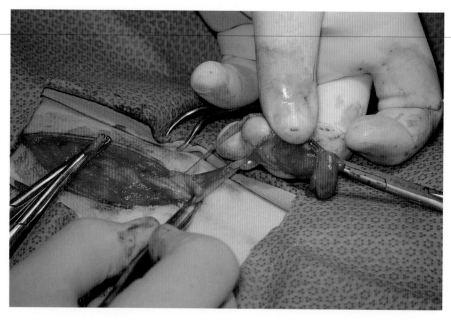

Figure 18.90   Extracting the left round ligament. An outward extraction force is applied to the round ligament to pull it out of the inguinal canal.

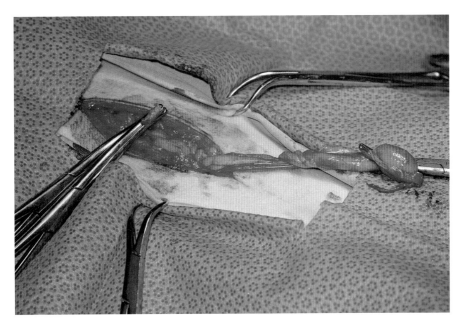

Figure 18.91   Completed left round ligament extraction. After extraction of the broad and round ligaments the left ovary and uterine horn are positioned caudally. Then, the left ovarian pedicle will be ligated.

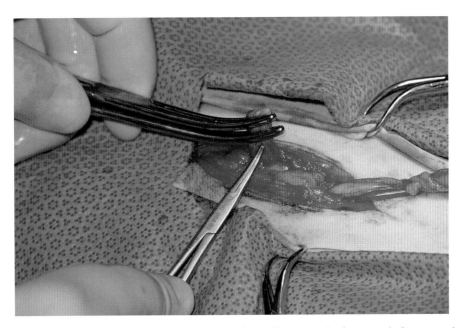

Figure 18.92   Location of first suture in left ovarian pedicle. The mosquito hemostatic forceps points to the first suture location immediately proximal to the first Rochester-Carmalt forceps.

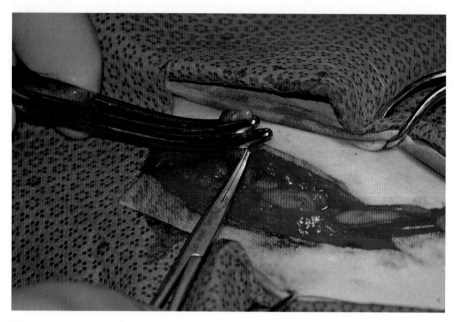

Figure 18.93 Passing a mosquito hemostatic forceps through left ovarian pedicle at the location for the first suture.

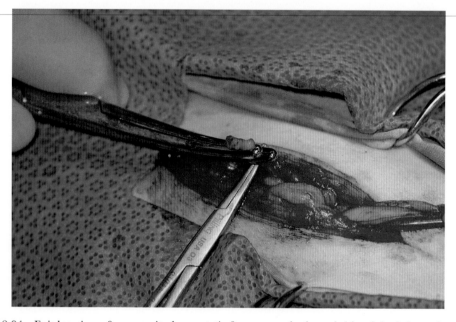

Figure 18.94 Exit location of a mosquito hemostatic forceps on the lateral side of the left ovarian pedicle.

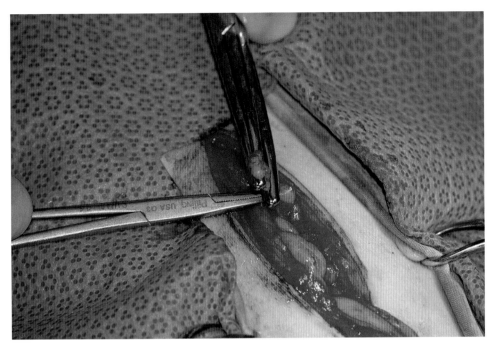

Figure 18.95   Continued advancement of a mosquito hemostatic forceps through the left ovarian pedicle immediately proximal to the first Rochester-Carmalt forceps.

end of the suture (Figures 18.96 and 18.97). Pull the suture through the pedicle and around one side for tying (Figures 18.98 and 18.99). Tie one half of a square knot (one throw) and bring the suture around the opposite side of the pedicle (Figures 18.100–18.104). Tie a surgeon's knot, removing the first (proximal) clamp as the first throw of the surgeon's knot is tightened (Figures 18.105–18.109). Most of the knot should be within the crimp of tissue where the proximal clamp had been. Tighten the surgeon's throw completely. Then, place three additional throws to complete a surgeon's knot followed by a square knot. A second circumferential ligature may be placed a few millimeters proximal to the transfixation suture (Figures 18.110–18.112). Then, the pedicle stump is grasped with thumb forceps as the remaining

clamp is removed (Figures 18.112 and 18.113). The stump is placed into the peritoneal cavity and withdrawn to see if tension relief results in hemorrhage (Figures 18.114 and 18.115). In some instances, the upward tension will prevent bleeding while the pedicle is exteriorized, but then bleeding will occur when the tension is reduced. If bleeding is noted, exteriorize the pedicle again and reapply hemostats prior to attempting another ligation. If the ligature is secure and no hemorrhage is noted, the stump is gently placed into the peritoneal cavity to allow the pedicle to slowly retract into the peritoneal cavity before it is released. If at any point in the procedure the pedicle slips into the peritoneal cavity before ligation is secure, methodically use knowledge of regional anatomy to locate the stump. Retract the descending colon

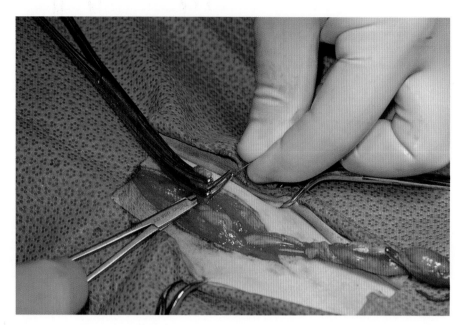

Figure 18.96 Opening a mosquito forceps after penetrating the left ovarian pedicle in order to introduce suture for ligation.

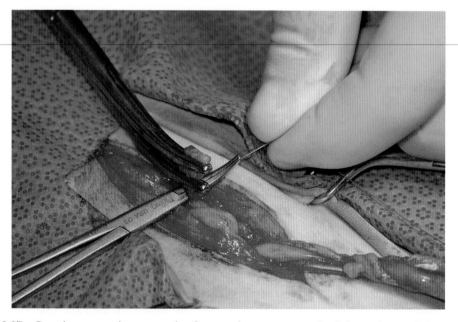

Figure 18.97 Grasping suture in a mosquito forceps that penetrates the left ovarian pedicle. The suture will be pulled through the ovarian pedicle. The suture material used for pedicle ligation in this case is 3–0 polyglactin 910.

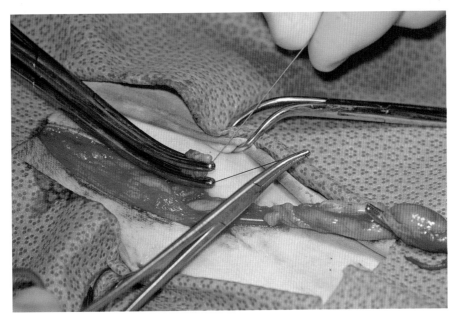

Figure 18.98   Passing the ligature suture around the caudal side of the left ovarian pedicle.

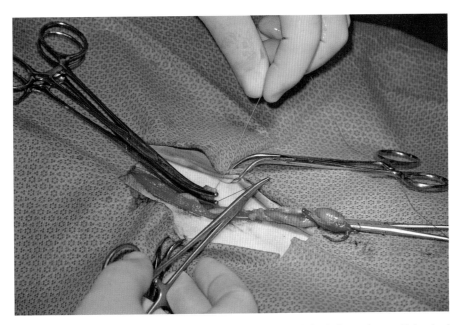

Figure 18.99   Preparing to tie the suture around the caudal side of the left ovarian pedicle. An instrument tie may be performed with the mosquito hemostatic forceps, or the surgeon may switch to a needle holder.

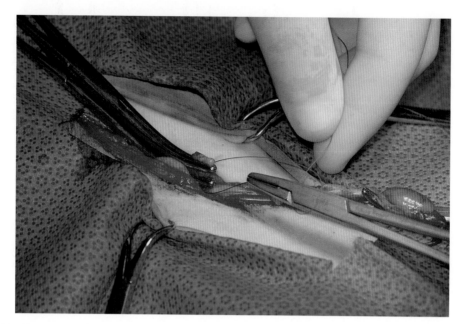

Figure 18.100 Tying the suture at the caudal aspect of the left ovarian pedicle with one throw (half of a square knot).

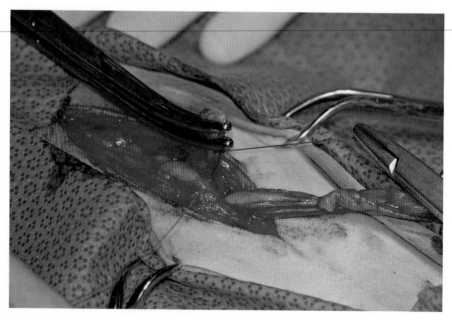

Figure 18.101 Positioning the first (and only) throw of a square knot at the caudal aspect of the left ovarian pedicle.

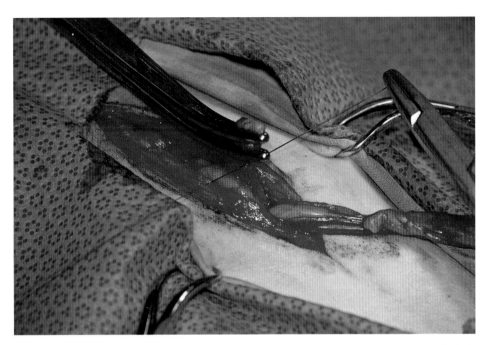

Figure 18.102 Securing the first (and only) throw of a square knot at the caudal aspect of the left ovarian pedicle.

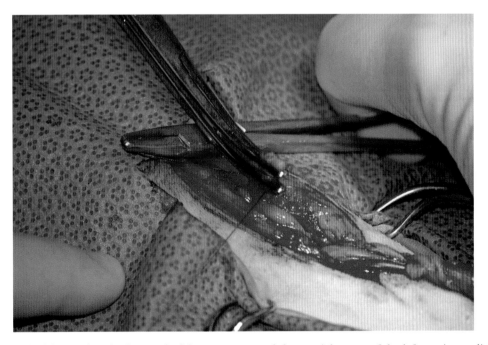

Figure 18.103 Passing the free end of the suture around the cranial aspect of the left ovarian pedicle.

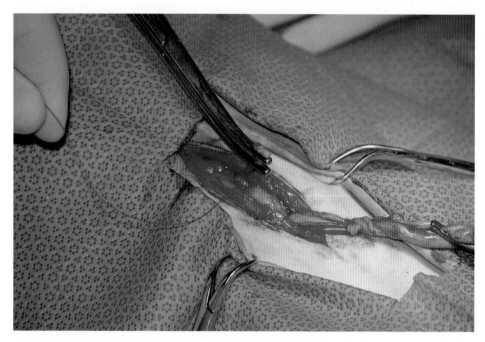

Figure 18.104   Preparing to tie the ligature around the cranial aspect of the left ovarian pedicle.

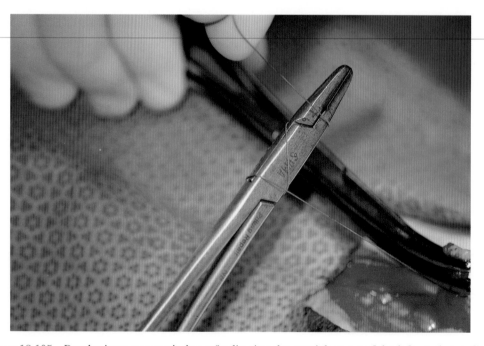

Figure 18.105   Developing a surgeon's throw for ligating the cranial aspect of the left ovarian pedicle.

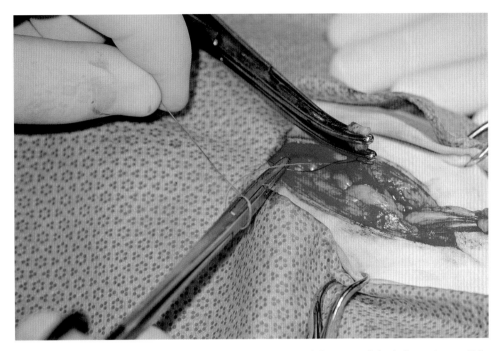

Figure 18.106   Positioning the surgeon's throw at the cranial aspect of the left ovarian pedicle.

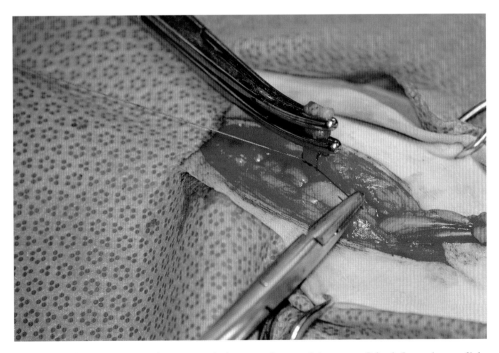

Figure 18.107   Tightening the surgeon's throw at the cranial aspect of the left ovarian pedicle.

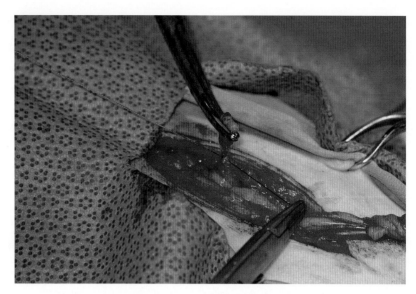

Figure 18.108 Securing the surgeon's throw at the cranial aspect of the left ovarian pedicle. As this throw tightens, the single throw in the caudal aspect of the pedicle is secured. Notice that the more proximal Rochester-Carmalt forceps is removed to allow full tightening of the ligature. Some surgeons attempt to have this surgeon's throw fall into the crimped tissue at the previous Rochester-Carmalt forceps site as the ligature is tightened; however, tightening proximal to the crimped tissue is also acceptable. The purpose of removing the proximal Rochester-Carmalt forceps is to allow the ligated tissue to collapse into a tubular shape. Not doing so can result in a loose ligature when the forceps is removed.

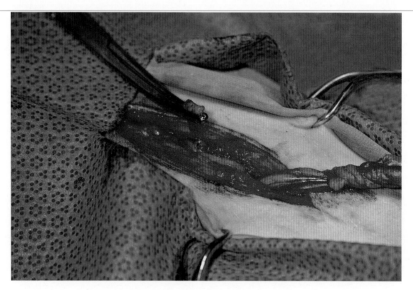

Figure 18.109 Completed transfixation suture on the left ovarian pedicle. The surgeon's knot was completed by placing a simple throw after the surgeons throw, and then the suture was cut. Some surgeons prefer to add a square knot on top of the surgeon's knot before cutting the suture.

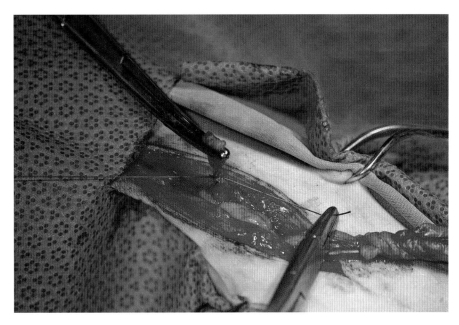

Figure 18.110   Preparing to place a second ligature applied circumferentially.

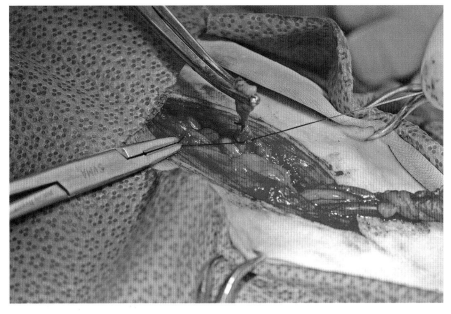

Figure 18.111   Placement of a circumferential ligature proximal to the transfixation suture. The first throw of a square knot is demonstrated. Typically, this ligature is accomplished with two square knots. Note that this second ligature is reasonably close to the transfixation suture.

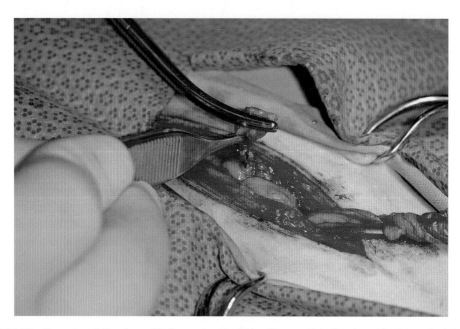

Figure 18.112 Completed ligation of left ovarian pedicle. The pedicle is grasped with a thumb forceps between the distal (transfixation) ligature and the remaining Rochester-Carmalt forceps in preparation for release of the pedicle.

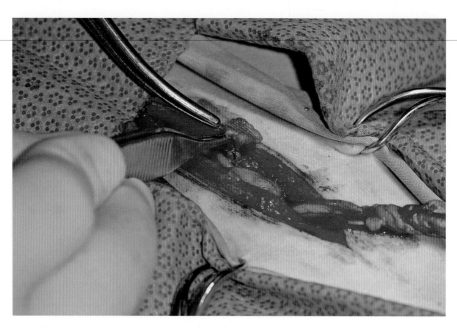

Figure 18.113 Preparing to release the ligated left ovarian pedicle. The Rochester-Carmalt forceps is released so that the pedicle may be gently placed into the peritoneal cavity with the thumb forceps.

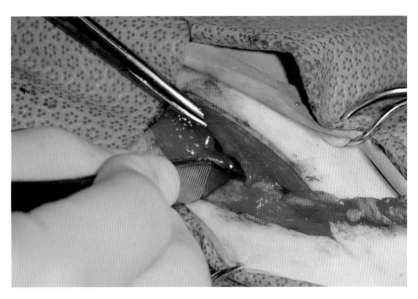

Figure 18.114   Placing the ligated left ovarian pedicle into the peritoneal cavity. The thumb forceps is used to gently place the ovarian pedicle into the abdomen, but the pedicle is not released from the thumb forceps until it is certain that the ligature will prevent bleeding.

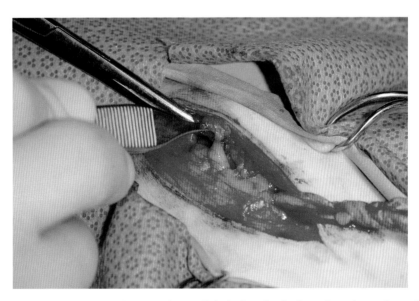

Figure 18.115   Checking the ligated left ovarian pedicle before final release into the peritoneal cavity. After gently placing the ovarian pedicle into the abdomen, without releasing the thumb forceps, the pedicle is exteriorized again to check its integrity. Tension on the pedicle, as occurs when forceps hold the pedicle exteriorized, can control hemorrhage by stretching the vessels, thereby decreasing their diameters. Removing the tension when the pedicle is placed into the abdomen will allow the vessels to fill with blood, and bleeding with occur if the pedicle ligatures are loose. If bleeding does not occur when the tension on the pedicle is relieved, then the pedicle may be released when it is replaced into the peritoneal cavity.

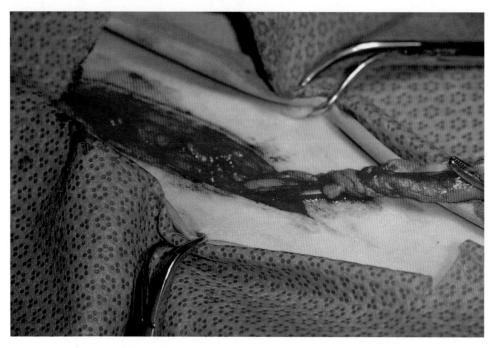

Figure 18.116 Preparing to find the right uterine horn. After the left ovarian pedicle is released the left ovary and uterine horn are pulled caudally to expose the uterine body. If the broad and round ligaments have not been removed, they must be removed at this point to adequately exteriorize the uterine body.

(left side) or descending duodenum (right side) medially, identify the pedicle at the caudal pole of the kidney, and grasp it with thumb forceps. Adequate exposure usually requires extension of the abdominal incision. Never apply crushing clamps until the pedicle has been isolated to avoid iatrogenic injury to the ureter.

Find the right ovary by tracing the left uterine horn to the uterine body to locate the right uterine horn. [Note: Use the ovariohysterectomy hook for retrieving only the first ovary. Using the hook for the second ovary frequently results in entangling the urinary bladder with the reproductive tract.] If the left broad and round ligaments have been removed, tracing from the left to right horn is easily achieved by pulling the left ovary caudally until the uterine body is exposed (Figures 18.116 and 18.117).

In small patients, a thumb forceps may be necessary to grasp the right uterine horn (Figure 18.118) to begin tracing it to the ovary (Figures 18.119 and 18.120). Once the ovary is located and the proper ligament clamped (Figure 18.121), the procedures of breaking the suspensory ligament, making a mesovarian window, applying three clamps, excising the ovary, removing the broad and round ligaments, transfixing the ovarian pedicle, and returning the pedicle to the peritoneal cavity are performed just as was done on the left (Figures 18.56–18.115). Both ovaries and uterine horns are pulled caudally (Figures 18.122 and 18.123) during transfixation and release of the ligated right pedicle into the peritoneal cavity. The uterus may remain in this position during ligation of the uterine body, or the horns may be pulled cranially and outward. The former

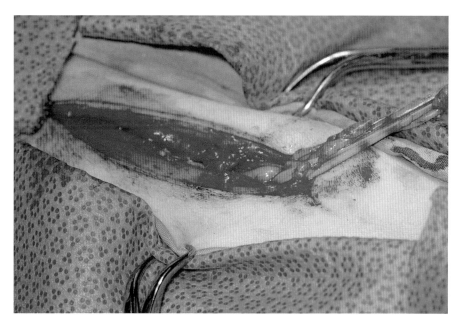

Figure 18.117   Exteriorizing the uterine body and right uterine horn. Caudal traction on the left ovary and uterine horn pulls the uterine body up through the caudal aspect of the incision.

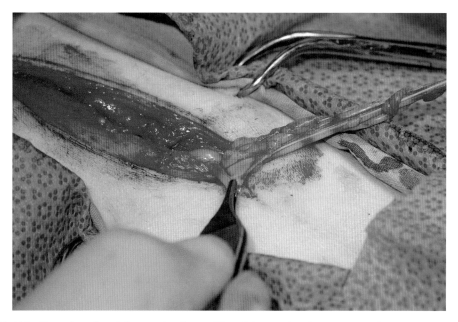

Figure 18.118   Exposing the right uterine horn. The right uterine horn is traced from the uterine body while the left uterine horn is pulled caudally. In small patients, it is helpful to first grasp the right uterine horn at its junction with the uterine body.

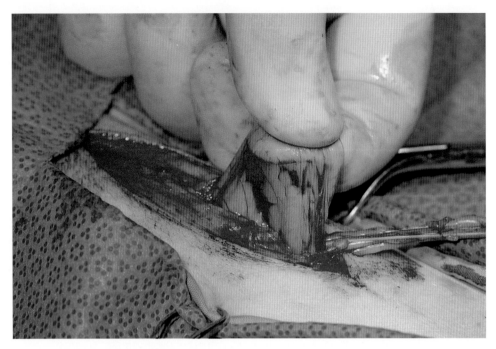

Figure 18.119 Tracing the right uterine horn toward the right ovary.

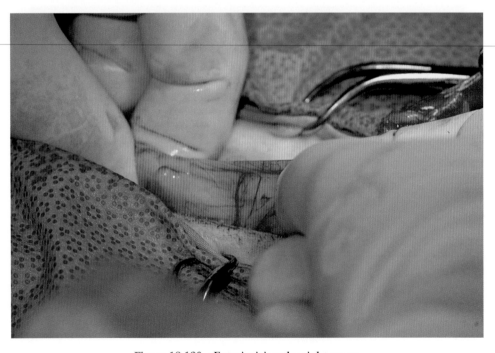

Figure 18.120 Exteriorizing the right ovary.

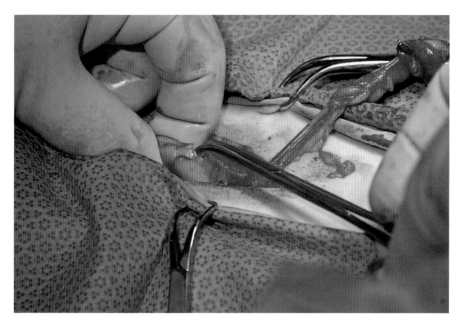

Figure 18.121   Applying a mosquito hemostatic forceps to the right proper ligament.

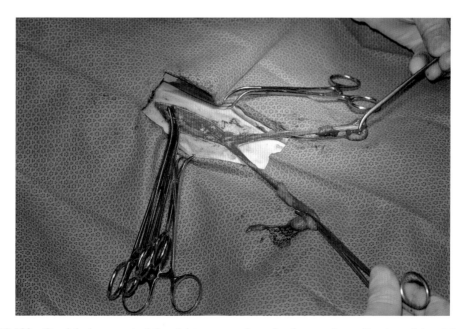

Figure 18.122   Caudal placement of the right ovary and uterine horn prior to ligation of the right ovarian pedicle. The broad and round ligaments have been manually torn and extracted so that the right ovary and uterine horn can be positioned caudally in preparation for uterine body ligation and extraction. At this point, the right ovarian pedicle will be ligated and replaced into the peritoneal cavity.

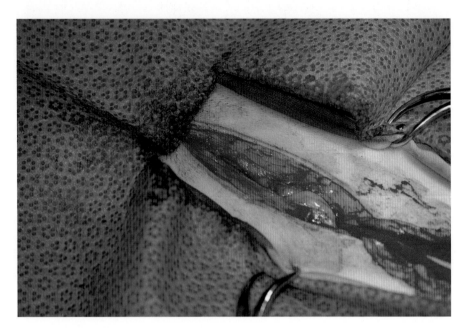

Figure 18.123   Completion of ovarian pedicle ligations. Both ligated ovarian pedicles have been replaced into the abdomen and the uterus is retracted caudally.

is preferred when the surgeon is operating without a scrubbed assistant, but for illustrative purposes the latter is shown in this chapter (Figures 18.124–18.155).

Ligation of the uterine arteries and veins may be done independently of the uterine body ligation, or the uterine blood vessels may be incorporated in the uterine body transfixation suture. Separate vessel ligation is advised when the uterine arteries are large and prominent. In large dogs, "stick tie" ligatures can be placed on the uterine arteries and veins. To place a "stick tie" ligature, take a small suture bite in the uterine wall adjacent to the uterine vessels and then ligate the vessels. As the ligature is tied, the knot is stuck against the uterine wall. When the uterus is small, circumferential uterine vessel ligatures can be placed rather than using "stick tie" ligatures. Most small- and medium- sized dogs, particularly those that have had few or no estrus cycles, do not require separate ligation of the uterine vessels; simple uterine body transfixa-

tion incorporating the uterine vessels as illustrated in this chapter will suffice. Transfixation begins with passage of the needle through the uterine body in forward fashion (Figures 18.125–18.129). There is no need to back the needle through the uterine body because, unlike the ovarian pedicle, the uterine vessels and branches can be easily seen and avoided. Place the first throw of a square knot (Figures 18.130–18.133) and then pass the suture around the opposite side of the uterus (Figures 18.134–18.136) and tie a surgeon's knot (Figures 18.137–18.143). A second (circumferential) suture may be placed proximal to the transfixation suture (Figures 18.144–18.146). Then, place a Rochester-Carmalt forceps across the uterus distal (cranial) to the transfixation suture (Figures 18.147 and 18.148) to control backflow bleeding from the uterus as it is cut. Place a mosquito hemostat on one edge of the uterine stump (Figure 18.149) to keep it from prematurely disappearing into the peritoneal cavity, and cut between the transfixation suture

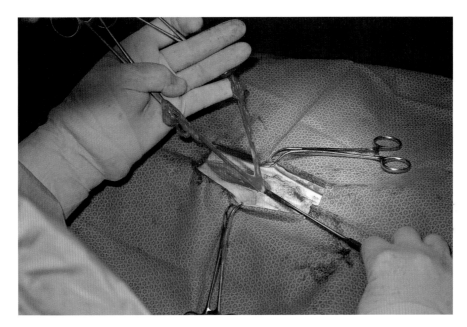

Figure 18.124   Preparing to ligate the uterine body. When operating without an assistant, the uterus may remain in the caudally retracted position for ligating the uterine vessels and uterine body. [For illustrative purposes, the uterus in this case is lifted upward and cranially for uterine body ligation.]

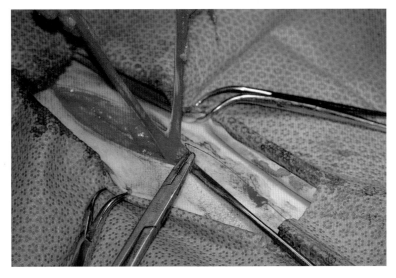

Figure 18.125   Location of transfixation suture in the uterine body. The suture needle points to the uterine body midway between the cervix and uterine bifurcation. The suture material used for uterine body transfixation in this case is 3–0 polyglactin 910.

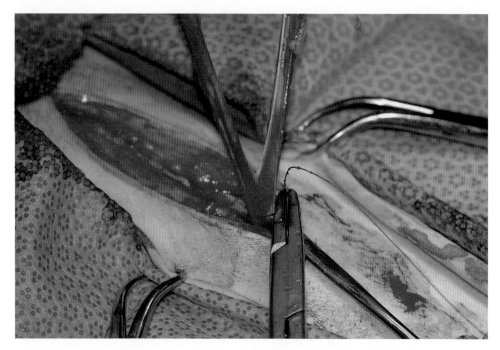

Figure 18.126   Passing transfixation suture needle through the midportion of the uterine body.

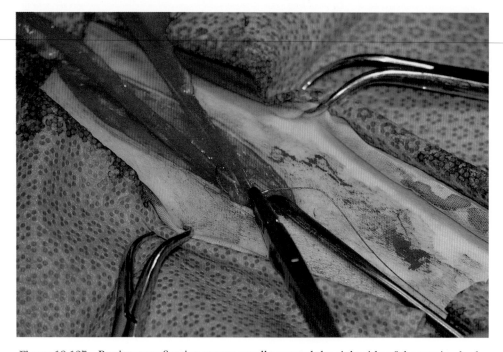

Figure 18.127   Passing transfixation suture needle around the right side of the uterine body.

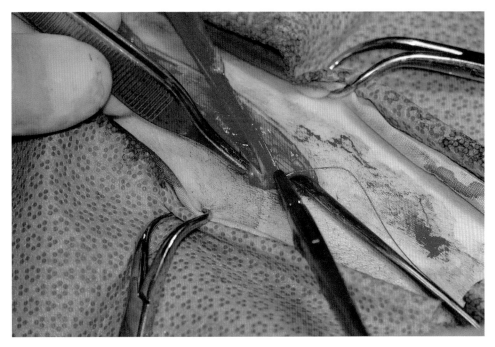

Figure 18.128   Grasping the transfixation suture needle with a Brown-Adson thumb forceps.

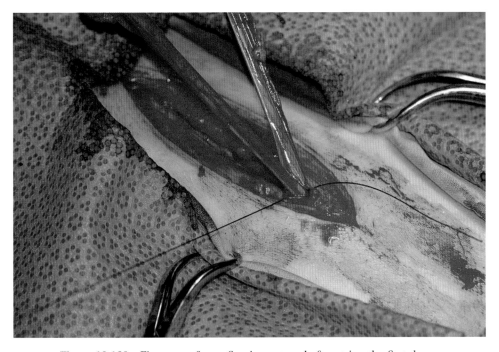

Figure 18.129   First pass of transfixation suture before tying the first throw.

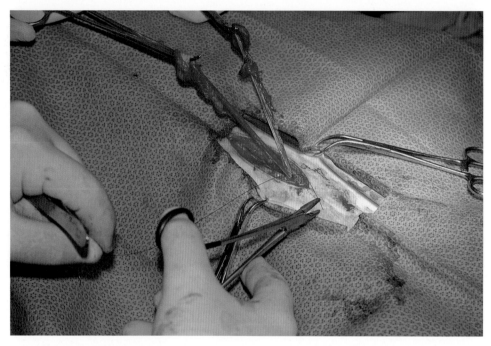

Figure 18.130   Preparing to tie the first throw of a transfixation suture in the uterine body.

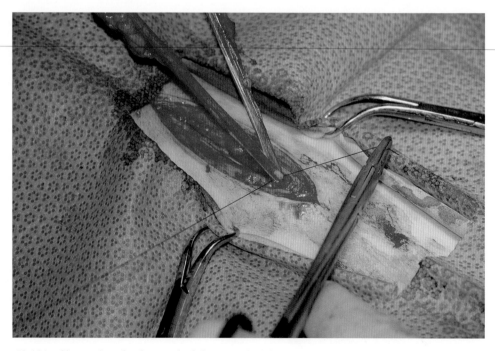

Figure 18.131   Shortening the free end of the strand of the uterine body transfixation suture before tying the first throw.

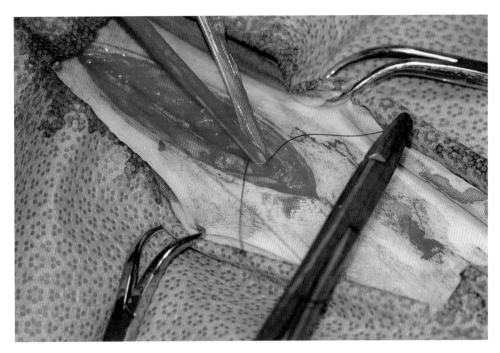

Figure 18.132 Developing first throw (half of a square knot) on the uterine body transfixation suture.

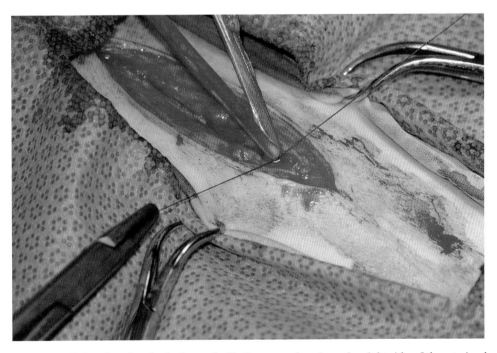

Figure 18.133 Tightening the single throw (half of a square knot) on the right side of the uterine body.

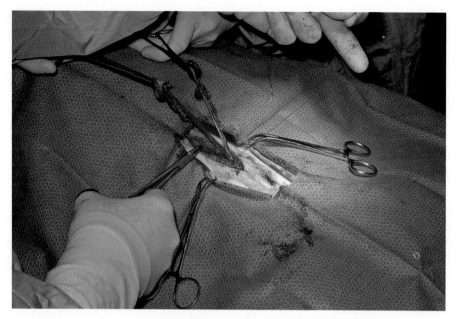

Figure 18.134 Preparing to pass the free end of the transfixation suture around the uterine body after the single throw has been tightened on the right side of the uterine body.

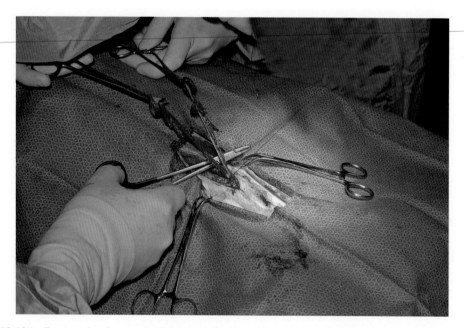

Figure 18.135 Passing the free end of the transfixation suture around the uterine body after the single throw has been tightened on the right side of the uterine body.

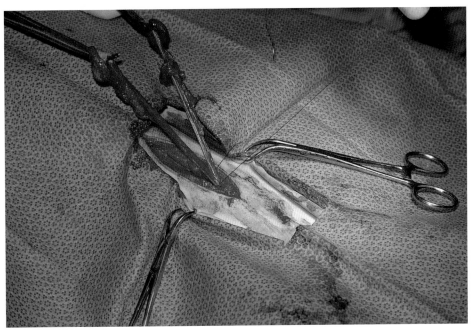

Figure 18.136 Both strands of the transfixation suture on the left side of the uterus prior to tying that side of the transfixation.

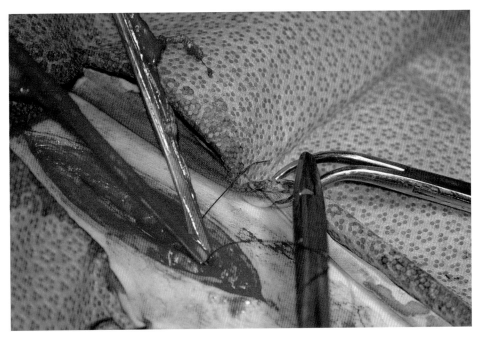

Figure 18.137 Developing a surgeon's throw as the first throw on the left side of the uterine body.

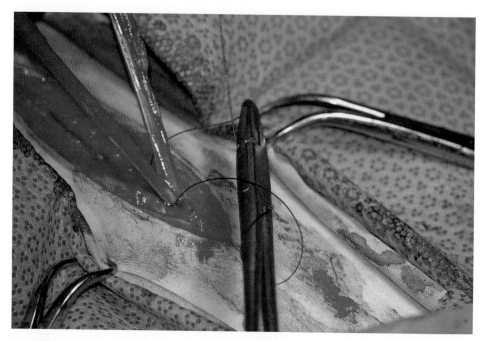

Figure 18.138   Grasping the free end of the suture to begin a surgeon's throw on the left side of the uterine body. [Notice the single throw on the right side of the uterine body.]

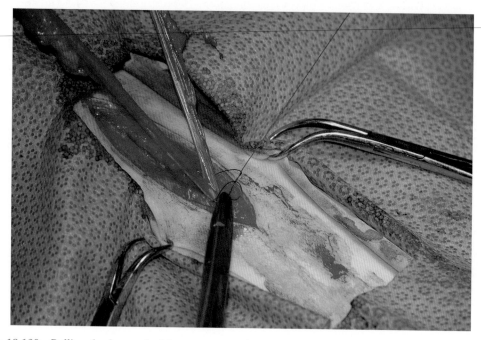

Figure 18.139   Pulling the free end of the suture strand toward the right side to continue a surgeon's throw.

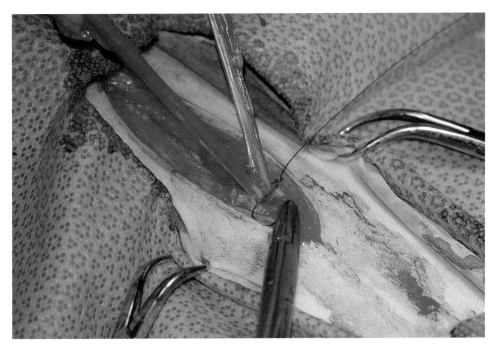

Figure 18.140   Advancing a surgeon's throw toward the uterine body.

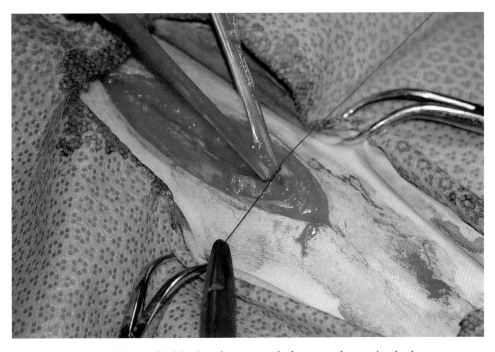

Figure 18.141   Positioning the surgeon's throw on the uterine body.

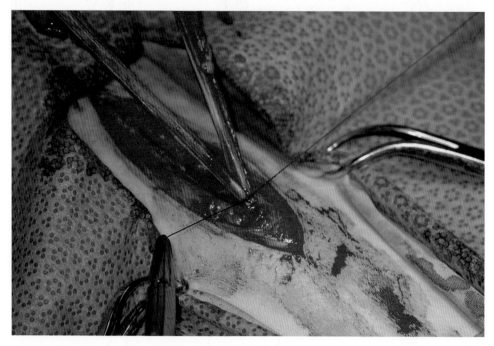

Figure 18.142   Tightening the surgeon's throw on the uterine body.

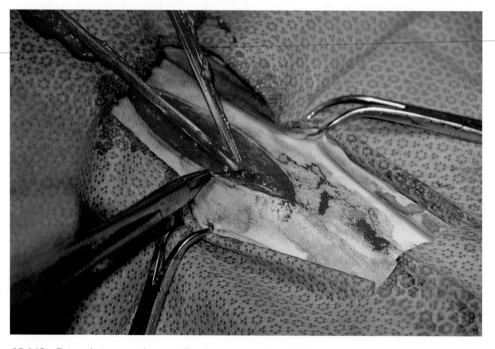

Figure 18.143   Preparing to cut the transfixation suture after finishing a surgeon's knot and covering it with a square knot.

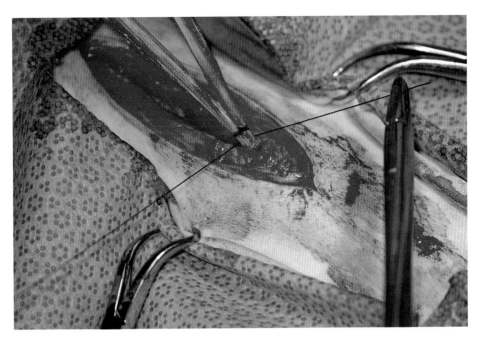

Figure 18.144   Preparing to place a circumferential square knot proximal (caudal) to the transfixation suture on the uterine body.

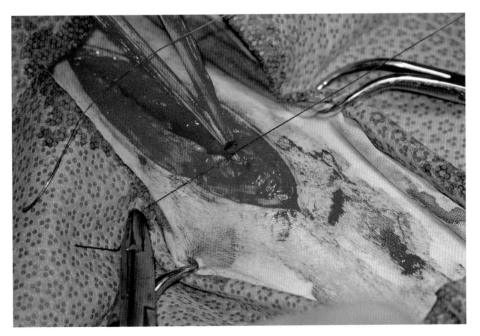

Figure 18.145   Tightening the first throw of a square knot proximal (caudal) to the transfixation suture on the uterine body.

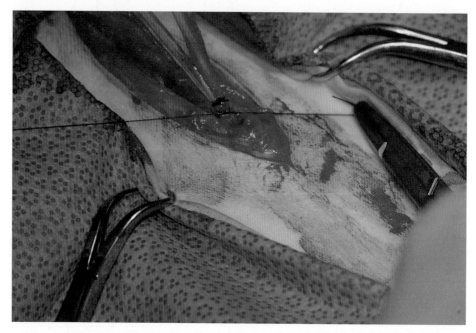

Figure 18.146   Finishing a square knot on the uterine body proximal (caudal) to the transfixation suture.

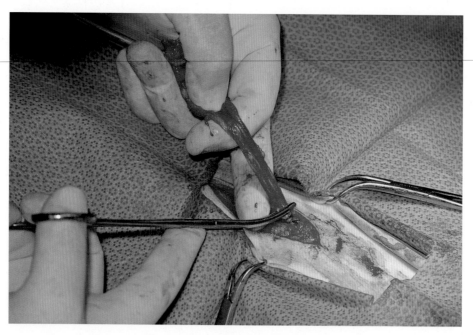

Figure 18.147   Placing a Rochester-Carmalt forceps on the portion of the uterus to be excised. The forceps is placed loosely close to the transfixation suture and moved away from the transfixation suture to milk blood away from site to be incised.

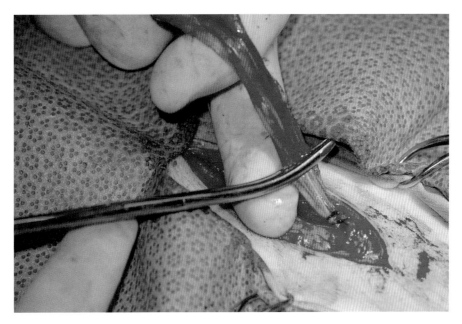

Figure 18.148 Securing the Rochester-Carmalt forceps on the uterus. Note the blanched appearance of the portion of the uterus to be incised.

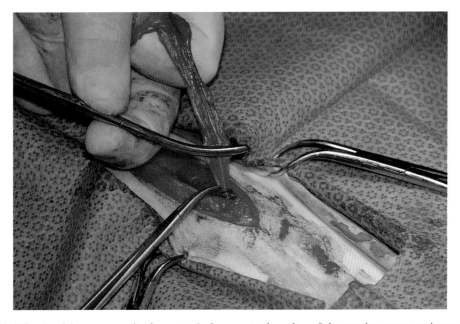

Figure 18.149 Applying a mosquito hemostatic forceps to the edge of the uterine stump prior to incising the uterine body. This maneuver is performed to prevent the uterine stump from disappearing into the abdomen when the uterus is incised and the horns and ovaries are removed.

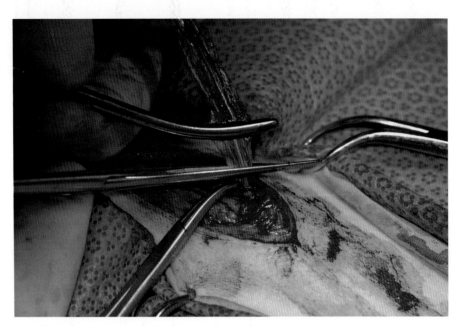

Figure 18.150 Incising the uterine body just distal (cranial) to the mosquito hemostatic forceps attached to the right edge of the uterine body.

and Rochester-Carmalt forceps (Figures 18.150 and 18.151) to complete the excision of the uterus and ovaries. Grasp the uterine stump with thumb forceps (Figure 18.152), remove the mosquito hemostat (Figure 18.153), and check for bleeding before carefully releasing the stump into the peritoneal cavity (Figures 18.154 and 18.155).

Abdominal closure begins as soon as the uterine stump is within the abdomen and there are no signs of bleeding that require inspection. The external rectus sheath must be securely closed to ensure that abdominal wall dehiscence does not occur. Proper closure necessitates good visualization of the external rectus sheath (Figure 18.156). If the initial surgical approach was properly performed, the external rectus sheath will be readily visible. If for any reason the external rectus sheath is not easily seen, the subcutaneous tissue obscuring it should be incised or excised. [Note: Incising or excising additional tissue at this time causes more tissue trauma and creates dead space; therefore, it is best to make a good surgical approach, optimally exposing the linea alba before incising into the abdomen, in order to facilitate a good closure.] Close the external rectus sheath using long-acting synthetic absorbable suture material in a simple continuous suture pattern (Figures 18.157–18.166). Suture size varies with the size of the patient, but general guidelines are 0 for large dogs, 2–0 for medium-sized dogs, and 3–0 for small dogs and cats. Tie three square knots (six throws) in each end of the continuous suture pattern. In general, suture bites should be 5 mm from the incision edge and 5 mm apart. Somewhat wider and longer bites can be used for large dogs. Suture bites less than 5 mm are more likely to cause ischemia of wound edges than wider and longer bites.

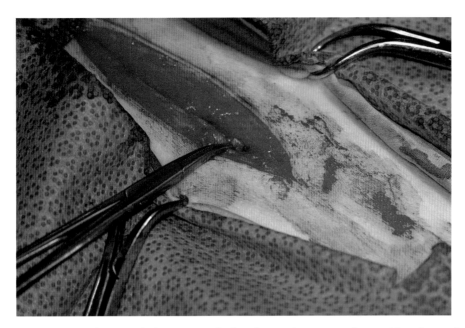

Figure 18.151 Mosquito hemostatic forceps attached to the uterine stump after excising the uterine horns and ovaries.

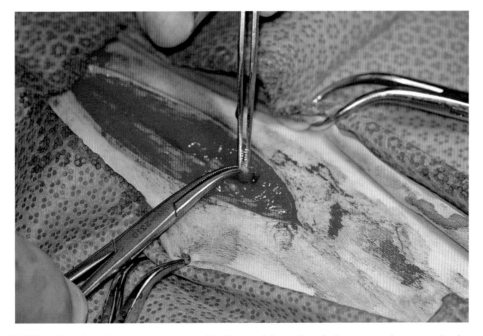

Figure 18.152 Grasping the uterine stump with Brown-Adson thumb forceps as the mosquito hemostatic forceps are released from the edge of the uterine stump.

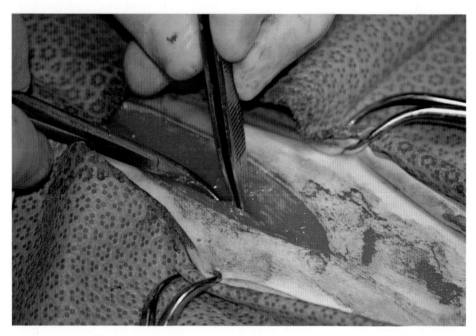

Figure 18.153   Placing the uterine stump into the abdomen to relieve tension on it and check for security of the ligatures.

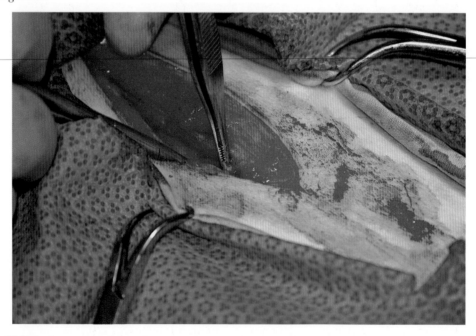

Figure 18.154   Inspecting the uterine stump for security of ligatures and absence of hemorrhage. The right abdominal wall is being retracted by mosquito hemostatic forceps to facilitate visualization of the uterine stump.

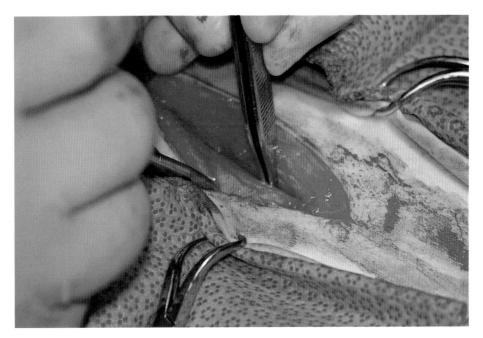

Figure 18.155   Final placement of uterine stump into the abdomen.

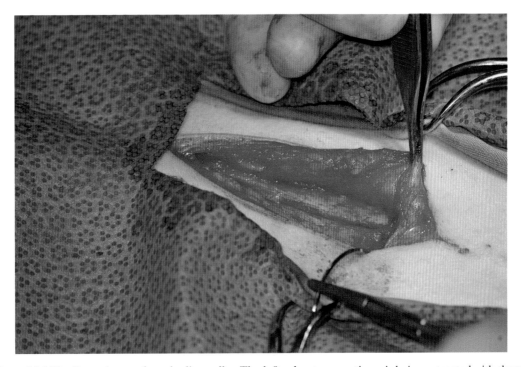

Figure 18.156   Preparing to close the linea alba. The left subcutaneous tissue is being retracted with thumb forceps, and the suture needle is retracting the right subcutaneous tissue to visualize the caudal extent of the linea alba incision.

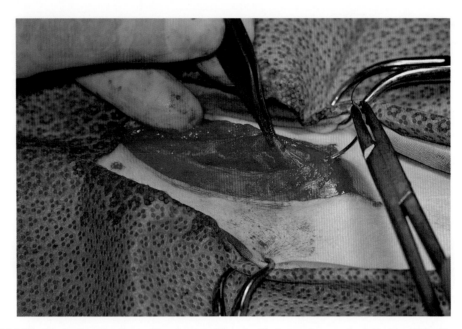

Figure 18.157   Beginning the linea alba closure. The needle is starting on the left side of the linea alba in the caudal aspect of the incision, approximately 5 mm from the incised edge. Linea alba closure is being achieved in this case with 2–0 polydioxanone suture.

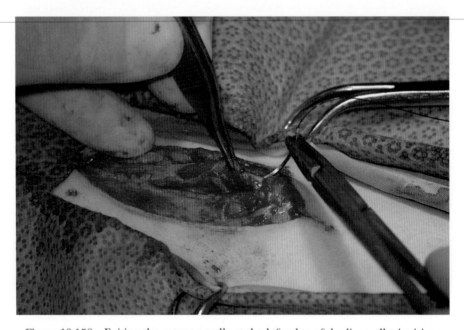

Figure 18.158   Exiting the suture needle at the left edge of the linea alba incision.

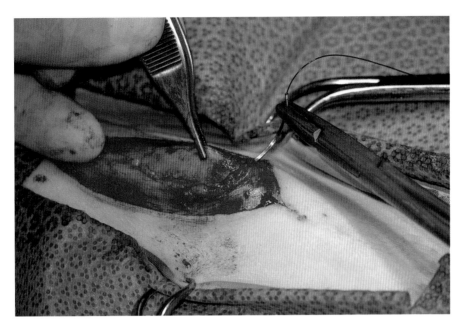

Figure 18.159   Lifting the right edge of the linea alba incision onto the suture needle that is engaging the left side of the linea alba.

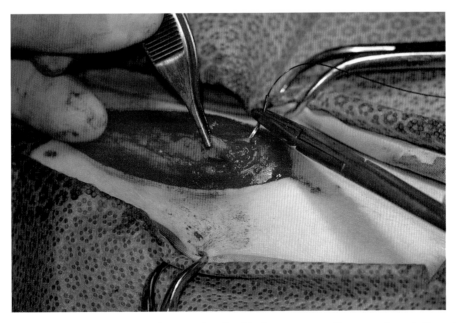

Figure 18.160   Penetrating the external rectus sheath with the suture needle approximately 5 mm from the linea alba incision.

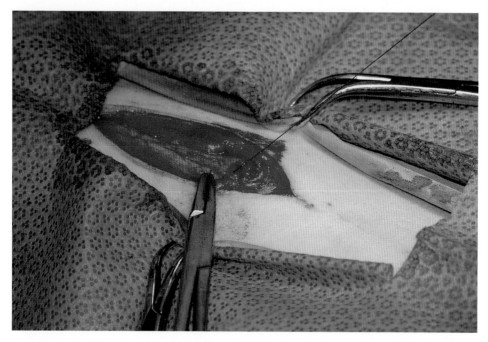

Figure 18.161 Tying three square knots at the caudal end of the linea alba incision.

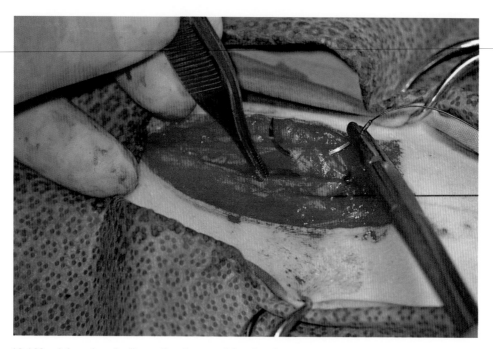

Figure 18.162 Advancing the linea alba closure with a simple continuous suture. A suture bite is being taken in the external rectus sheath approximately 5 mm from the left incision edge and exits at the incision edge.

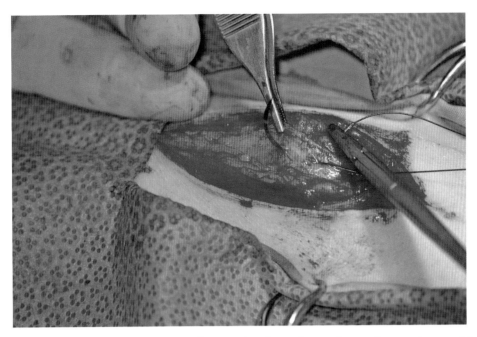

Figure 18.163 Penetrating the right external rectus sheath to advance the continuous closure of the linea alba.

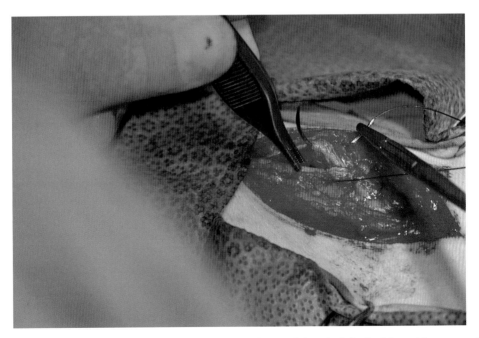

Figure 18.164 Finishing the linea alba closure toward the cranial end of the incision with a suture bite in the left external rectus sheath.

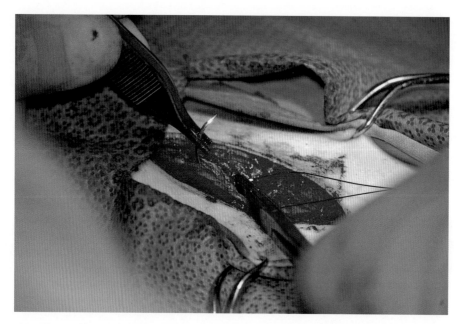

Figure 18.165   Finishing the linea alba closure toward the cranial end of the incision with a bite in the right external rectus sheath. The next bite will preserve a suture loop for tying.

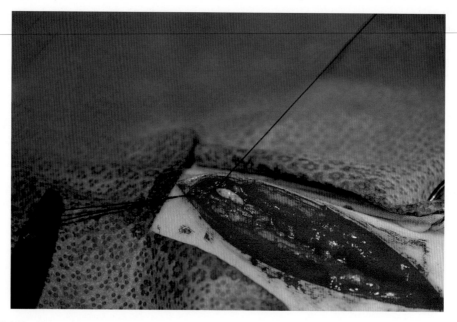

Figure 18.166   Tying the continuous suture pattern at the cranial edge of linea alba incision. Three square knots are recommended.

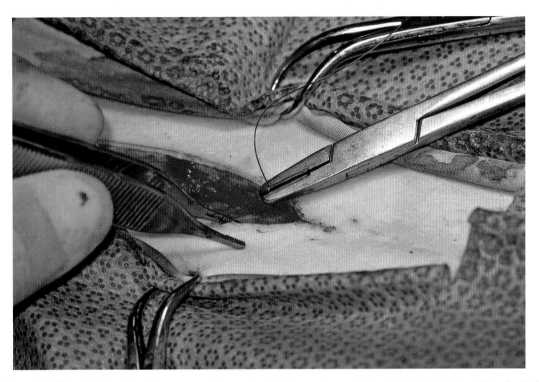

Figure 18.167 Closing the subcutaneous tissues, beginning at the caudal end of the incision with a buried knot. The first bite is taken deep in the wound, in the external rectus sheath, and is directed toward the right side. The subcutaneous tissue is being closed in this case with 3–0 poliglecaprone 25.

After completing the external rectus sheath closure, the subcutaneous tissue is closed with short-acting synthetic absorbable suture material in a simple continuous suture pattern, burying the knots on each end. Suture size varies with the size of the patient, but general guidelines are 2–0 for large dogs, 3–0 for medium-sized dogs, and 4–0 for small dogs and cats. Some surgeons prefer to perform a strictly subcutaneous closure followed by skin sutures to complete the skin apposition. Others prefer to perform an intradermal (also called subcuticular) technique to close the skin edges without the need for skin sutures. Demonstrated in this chapter is a subcuticular pattern that closes the skin edges so that skin sutures are supportive and are not dependent upon to bring the dermal edges into apposition (Figures 18.167–18.210). If performed meticulously, skin sutures may not be necessary for this subcuticular pattern. Whichever subcutaneous closure is used, take a bite down into the external rectus sheath every third or fourth suture passage to eliminate dead space. When skin sutures are used, an interrupted pattern is preferred. Common skin suture patterns include simple interrupted, cruciate, and figure-of-eight sutures (Figure 18.211). Synthetic nonabsorbable monofilament suture is preferred for skin sutures.

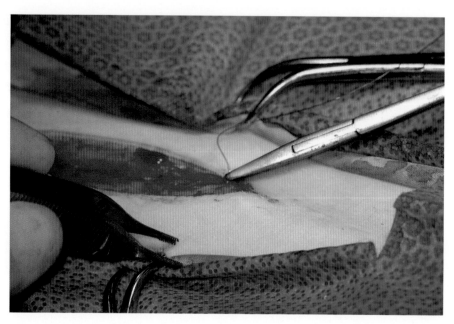

Figure 18.168 Bringing the suture needle up from the bite in the external rectus sheath toward the skin edge at the caudal end of the incision.

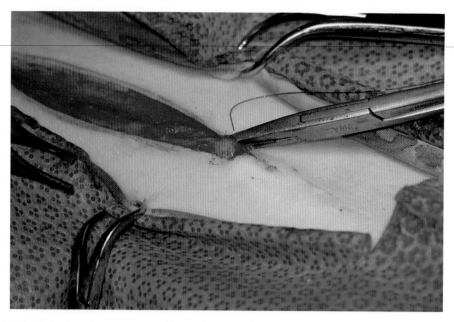

Figure 18.169 Bringing the suture needle up from the bite in the external rectus sheath, through the subcutaneous fat, and out of the wound at the skin edge, engaging the dermis at the caudal end of the incision.

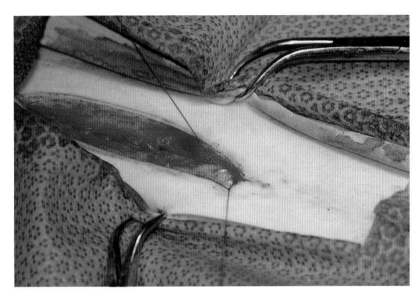

Figure 18.170 Completion of first suture pass in the process of burying the knot at the beginning of subcutaneous closure in the caudal aspect of the incision. The needle portion of the strand is toward the right (lower portion of the photograph) and the needleless portion of the strand is toward the left and cranial (upper portion of the photograph).

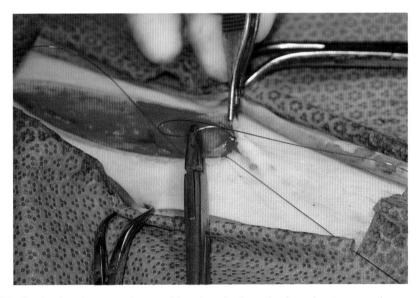

Figure 18.171 Beginning the second pass of burying the knot in the subcutaneous closure at the caudal aspect of the incision. The needle engages the dermis under the left skin edge across from the exit on the opposite skin edge.

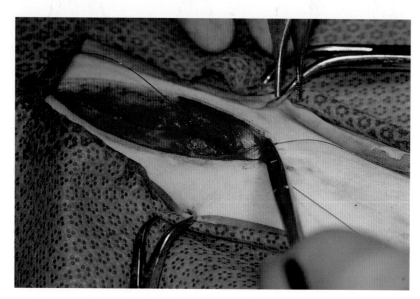

Figure 18.172   Finishing the second pass of burying the knot in the subcutaneous closure on the left side at the caudal aspect of the incision. The needle comes out in the deep tissues and will be tied to the opposite strand that engages the external rectus sheath.

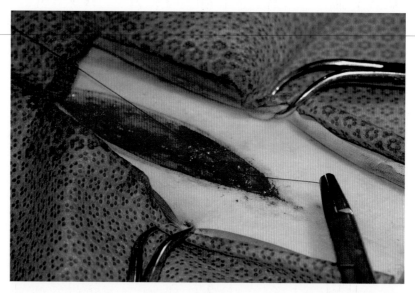

Figure 18.173   Beginning to tie the buried knot in the subcutaneous closure at the caudal aspect of the incision. The first throw of a square knot is being tied. Note that the strands are pulled parallel to the incision, instead of the usual perpendicular orientation, in order to help sink the knot deep under the subcutaneous fat.

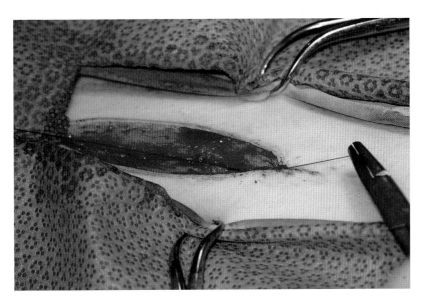

Figure 18.174 Tightening the first throw of the buried knot in the subcutaneous closure at the caudal aspect of the incision. Note that the strands are pulled parallel to the incision to help sink the knot deep under the subcutaneous fat.

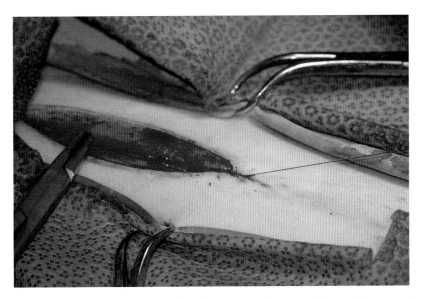

Figure 18.175 Finishing the buried knot in the subcutaneous closure at the caudal aspect of the incision. Note that the strands are pulled parallel to the incision to sink the knot deep under the subcutaneous fat. Three square knots are recommended.

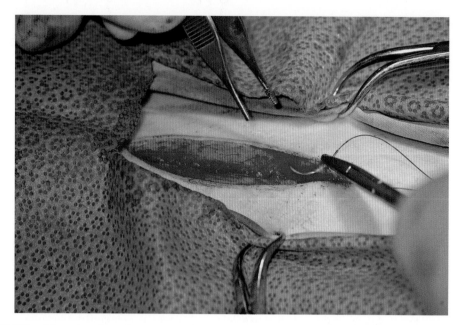

Figure 18.176 Advancing the subcutaneous closure by engaging the dermis just under the skin edge on the left and avoiding the bulk of the subcutaneous fat.

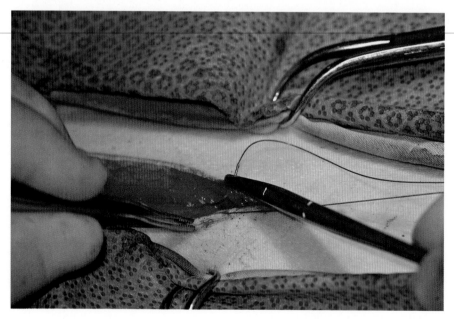

Figure 18.177 Continuing the subcutaneous closure by engaging the dermis just under the skin edge on the left, avoiding the bulk of the subcutaneous fat, and preparing to engage the dermis on the right.

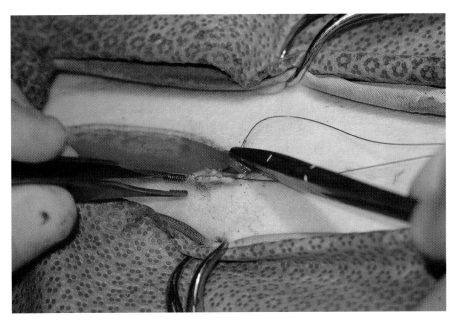

Figure 18.178 Continuing the subcutaneous closure by engaging the dermis just under the skin on both sides. Note how minimal subcutaneous fat is incorporated in the needle.

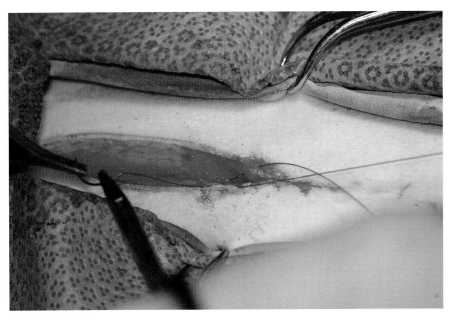

Figure 18.179 Pulling the suture that engages only dermis on each side. Note how this pattern apposes the skin edges in the completed portion of the closure in the caudal aspect of the incision.

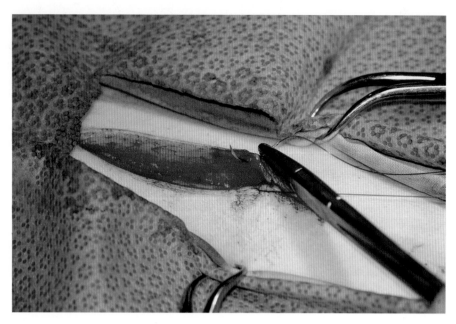

Figure 18.180 Continuing the subcutaneous closure by engaging the dermis just under the left skin edge and preparing to obliterate dead space.

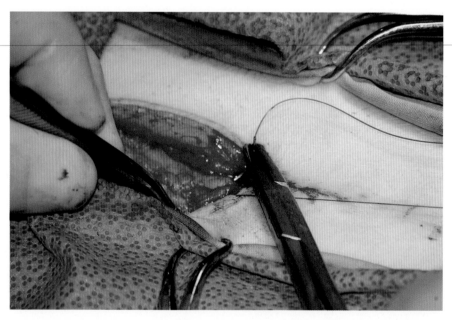

Figure 18.181 Engaging external rectus sheath as the suture needle passes toward the right side. This maneuver is done approximately every third pass in order to obliterate dead space. Note that the needle passes over the subcutaneous fat, instead of through it, before engaging the external rectus sheath.

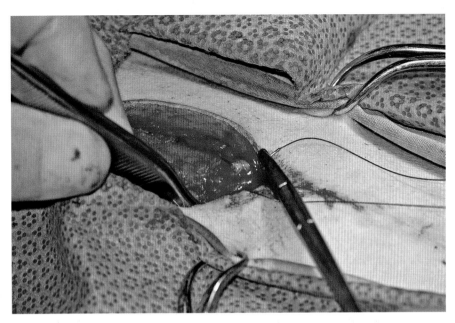

Figure 18.182 Needle exiting the external rectus sheath after engaging the dermis under the left skin edge to obliterate dead space. The needle will then pass over the right subcutaneous fat to engage the dermis under the right skin edge.

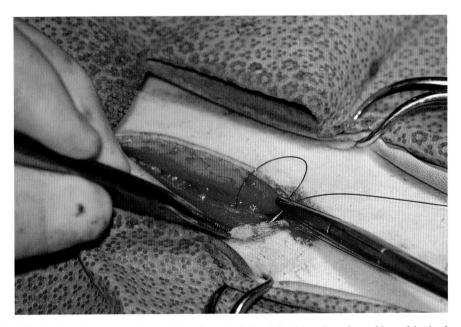

Figure 18.183 Passing the suture through the dermis of the right skin edge after taking a bite in the external rectus sheath to obliterate dead space.

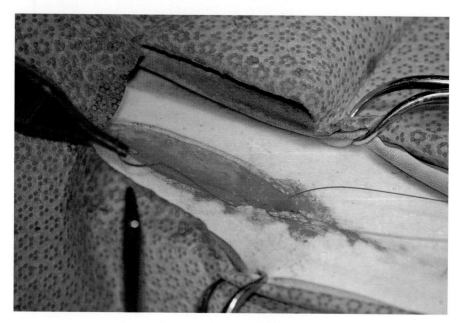

Figure 18.184 Pulling the suture that engages dermis on each side and the underlying external rectus sheath.

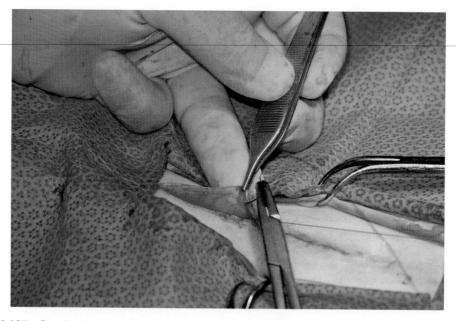

Figure 18.185 Continuing the subcutaneous closure in the mid portion of the incision on the left. Note where the needle enters the dermis and how the ring finger of the nondominant hand can be used to facilitate needle placement.

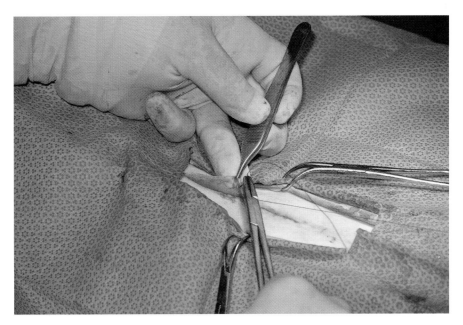

Figure 18.186 Passing the suture needle through the dermis on the left in the midportion of the incision.

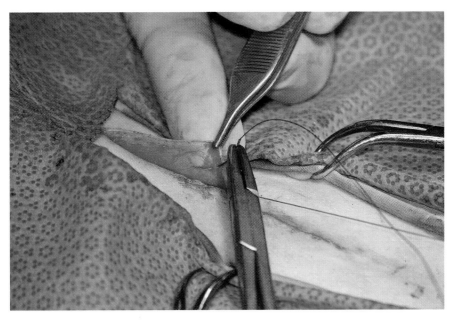

Figure 18.187 Closeup view of passing the suture needle through the dermis on the left in the midportion of the incision. Note that the thumb forceps must be used with a gentle touch to avoid excessive trauma to the skin edge.

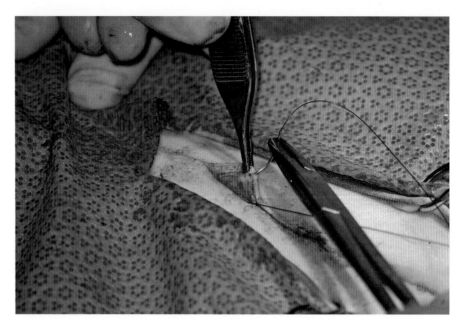

Figure 18.188   Preparing to tie a knot at the cranial end of the incision. Planning for this knot requires saving enough room for what would ordinarily be two more suture passes.

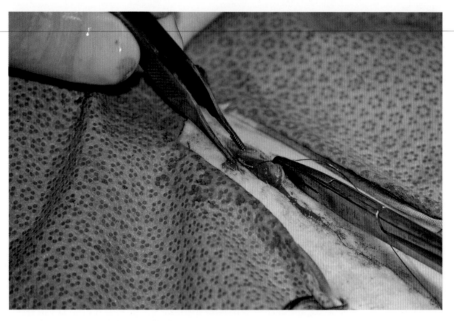

Figure 18.189   First passage of the needle in preparation for a buried knot at the cranial end of the incision. After engaging dermis just under the left skin edge, the needle is directed into the deep tissues.

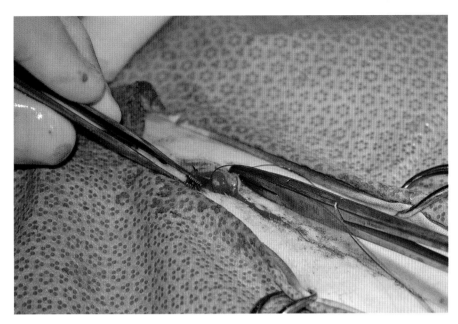

Figure 18.190 Ensuring engagement of deep tissue with the first needle passage for burying a knot at the cranial end of the incision. The deep bite is taken in the external rectus sheath.

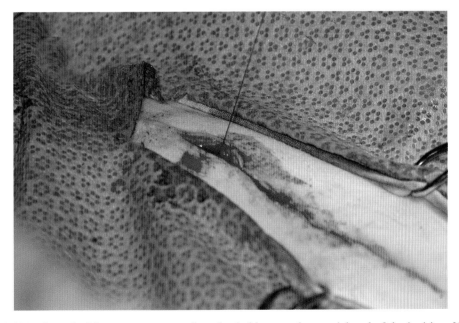

Figure 18.191 Strand of first suture passage for a buried knot at the cranial end of the incision. Note that this strand emerges from the deep tissues and will eventually be one side of a loop to which the free strand of suture will be tied.

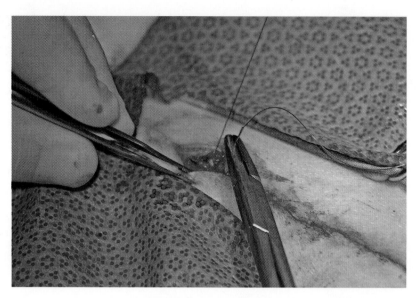

Figure 18.192   Second passage of the needle in preparation for a buried knot at the cranial end of the incision. The first strand is lifted with mild tension to somewhat exteriorize the external rectus sheath to facilitate taking a needle bite in the fascia. After engaging the sheath, the needle will engage the dermis just under the right skin edge and the resultant loop of suture will be preserved for tying.

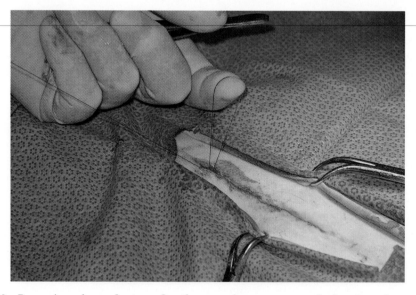

Figure 18.193   Preserving a loop of suture after the second suture passage for burying a knot at the cranial end of the incision. Note that both strands of the loop emerge from the depths of the wound and the free strand exits just under the right skin edge. One more needle pass will be necessary before the knot can be tied.

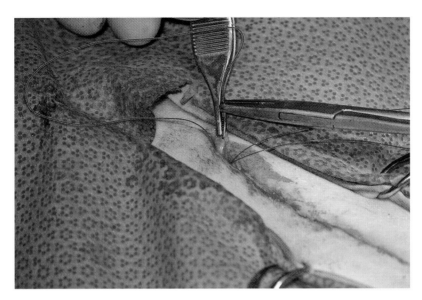

Figure 18.194   Third and final needle pass in preparation for a buried knot at the cranial edge of the incision. Note that dermis is engaged just under the left skin edge so that when the knot is tied, the skin edges will be apposed between this location and the right skin edge where the opposite strand is emerging. After engaging the dermis, the needle will be directed into the deep tissues to engage the external rectus sheath next to the loop strands.

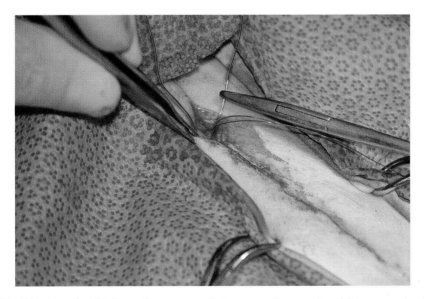

Figure 18.195   Directing the third needle pass toward the external rectus sheath in preparation for a buried knot at the cranial edge of the incision. The needle has engaged the dermis and is angled slightly caudally toward the loop strands.

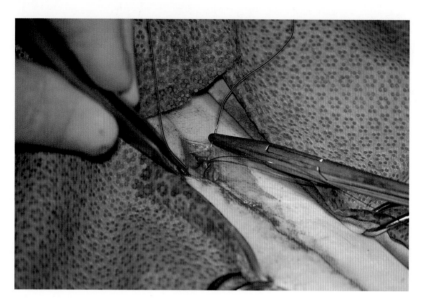

Figure 18.196   Engaging the external rectus sheath with the final needle pass in preparation for a buried knot at the cranial edge of the incision. Note that the needle engages the external rectus sheath just cranial to the preserved deep loop. Care is taken to make sure the needle will exit the wound between the deep loop (retracted caudally) and the final appositional strands (located cranially). Otherwise, the appositional strands will prevent the knot from sinking deeply.

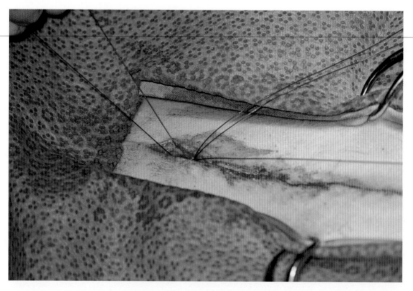

Figure 18.197   Location of strands immediately prior to tying a buried knot at the cranial end of the incision (as viewed by the surgeon). The deep loop is being retracted caudally and to the dog's left and the free strand (also deep) that will be tied to that loop is being pulled caudally parallel to the incision. The two strands in the cranial aspect of the wound will appose the skin edges when the free strand is pulled and tied to the deep loop.

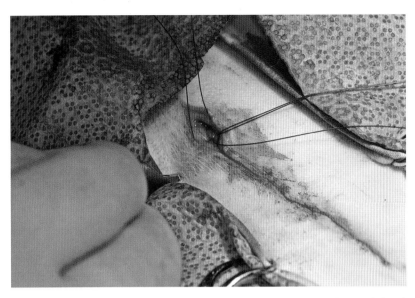

Figure 18.198 Location of strands immediately prior to tying a buried knot at the cranial end of the incision (ventral view). Note how the deep strand and deep loop are located between the last two appositional suture passages. The last appositional suture passage is the superficial loop in the cranial aspect of the incision. It is important that the deep strand and deep loop are both on the same side of the superficial loop, or else the superficial loop will prevent the knot from sinking into the deep portion of the wound when the deep strand and loop are tied.

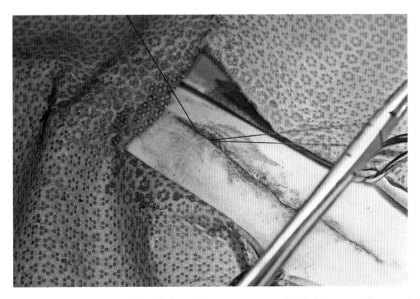

Figure 18.199 Tying the deep strand and deep loop to create a buried knot at the cranial end of the incision. Note that the strand and loop are pulled parallel to the incision to facilitate sinking the knot within the wound. Also note how equal tension is applied to each strand of the deep loop.

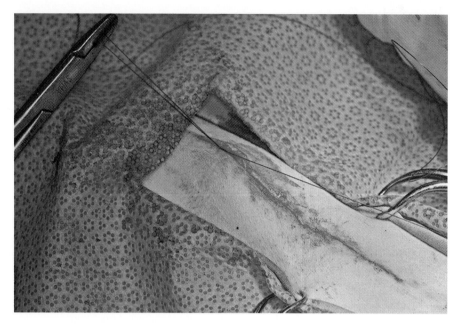

Figure 18.200 Completing the buried knot at the cranial end of the incision. Three square knots have been placed.

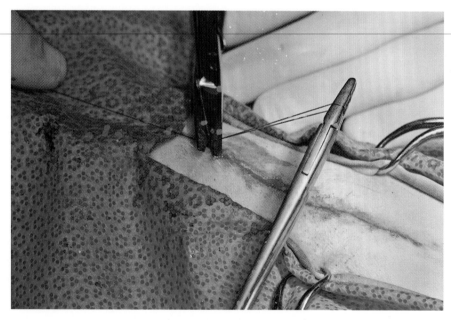

Figure 18.201 Cutting the loop of the knot at the cranial end of the incision in preparation to sink the knot. The loop is cut as close to the knot as possible. "On the knot, but not the knot."

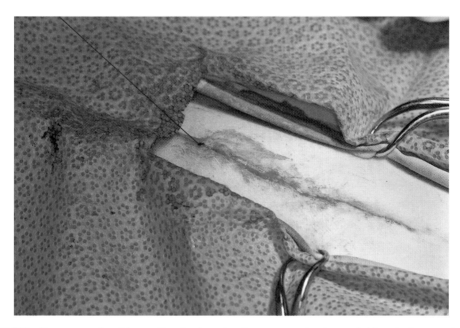

Figure 18.202   Deep strand and knot after the loop has been cut and prior to sinking the knot at the cranial end of the incision.

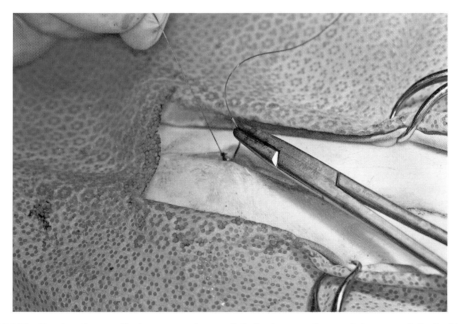

Figure 18.203   Passing the needle in preparation to sink the knot at the cranial aspect of the incision. The deep strand is elevated to visualize the knot and place the needle into the deep tissue immediately adjacent to the knot.

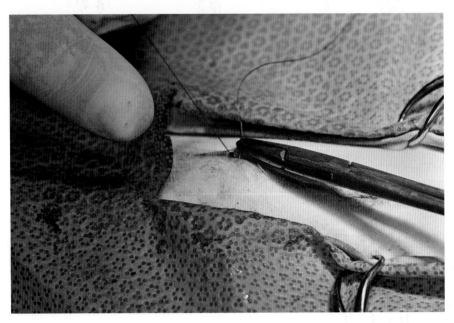

Figure 18.204 Passing the needle laterally for sinking the knot at the cranial aspect of the incision. The needle is passed up from the deep tissues toward the skin on the right side of the incision (toward the right-handed surgeon).

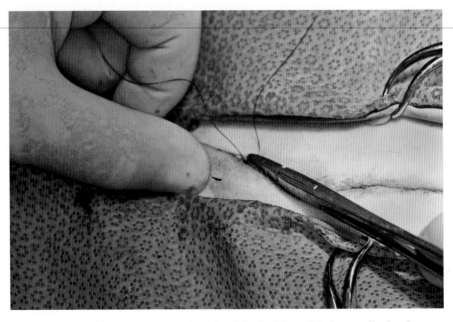

Figure 18.205 Penetrating the skin on the right side of the incision with the needle that has engaged deep tissues near the knot.

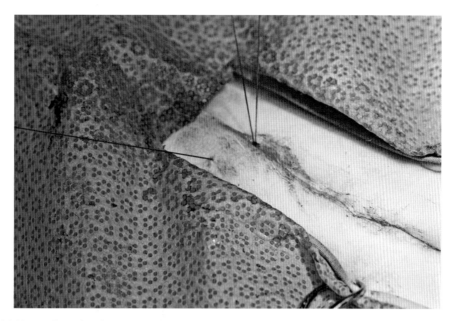

Figure 18.206   Pulling the deep suture strand through the skin to the right of the incision in preparation to sink the knot at the cranial aspect of the incision. When the strand is pulled completely, the loop that is apparent over the knot will disappear as will the knot.

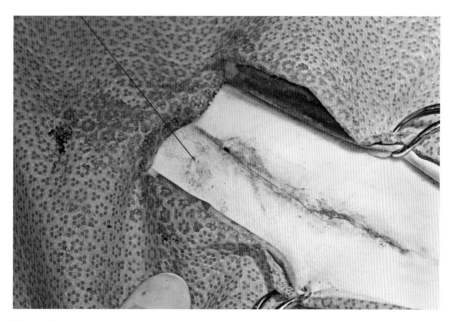

Figure 18.207   Pulling the deep suture strand through the skin on the right side of the incision to make the loop attached to the knot disappear in preparation to sink the knot at the cranial aspect of the incision.

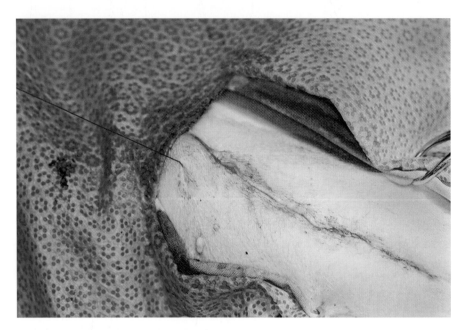

Figure 18.208 Sinking the suture knot at the cranial aspect of the incision by pulling snugly on the deep suture strand exiting to the right of the incision.

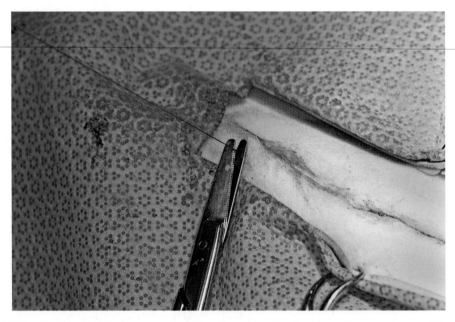

Figure 18.209 Cutting the deep suture strand that is attached to the buried knot at the cranial end of the incision. Tension is held on the strand while suture scissors cut the strand at skin level so that the end of the suture retracts under the skin.

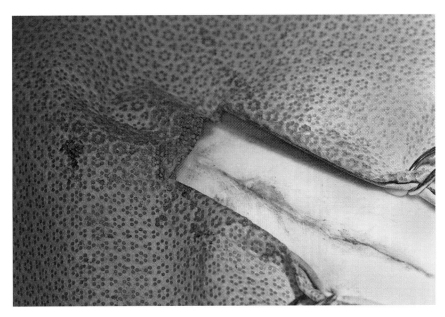

Figure 18.210   Final appearance of ovariohysterectomy incision after subcutaneous closure. If there is good skin edge apposition without gapping when lateral tension is applied by the surgeon's fingers, then skin sutures are optional.

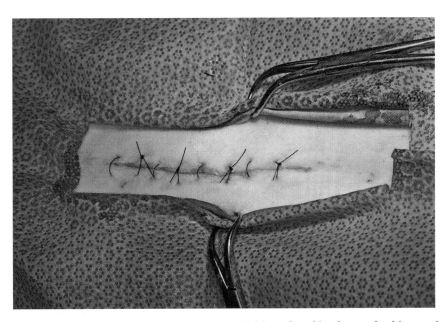

Figure 18.211   Final appearance of ovariohysterectomy incision after skin closure. In this case, interrupted figure-of-eight 3–0 nylon sutures have been used.

ADDITIONAL RESOURCES

Additional information about ovariohysterectomy in small animal surgery can be found in the following textbooks:

1. Bojrab MJ, ed. *Current Techniques in Small Animal Surgery*, 4th ed. Baltimore, Maryland: Williams & Wilkens, 1998.

2. Fossum TW, ed. *Small Animal Surgery*, 3rd ed. St. Louis, Missouri: Mosby Elsevier, 2007.

3. Slatter D, ed. *Textbook of Small Animal Surgery*, 3rd ed. Philadelphia, Pennsylvania: Saunders, 2003.

Chapter 19

POSTOPERATIVE PAIN MANAGEMENT

John P. Punke and Fred Anthony Mann

Dying is nothing, but pain is a very serious matter
HENRY JACOB BIGELOW, 1871

Henry J. Bigelow, MD (1818–1890) was a surgeon and anesthesiologist in the days when opium and hemp were common analgesics. He realized the importance of sound pain management as the basis of quality medicine and surgery and the need for improvement in his time. The importance of adequate pain management in veterinary patients cannot be stressed enough today.

A textbook on surgery could not be complete without a chapter addressing pain management. The degree of pain induced by surgery is dependent on the underlying disease process, anatomic location, invasiveness of the procedure, and concurrent disease. For example, one would expect a fracture repair to induce more pain than a routine castration. In general, orthopedic pain is considered to be more severe than soft tissue pain. And, premedicating patients before they experience injury and pain (i.e., preemptive analgesia) has been shown to significantly decrease postoperative discom-

fort. Analgesic plans should be tailored to each patient's disease, behavior, and pain tolerance, and modified based on response to treatments.

Performing an indicated surgery is in the patient's best interest, but every surgery induces pain to some degree, and that pain must be abated for the patient's wellbeing. Cessation of pain is obviously important for patient comfort, but is also beneficial to the overall healing process. Studies in human beings have shown that appropriate analgesic use speeds healing, decreases hospital stays, and decreases postoperative complications and mortality rates. Patients with adequate pain control eat sooner after surgery, heal faster, and have fewer complications.[1,2] The mechanisms behind these results are complicated and are not fully understood. Pain is a complex entity that involves physical, emotional, and psychological components. The effects of pain on future emotions and perception of future pain can be long lasting. Studies have shown that men who were circumcised as infants without pain control have a significantly decreased pain tolerance compared to uncircumcised adults, or those with adequate pain control at the time of circumcision.[3–5] This effect is independent

Fundamentals of Small Animal Surgery, 1st edition.
By Fred Anthony Mann, Gheorghe M. Constantinescu and Hun-Young Yoon.
© 2011 Blackwell Publishing Ltd.

of conscious memory since these procedures were performed within days of birth. Perhaps puppies and kittens with adequate pain control at the time of castration or ovariohysterectomy would be better pets and patients with an increased tolerance for pain in the future as well.

In addition to the obvious immediate and potential long-term benefits to the patient, appropriate analgesic use can be considered good practice management and business as well. Veterinary technicians and staff are compassionate people. Morale is quickly injured when a patient under their care is thought to be suffering without adequate pain control. Similarly, today's pet owners increasingly see their pets as family members. They do not want their family members to suffer unnecessarily and will readily invest in analgesic therapy for their pets.

Postoperative analgesic therapy should not be optional for pet owners. The price of appropriate analgesia should be included in the cost of a given procedure without question. A veterinarian would not offer a client the option of ligating an ovarian pedicle or not during an ovariohysterectomy due to the severe potential complications for the patient. Why make analgesia care optional given all of its advantages to patient care?

PATHOPHYSIOLOGY OF ACUTE PAIN

It is beyond the scope of this chapter to delve deeply into the pathophysiology and modulation of pain. There are numerous textbooks dedicated to the physiology of pain alone. It is necessary, however, for a clinician to realize that there are many processes that intertwine and overlap to result in the sensation of pain. Addressing only one mechanism of pain or inflammation may alleviate some of the negative sensation, but may not completely resolve the pain, depending on the pain's source and severity.

Pain is a complex entity that begins with *nociception*. Nociception is the process by which an insult results in the stimulation of special-ized nerve fibers termed nociceptors. Nociceptors come in three forms determined by the noxious stimulus that they detect: mechanosensitive, thermosensitive, and chemosensitive. Mechanoreceptors respond to stretching, compression, and crushing. Thermoreceptors respond to heat and cold. Chemoreceptors respond to a large number of compounds, including neurotransmitters (acetylcholine, neurokinin-1, and others), prostaglandins ($A_{2\alpha}$, thromboxane, and others), bradykinin, histamine, proteolytic enzymes, acids, cytokines (tumor necrosis factor, interleukins, and others), and leukotrienes. Once nociceptors have been stimulated beyond their threshold potential, an action potential is propagated from a peripheral nerve to the spinal cord. Peripheral nerves can be of two general types: myelinated A fibers and nonmyelinated C fibers. Type A fibers are fast conducting and result in an acute, localized, sharp, and rapid onset of pain. Type C fibers when stimulated result in a diffuse, chronic, dull, throbbing pain. Both A and C peripheral fibers terminate in the dorsal horn of the spinal cord before ascending to the brain for conscious perception. Conscious perception of nociception is the sensation of pain. Other concurrent sensations or observations (the classical signs of inflammation) may be present as a result of cytokine-induced inflammation at the site of injury: redness (rubor), heat (calor), swelling (tumor), pain (dolor), and loss of function (functio laesa). Withdrawal reflexes can be stimulated from nociception at the level of the spinal cord before pain is registered. And, in the brain, the reticular activating system is stimulated by nociception to cause increased awareness, cardiopulmonary effects, and stress responses.

Pain results from an intricate interaction of events, and as such, can be addressed at multiple levels. When pain is inhibited by multiple mechanisms simultaneously utilizing multiple classes of analgesics, an exponential increase in analgesic efficacy results. This is termed *multimodal analgesia*. Multimodal analgesic techniques are the basis of modern pain management, and should be used in every clinical case where anything above very mild pain exists. A common example of multimodal analgesia is to use a nonsteroidal anti-inflammatory drug (NSAID), opioid, and local analgesic technique in combination. The resulting effect would be almost complete elimination of pain in the immediately postoperative period by the local analgesic drug, and persistently lower levels of pain sensation in the following hours and days due to inhibition of prostaglandins (NSAID) at the tissue level and blockade of mu receptors (opioid) in the brain and dorsal horn of the spinal cord.

Another major principle in modern analgesic therapy is that of *preemptive analgesia*. The rationale for preemptive analgesia is that once pain has occurred, higher doses of analgesics are required to control that pain. Waiting for pain to occur is not desirable because of the decreased ability to control the pain, and because the risk for drug side effects is increased as increased dosages of drugs are used. Therefore, it is more desirable to treat pain before it occurs. In other words, the best time to start treating *postoperative* pain is *preoperatively*.

The need for preemptive analgesia comes from the physiologic process of *central sensitization*, also known as the "windup phenomenon." Intense pain activates amino-hydroxy-methyl-isoxazolepropionate/kainate and N-methyl-D-aspartate (NMDA) receptors. In response, signaling pathways alter gene expression and increase the responsiveness of the central nervous system to further noxious stimuli. Thus, future pain levels are increased over what they would be otherwise, making control with analgesic therapy more difficult.

LOCAL ANESTHETICS

Of all the analgesics available to veterinarians, local anesthetics are the only class that completely blocks pain sensation. They do so by reversibly blocking the transduction of nociception by peripheral nerves. Normally, nerve fibers send sensory signals to the central nervous system by depolarization of nerve membranes via a rapid inward intracellular flux of sodium ions from the extracellular space. Local anesthetics block this process by inhibiting the conformational change of the sodium ion channels, thus preventing sodium ion influx and signal transduction.

Traditionally, local anesthetics have been more commonly used in large animal veterinary practice than small animal practice. However, there are many opportunities for their increased usage in small animals as well. In regard to postoperative pain management, the utility of local anesthetics is greater when used in a preemptive manner. Since the majority of effects occur locally, local anesthetics can be used in a variety of methods with high efficacy and little to no systemic side effects (Table 19.1). Local anesthetics are most effective when directly applied to the nerve or nerves that would transmit the nociceptive signal to the central nervous system, as with specific nerve blocks and epidurals. However, local anesthetics can also be used regionally, as with lidocaine patches, line blocks, intra-articular injections, and regional limb perfusions. Further reading of anesthesia textbooks is recommended for instructional purposes, especially in regard to specific nerve blocks techniques and epidural administration. Dosages for local and intravenous (lidocaine only) use are given in Table 19.2.

Lidocaine is the local anesthetic drug used for constant rate infusion (CRI) because it has the highest safety margin for intravenous administration. Constant rate infusion calculations are described later in this chapter. When administering intradermal or local infusions of local anesthetics, one should always aspirate first before injection to avoid inadvertent intravenous or intra-arterial administration. Similarly, lidocaine and bupivacaine are sometimes supplemented with epinephrine (5 µg/mL) to cause local vasoconstriction and prolong

Table 19.1 Potential routes for local anesthetic administration

Route	Technique	Examples
Nerve block	Injected adjacent to the specific nerve of interest	Onychectomy, dental nerve blocks
Incisional line block	Injected over the planned incision, or around the lesion	Prior to any skin incision, laceration repair
Splash block	Applied directly on a wound or exposed nerve	Open wound care, nerves exposed during amputation
Transdermal	Application of lidocaine patches directly to or around a lesion	Around celiotomy incision
Regional limb perfusion	Injected into the vein of a limb distal to an applied tourniquet	For complete nerve blockade of a distal limb to facilitate toe amputation
Epidural	Injected directly into the epidural space	Prior to pelvic limb orthopedic surgery
Intra-articular	Directly injected into the joint of interest (Do not use bupivacaine)	Intraoperatively for joint surgery
Constant rate intravenous infusion	Given as a continuous infusion as an adjunctive analgesic (lidocaine only; avoid lidocaine infusion in cats)	Postoperatively for major orthopedic or soft tissue surgery

anesthetic effect. Intravascular injection could cause untoward cardiovascular effects. Either lidocaine or mepivacaine can be used for intra-articular injection, but lidocaine has been shown to enhance methylprednisolone-induced chondrocyte death in vitro. Bupivacaine has been associated with chondrocyte death when given intra-articularly in both people and dogs.

Local analgesics can also be given epidurally to completely block motor function and sensation through the spinal nerve roots bilaterally. Epidural administration provides profound pain control and motor blockade of most of the anatomy caudal to the umbilicus including the pelvic limbs, perineum, and tail. When combined with an opioid (usually preservative-free morphine), the epidural drug combination is synergistic and is an excellent option for patients requiring surgery caudal to the umbilicus. The spread of local anesthetic in the epidural space is a function of both concentration and volume of the drug administered. The reader is referred to other resources to learn technique and relevant anatomy involved in performing epidural anesthesia, but epidural administration can be easily and safely performed in experienced hands.

Increased systemic concentrations of local anesthetics have a predictable pattern of central nervous toxicity characterized by central nervous system excitement followed by depression, apnea, and cardiovascular collapse. When given intravenously, bupivacaine can cause cardiac arrhythmias and ventricular fibrillation. The neurologic side effects of local anesthetics occur in cats at lower concentrations than in dogs. Allergic-type reactions to local anesthetics are rare, and more often associated with the preservative (methylparaben) than the anesthetic itself.

OPIOIDS

Opioid analgesics are some of the safest and most effective analgesic drugs available to the

Table 19.2   Dosages (mg/kg, unless otherwise noted) and some unique properties of local anesthetics, N-methyl-D-aspartate receptor antagonists, and alpha-two agonists usedin veterinary medicine

Drug	Dog dosages	Cat dosages	Unique properties
Local anesthetics			
Bupivacaine	Up to 2 for local infusion 1–1.5 for epidural administration	Up to 1 for local infusion 1–1.5 for epidural administration	Not for intravenous use
Lidocaine	Up to 6 local infusion 2–4 IV bolus, then 0.15–0.45 mg/kg/h CRI 4.4 for epidural	Up to 3 local infusion 0.25–1 IV bolus, then 0.06–0.24 mg/kg/h CRI* 4.4 for epidural	Take care to not give the local infusion dosage intravenously. *Although a dosage is given, avoid intravenous use in cats.
Mepivacaine	Up to 6 local infusion	Up to 3 local infusion	Not for intravenous use
N-methyl-D-aspartate Receptor Antagonists			
Ketamine	0.5 IV for induction 0.6 mg/kg/h CRI intraoperatively 0.12 mg/kg/h CRI for postoperative analgesia	0.5 IV for induction 0.6 mg/kg/h CRI intraoperatively 0.12 mg/kg/h CRI for postoperative analgesia	
Tiletamine	6–10 IM for short duration 9–13 IM for induction of anesthesia	6–10 IM for short duration 9–13 IM for induction of anesthesia	Only available in combination with zolazepam
Amantadine	3–5 PO q 24	3–5 PO q 24	Literature only supports usage for chronic pain.
Alpha-two Agonists			
Xylazine	0.5–1 IV 1.1–2.2 IM, SC	0.5–1 IV 1.1 IM	
Medetomidine	0.01–0.02 IV for short sedation and analgesia use 0.001–0.002 mg/kg/h CRI for extended sedation and analgesia	0.015–0.03 IV for short sedation and analgesia use	
Dexmedetomidine	0.005–0.01 IV for short sedation and analgesia use 0.0005–0.001 mg/kg/h CRI for extended sedation and analgesia	0.008–0.015 IV for short sedation and analgesia use	

CRI, constant rate infusion; IV, intravenous; IM, intramuscular; PO, by mouth; SC, subcutaneous.

veterinarian for managing acute and postoperative pain. They rapidly act to provide analgesia without loss of consciousness or mobility. Opioids exert their effect by binding to one of four opioid receptors: mu, delta, kappa, or nociceptin opioid peptide. Mu receptors are thought to be the receptor most relevant to opioid activity. Traditionally, mu receptors were thought to only exist in the central nervous system. However, there is recent evidence that mu receptors may also exist in peripheral tissues as well. The significance of their peripheral location is not known.

There are four general categories of opioids: full agonists, partial agonists, agonist/antagonists, and antagonists. Examples and dosages of each are listed in Table 19.3. Full mu agonists exert maximal activation of the mu receptor when bound. In general, these opioids are best used for moderate to severe pain control. Morphine is the prototypical full agonist and is generally the basis to which all other opioids are compared. Morphine is inexpensive and routinely used subcutaneously, intramuscularly, intravenously either as a bolus or constant rate infusion, or epidurally. Other examples of full mu agonists include codeine, fentanyl, hydrocodone, hydromorphone, meperidine, methadone, and oxymorphone. Each varies in its duration of action, unique side effects, availability and cost. For example, morphine can cause mast cell degranulation as an adverse side effect in dogs. Dogs with mast cell tumors should be treated with a different opioid for premedication and postoperative care. Methadone is not widely available for clinical usage in the United States; however, it has the unique property of additional analgesia and prevention of central sensitization by inhibition of the NMDA receptor as well as acting as an opioid.

Partial mu agonists bind to the mu receptor like a full agonist, but produce limited clinical effect. As a result, mu receptor partial agonists have a ceiling effect at which they maximally produce analgesia and adverse side effects as well. Buprenorphine is the best example of a mu receptor partial agonist. It has the unique ability to be given transbuccally in cats with almost identical pharmacokinetics as if given intravenously. Buprenorphine is also used commonly as a CRI with lidocaine for moderate to severe postoperative pain with seemingly less appetite suppression than morphine CRIs.

Agonist/antagonists are opioids that may stimulate and exert their effects on one opioid receptor (usually the kappa receptor) while simultaneously binding and inhibiting another opioid receptor (usually the mu receptor). Butorphanol and nalbuphine are the prototypical agonist/antagonists. Analgesia provided by butorphanol and nalbuphine is moderate at best and short lived. The duration of effect is only 1–3 hours, while sedative effects last longer. Butorphanol tends to be one of the more expensive opioids used in veterinary practice.

Antagonists have high affinity for the mu and kappa opioid receptors. They "reverse" the effects of full agonists by competitively displacing them from the receptors. Antagonists, however, do not activate receptors, thus preventing opioid activity. Antagonists are particularly useful in cases of opioid overdosage; however, the antagonist will reverse all opioid effects, including analgesia. Agonist/antagonists may be a better first choice for mild overdose. Naloxone and naltrexone are examples of full antagonists. Naloxone's clinical effects last about half the duration of naltrexone. Therefore, naltrexone may be a better antidote for longer lasting opioids.

Side effects of opioids include a variety of systems. Central nervous system depression may be a desirable side effect. However, cats may become excitable when given opioids, especially morphine. Dysphoria may also be seen in dogs, especially malamute and husky-type breeds. Bradycardia secondary to increased vagal tone may be seen in nonpainful patients. Fortunately, other cardiovascular effects of opioids are minimal. In people, respiratory depression can be profound and life-threatening.

Table 19.3   **Dosages (mg/kg) and some unique properties of opioids used in veterinary medicine**

Drug	Dog dosages	Cat dosages	Unique properties
Pure Agonists			
Codeine	1–2 PO	0.1–1 PO	Do *not* give the preparation with acetaminophen to cats
Fentanyl	0.002–0.005 IV 0.002–0.06/h IV CRI	0.001–0.005 IV 0.002–0.03/h IV CRI	Profound analgesic effects, Recommended as a CRI due to short half life, Decreases anesthesia requirements
Hydromorphone	0.05–0.2 IV, IM, SC 0.05–0.1/h CRI	0.05–0.2 IV, IM, SC 0.05–0.1/h CRI	May cause hyperthermia in cats, May elicit panting in dogs
Methadone	0.05–1.5 IM, SC, PO	0.05–0.5 IM, SC, PO	Also has NMDA receptor antagonist properties
Morphine[a]	0.3–2.0 IM, SC 0.1–0.5 IV 0.05–0.3/h CRI 0.1–0.2 epidural	0.05–0.2 IM, SC 0.1–0.2 epidural	May cause emesis, May cause mast cell degranulation
Partial Agonists			
Buprenorphine	0.005–0.03 IV, IM, SC 0.04/day CRI	0.005–0.03 IV, IM, SC 0.01–0.03 PO[b] 0.04/day CRI	Ceiling effect with analgesia and adverse side effects
Agonist-Antagonists			
Butorphanol	0.1–0.4 IV, IM, SC 0.5–2.0 PO	0.1–0.8 IV, IM, SC 0.5–1.0 PO	1–3 hours duration of analgesia
Nalbuphine	0.3–0.5 IM, SC 0.1–0.3 IV	0.2–0.4 IM, SC 0.1–0.2 IV	1–3 hours duration of analgesia
Antagonists			
Naloxone	0.002–0.04 IV	0.002–0.02 IV	Effects last up to 45 minutes
Naltrexone	0.0025–0.003 IV	0.0025–0.003 IV	Approximately twice the duration of effect as naloxone

CRI, constant rate infusion; IV, intravenous; IM, intramuscular; NMDA, N-methyl D-aspartate; PO, by mouth; SC, subcutaneous.

[a]Morphine without preservatives is recommended for epidural administration.

[b]Buprenorphine as an injectable formulation has been shown to be effective when given transbuccally to cats.

However, veterinary patients rarely suffer respiratory depression from opioid administration alone. As mentioned earlier, morphine has been associated with histamine release in dogs, especially when given intravenously. Histamine release can cause profound vasodilatation, hypotension, and cardiovascular collapse. Nausea, vomiting, and defecation are common after administration of opioids. Vomiting is more likely with subcutaneous or intramuscular administration than with intravenous boluses. With long-term use, opioids may cause constipation. Urinary retention may occur with morphine use secondary to decreased detrusor muscle tone and increased urinary bladder sphincter tone. Urinary catheterization or manual urinary bladder expression may be necessary.

NONSTEROIDAL ANTI-INFLAMMATORY DRUGS

Nonsteroidal anti-inflammatory drugs are an extensively researched drug class and the most prescribed pharmaceutical in veterinary medicine.[6] Nonsteroidal anti-inflammatory drugs act to reduce inflammation and pain by inhibition of prostaglandin synthesis. They exert their action locally at the site of tissue damage where there is release of arachidonic acid from cell walls secondary to cellular injury. They also have been shown to act within the central nervous system. Nonsteroidal anti-inflammatory drugs have been given epidurally with the same clinical effect as systemic administration.

Current research and development of NSAIDs has been guided by the COX-1:COX-2 theory of NSAID efficacy and side effects. There are multiple isoforms of the cyclooxygenase (COX) enzyme that eventually convert arachidonic acid to functional eicosanoids called prostaglandins. The two major COX enzymes are COX-1 and COX-2, though a third,

termed COX-3 (actually a splice variant of COX-1), has been identified in some species including man and the dog. In general, COX-1 is the "house-keeping" COX isoform responsible for normal homeostasis in tissues including the stomach, intestines, kidneys, platelets, and reproductive tract. Theory holds that COX-2 is produced in response to local tissue injury to promote inflammation. Working on this theory, pharmaceutical companies have developed NSAIDs that are more selective for the COX-2 enzyme in an effort to inhibit inducible COX-2 production to reduce inflammation, while minimizing NSAID side effects thought to be caused by COX-1 inhibition.

However, in opposition to the COX-1:COX-2 paradigm, COX-2 has been found to be produced at basal levels in endothelial cells, synovial cells, chondrocytes, smooth muscle cells, fibroblasts, monocytes, and macrophages. Additionally, while COX-2 selective NSAIDs have a side effect rate about 50% of the nonselective NSAIDs, severe and potentially fatal side effects still occur with COX-2 selective NSAIDs.

In addition to the COX pathway, arachidonic acid can be metabolized by the 5-lipoxygenase (5-LOX) enzyme to produce another group of eicosanoid compounds called leukotrienes. Leukotrienes are proinflammatory in their own right, and have been shown to be potent chemical attractants and activators of neutrophils. When the COX pathways are inhibited by nonselective NSAIDs, arachidonic acid metabolism may be shunted preferentially through the 5-LOX pathway. Combined COX/LOX inhibitors have been developed to block both pathways simultaneously. Simultaneous COX/LOX blockade has the theoretical advantages of increasing analgesic efficacy and decreasing adverse side effects that may be present due to leukotriene production. There may be merit in this theory. Tepoxalin is the only COX/LOX inhibitor currently on the veterinary market. It is a nonselective inhibitor of the COX enzymes. However, preliminary studies show that tepoxalin has a safety profile that is similar to the selective COX-2 inhibitors. In a single dose surgical model, tepoxalin did not alter hemostatic, hepatic, or renal function.[7] In a separate study, dogs with gastric ulcers healed faster on tepoxalin compared to firocoxib (a highly COX-2 selective NSAID), which significantly delayed gastric healing.[8] Both of these studies and early clinical results support the theoretical advantage of combined COX/LOX inhibition over COX-2 inhibition alone.

For postoperative pain management, NSAIDs have better effect when given preemptively. There are injectable forms of both carprofen and meloxicam that can be given at anesthetic induction. The oral formulations can then be continued postoperatively for continued pain control. Loading doses at twice the daily dose of meloxicam, carprofen, and tepoxalin have been recommended, but are not entirely necessary (see Table 19.4). Some authors have recommended screening renal and hepatic function by performing serum chemistries prior to administration, but no specific guidelines have been evaluated scientifically.

Nonsteroidal anti-inflammatory drugs are highly efficacious and should be considered whenever possible as part of a complete analgesic protocol. However, there are a number of contraindications to NSAID use, and NSAID side effects can be fatal. Nonsteroidal anti-inflammatory drugs should *not* be used in patients receiving concurrent systemic corticosteroids because of an unacceptably high risk of gastrointestinal ulceration and perforation. Nonsteroidal anti-inflammatory drugs should also be avoided in patients with renal or hepatic dysfunction, hypovolemia (dehydration, hypotension, shock, or ascites), hemorrhage, coagulopathy, pulmonary disease, or gastrointestinal disease, and should not be used in pregnant or actively breeding females. Different NSAIDs should not be used concurrently. Pharmaceutical companies recommend a 3–4 half-life wash out period between administrations of differ-

ent NSAIDs. Finally, NSAIDs should always be used within or below their recommended therapeutic dose range. Chronically, NSAIDs should be tapered to the lowest effective dose. Nonsteroidal anti-inflammatory drugs should be given with food.

Nonsteroidal anti-inflammatory drug side effects have been associated mostly with the gastrointestinal tract and include vomiting, diarrhea, hematemesis, melena, and perforation of the stomach or duodenum. Perforating ulcers can be silent and occur with no prior clinical signs. Aspirin is unique in having a local erosive effect on gastric mucosa in addition to systemic COX-1 inhibition. Renal disease has occurred secondary to NSAID administration; however, most reports of renal dysfunction have occurred when NSAIDs were given to hypovolemic patients or those with underlying renal disease. Hepatotoxicosis has also been reported with NSAIDs, but is largely an idiosyncratic effect. Idiosyncratic hepatotoxicosis usually occurs within the first 21 days of administration, but has been reported up to 180 days later. Most dogs recover from hepatic toxicity once the NSAID is discontinued. The hypercoagulability syndrome that has been seen in people with COX-2 selective NSAIDs does not seem to be a concern with any of the NSAIDs used in dogs and cats. Similarly, aspirin and ketoprofen are the only NSAIDs commonly used in veterinary patients that have been shown to delay clinical bleeding times by their inhibition of platelet thromboxane production.

With the numerous choices for NSAID selection, the question is often asked about which specific NSAID to choose. The COX-2 selective NSAIDs have been shown to result in fewer adverse side effects. However, side effects seem to be idiosyncratic and individualistic. So, an individual may tolerate a nonselective NSAID better than a selective one. For postoperative usage, the injectable formulation is convenient to administer. Following injection, the same drug

Table 19.4 Recommended oral dosages (mg/kg, unless otherwise noted) of nonsteroidal anti-inflammatory drugs (NSAIDs) for usage in veterinary medicine[a]

Drug	Dog dosages	Cat dosages	Comments
Nonselective NSAIDs[b]			
Aspirin	10–25 q 12 hours	10 q 48–72 hours	Causes irreversible platelet inhibition
			Avoid usage if possible
Etodolac	10–15 q 24 hours	Not for use in cats due to lack of research on dosage in cats	Has narrow therapeutic window; great care in dosage must be taken
Cycloxygenase-2 (COX-2) Selective NSAIDs[b]			
Carprofen	2.2 q 12 hours, 4.4 q 24 hours	2–4 once	Available in an injectable formulation for use at the same dosage
Deracoxib	1–2 q 24, 3–4 in postoperative period (no more than 7 days)	No recommended dosages	May be a useful alternative to piroxicam for dogs with transitional cell carcinoma
Firocoxib	5 q 24 hours	No recommended dosages	Reported to be the most selective NSAID for the COX-2 enzyme
Meloxicam	0.2 once, 0.1 q 24 hours	0.1 once, 0.05–0.1 q 24 hours, 0.1 mg/cat[c] chronically	Accurate dosage is made easier by liquid formulation; available in an injectable formulation for use at the same dosage
Piroxicam	0.3 mg/kg q 48 hours	No recommended dosages	Dose accurately due to narrow therapeutic index
COX/Lipoxygenase (LOX) Inhibitors			
Tepoxalin	10–20 once, 10 q 24 hours	No recommended dosages	Mucosal disk formulation commercially available

[a] NSAIDs that are not currently recommended for usage in veterinary medicine are not listed.
[b] Based on in vitro testing in dogs.
[c] Note this dosage is per entire cat, *not* mg/kg, due to the highly variable and potentially extended half-life of meloxicam in cats.

should be used in its oral formulation. Initial NSAID selection is usually based on clinician preference and experience, rather than one NSAID being "better" than another. Specific NSAIDs used are then changed based on patient tolerance. So, if a patient has a history of good tolerance on one particular NSAID, it may be wise to continue using that one. However, for patients with no prior NSAID history, drug selection can be made on drug availability, cost, formulation (chewable tablet, liquid, injectable, etc.), and clinician preference.

N-METHYL-D-ASPARTATE RECEPTOR ANTAGONISTS

Ketamine and tiletamine are dissociative anesthetics that are commonly used in veterinary medicine. In addition to anesthesia, they provide good somatic pain control. As a third beneficial trait, ketamine and tiletamine have been shown to be good preemptive analgesics by preventing "wind up" via antagonism of the NMDA receptor. So, in patients in which dissociative anesthetics are a good choice, usage of these drugs enhances intraoperative and postoperative pain control. Tiletamine is only commercially available in combination with the benzodiazepine zolazepam. Ketamine is less expensive than the tiletamine–zolazepam combination and can be used as a sole agent. In recent years, ketamine CRIs have come into vogue for treatment of severe traumatic and postsurgical pain. Ketamine CRIs (often in combination with an opioid and lidocaine) are highly efficacious for pain control, but can cause dramatic sedation, which may or may not be desirable depending on patient circumstances (see Table 19.2).

Dissociative analgesics give poor muscle relaxation and may cause tremors or seizures when given alone. They are most often administered in combination with a benzodiazepine. Dissociatives are contraindicated in patients with increased intracranial pressure or head injury.

Amantadine is an NMDA receptor antagonist that has been shown to have beneficial analgesic properties in dogs with chronic pain when given for 60 days. Its efficacy in postoperative patients has not been evaluated or shown as of the time of this writing.

ALPHA-TWO AGONISTS

Alpha-two agonists are mostly known in veterinary medicine for their sedative and muscle relaxant effects; however, they have potent analgesic effects as well. There are a number of alpha-two receptor subtypes (alpha-two A, alpha-two B, alpha-two C, and alpha-two D) in the central nervous system and peripherally. Differences in affinity for each receptor subtype account for the differences in alpha-two agonist effects and dosages in each species. Side effects of alpha-two agonist administration are primarily cardiovascular in nature and include severe bradycardia, bradyarrhythmias, and hypotension. With initial administration, an increase in peripheral vascular tone causes a physiologic hypertension and bradycardia. Hypotension can occur subsequently. Alpha-two agonists are contraindicated in patients with cardiovascular disease and should be used cautiously in very young, old, or debilitated patients. However, alpha-two agonists are highly synergistic with other analgesics and can make a nice adjunct in combination with opioids or other analgesics to provide good multimodal pain control. Alpha-two agonists should be used at the lowest dose necessary and in combination with other analgesics to achieve the desired effect (see Table 19.2). A major advantage of alpha-two agonists is that they are rapidly and completely reversible with the administration of alpha-two antagonists. Yohimbine and atipamezole are the two most common alpha-two antagonists.

Xylazine was the first alpha-two agonist synthesized. Xylazine is effective, readily available, and inexpensive, but may be associated with increased cardiovascular side effects compared with newer alpha-two agonists. Medetomidine was the most commonly used sedative in small animal practice when it was taken off the market. Medetomidine was more highly selective for the alpha-two receptor, and thus more potent than xylazine. It was supplied as a racemic mixture of two optical enantiomers of the same compound, levomedetomidine and dexmedetomidine, the latter being the only active enantiomer. A purified dexmedetomidine formulation has replaced medetomidine. Dexmedetomidine is an alpha-two agonist

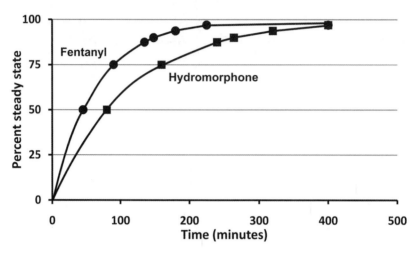

Figure 19.1   Example graph of the time to steady state drug concentrations for a healthy adult dog on a hydromorphone (half-life = 80 minutes) constant rate infusion (CRI) compared to a fentanyl (half-life = 45 minutes) CRI without administration of a loading dose. Circles and boxes represent successive half-life times for fentanyl and hydromorphone, respectively, for up to five half-lives.

currently on the market in the United States, but has not been shown to have clinical benefits (besides being twice as potent) over the racemic mixture.

CONSTANT RATE INFUSION

Constant rate infusion (CRI) of various analgesics can provide effective, reliable, steady-state analgesic drug concentrations for postoperative patients. Constant rate infusions avoid fluctuations in blood concentrations of analgesics so that the risk of toxicity at peak concentrations and potential loss of analgesia at trough concentrations are avoided. Except for NSAIDs, all of the previously listed drug classes can be administered by CRI for pain control. Basic knowledge of CRI pharmacology is important for effective use.

When CRIs are initiated without giving a loading dose, the time required for the drug to reach steady state is dictated solely by the half-life of that drug in the patient. Increases in the serum concentration of a drug occur in logarithmic fashion. In one half-life, the drug

will be at 50% of steady state, 75% at two half lives, 87.5% at three half-lives, and so on. After five half-lives, the serum drug concentration will only be at 97% of steady state. In clinical terms, if a healthy adult dog is not given a loading dose of hydromorphone (half-life = 80 minutes), but solely placed on a hydromorphone CRI postoperatively, it would take 6 hours and 40 minutes for that patient to reach 97% of the steady state level of hydromorphone (see Figure 19.1). To provide immediate postoperative pain control from hydromorphone, a loading dose should be given when the CRI is initiated to bring the patient to steady state drug concentrations and adequate analgesia. More simply, the purpose of the CRI is not to initiate analgesic concentrations of a drug, but to maintain them at that level once a loading dose is given. In the same regard, once the infusion rate is changed (increased or decreased) after the drug is at steady state, it would then take another five half-lives to reach 97% of the new steady state level. As an illustration of how serum drug concentrations change in a logarithmic fashion, morphine can be detected in the urine of healthy adult dogs 6 days after a single intravenous dose even though

Method A:
In order to calculate the rate a full strength drug should be given to a patient for a given CRI rate:

$$\frac{Patient\ Weight\ (kg)\ X\ CRI\ rate\ (mg/kg/hr)}{drug\ concentration\ (mg/ml)}$$

To administer undiluted morphine (10 mg/ml) as a CRI to a 25 kg patient at 0.1 mg/kg/hr:

$$\frac{25\ kg\ X\ 0.1\ mg/kg/hr}{10\ mg/ml} = 0.25\ ml/hr$$

The syringe pump should be set for 0.25 ml/hr (which is 2.5 mg/hr).

Method B:
In order to calculate the amount of analgesic to be added to a 250 mL bag of 0.9% sodium chloride to make a CRI to be given to a patient at 10 mL/hr, the following formula is used:

$$\frac{Patient\ weight\ (kg)\ X\ CRI\ rate\ (mg/kg/hr)}{drug\ concentration\ (mg/ml)} \quad X \quad \frac{volume\ of\ fluid\ to\ be\ diluted\ (ml)}{desired\ rate\ of\ infusion\ (ml/hr}$$

= volume of fluid to be replaced with drug

For the same scenario in Method A:

$$\frac{25\ kgs\ X\ 0.1\ mg/kg/hr}{10\ mg/ml} \quad X \quad \frac{250\ ml}{10\ ml/hr}$$

= 6.25 ml of morphine (10 mg/ml)

So, 6.25 ml of 0.9% sodium chloride should be removed from the 250 ml bag and replaced with 6.25 ml of morphine (10 mg/ml). The resulting solution will provide morphine at 0.1 mg/kg/hr when given at 10 ml/hr.

Figure 19.2   Formula and example calculations for a constant rate infusion (CRI).

analgesic effects are gone by 6 hours or so. A CRI of fentanyl (half life = 45 minutes) is graphed as well in Figure 19.1 to illustrate the difference half-life makes in CRI management.

The easiest way to administer a CRI in the clinical setting is to use an electronic syringe pump. Many of the newer syringe pump models calculate and administer the drug at the appropriate rate after the following information is entered: the patient's body weight, concentration of drug, and rate of CRI administration (mg/kg/h, micrograms/kg/min, etc.). It is possible to do the calculations by hand (Method A in Figure 19.2) and set a syringe pump to administer the drug at the desired rate (mL/h, mL/min, etc.). An alternative method for CRI administration (Method B in Figure 19.2) is to resuspend the drug in a volume of physiologic intravenous fluids (usually 0.9% sodium chloride) so that the fluids can be given at a desired rate that also gives appropriate drug administration. If this second method is used, care must be taken to not fluid overload smaller patients by making the CRI fluid rate higher than physiologically tolerable. Regardless of which method is used, careful attention should be made to be sure that the appropriate units are used in calculation. All weights should be in kilograms, and CRI rates should be converted to mg/kg/hour. Constant rate infusion doses can be listed in reference texts as drug units of micrograms per kilogram, and time can be expressed per minute, hour, or day.

CONCLUSIONS

In summary, veterinary patients are fortunate to have many analgesic drugs and protocols available to ease the inevitable discomfort that occurs with surgical intervention. It is the veterinarian's responsibility to choose the appropriate options to prevent and manage surgically induced pain for each individual patient while avoiding adverse drug effects. The analgesic drugs available today have levels of anal-gesic efficacy and side effects unique to the drug class. It is vitally important that the veterinary clinician knows and understands the analgesics available and their limitations. The importance of multimodal analgesia and its ability to minimize adverse drug effects by using lower dosages of different drug classes in combination to maximize efficacy and minimize adverse effects cannot be stressed enough. Likewise, the concept of maximizing pain control by giving analgesics preemptively should be utilized at every opportunity. In this way, veterinarians can provide the best possible postoperative care for their patients.

REFERENCES

1. Bonnet F, Marret E. Postoperative pain management and outcome after surgery. *Best Pract Res Clin Anaesthesiol* 2007;21:99–107.
2. Kehlet H. Effect of postoperative pain treatment on outcome: current status and future strategies. *Langenbecks Arch Surg* 2004;389:244–249.
3. Fitzgerald M, Millard C, McIntosh N. Cutaneous hypersensitivity following peripheral tissue damage in newborn infants and its reversal with topical anaesthesia. *Pain* 1989;39:31–36.
4. Geyer J, Ellsbury D, Kleiber C, et al. An evidence-based multidisciplinary protocol for neonatal circumcision pain management. *J Obstet Gynecol Neonatal Nurs* 2002;31:403–410.
5. Weisman SJ, Bernstein B, Schechter NL. Consequences of inadequate analgesia during painful procedures in children. *Arch Pediatr Adolesc Med* 1998;152:147–149.
6. Bergh MS, Budsberg SC. The coxib NSAIDs: potential clinical and pharmacologic importance in veterinary medicine. *J Vet Intern Med* 2005;19:633–643.
7. Kay-Mugford PA, Grimm KA, Weingarten AJ, et al. Effect of preoperative administration of tepoxalin on hemostasis and hepatic and renal function in dogs. *Vet Ther* 2004;5:120–127.
8. Goodman L, Torres B, Punke J, et al. Effects of firocoxib and tepoxalin on healing in a canine gastric mucosal injury model. *J Vet Intern Med* 2009;23:56–62.

ADDITIONAL RESOURCES

Additional information about analgesic drugs and postoperative pain management in small animal surgery can be found in the following textbooks:

1. Gaynor JS, Muir III. WW. *Handbook of Veterinary Pain Management*. St. Louis, Missouri: Mosby Elsevier, 2009.

2. Plumb DC. *Veterinary Drug Handbook*, 5th ed. Ames, Iowa: Blackwell Publishing, 2005.
3. Tranquilli WJ, Thurmon JC, Grimm KA. *Lumb & Jones' Veterinary Anesthesia and Analgesia*. Ames, Iowa: Blackwell Publishing, 2007.

[**Note**: Drug dosages and other information in the tables and figures in this chapter are based on individual drug package inserts and the above three additional resources.]

Chapter 20

PATIENT AFTERCARE AND FOLLOWUP

Elizabeth A. Swanson and Fred Anthony Mann

Postoperative care and followup are just as important as the care and attention to detail afforded before and during surgery. Good care in the immediately postoperative period will facilitate a smooth recovery from anesthesia and keep the patient comfortable, whether the procedure was a simple feline castration or a complicated liver lobe resection or fracture repair. Providing warmth, maintaining adequate perfusion and ventilation, providing good nursing care and analgesia, maintaining a positive nutritional status, and restricting activity to allow proper wound healing are all important factors that will be discussed in this chapter. Followup after the patient is released from the hospital is essential to maintaining open communications with the client. Followup communications and examinations allow the surgeon to monitor the healing process, determine if additional care is needed, and decide when it is appropriate for the patient to return to normal activity.

Fundamentals of Small Animal Surgery, 1st edition.
By Fred Anthony Mann, Gheorghe M. Constantinescu and Hun-Young Yoon.
© 2011 Blackwell Publishing Ltd.

IMMEDIATELY POSTOPERATIVE CARE

A patient first entering the recovery ward or intensive care unit is usually still awakening from anesthesia. A patent airway should be maintained with the endotracheal tube until a strong swallow reflex has returned. Because flaccid, redundant soft tissue structures may interfere with normal respiration in brachycephalic breeds, it is best in these breeds to wait to extubate until the animal is lifting its head and starting to chew the tube. Recovering patients with endotracheal tubes in place must be monitored closely so that the tube is not accidently severed. After extubation, ascertain that the patient is breathing in an unobstructed manner before leaving the area.

Basic postoperative monitoring for all patients regardless of procedure performed includes measuring body temperature and assessing cardiovascular parameters, respiratory function, level of consciousness, and pain status. Most patients are cold by the time they reach the recovery area. An anesthetized patient is unable to regulate its body temperature and will lose heat quickly on transfer from the operating table. Small patients have a higher surface area to body mass ratio and will dissipate body heat faster than larger patients. Body temperature should be checked every 30–60 minutes until it has reached 100°F (37.8°C). Once the body temperature is normal, a stable, awake patient can be moved from the recovery area to the regular wards. External heat sources should be turned off or removed from patients who are able to regulate their body temperature.

The simplest parameters used to monitor adequacy of perfusion and ventilation are heart rate, pulse quality, respiratory rate and effort, mucous membrane color, and capillary refill time. These parameters should be monitored hourly until the patient is awake and alert after anesthesia, then every 6–12 hours thereafter, depending on the nature of the case. Critical patients require more frequent monitoring. For example, a patient recovering from thoracotomy should be checked hourly for changes in respiratory rate or character. Heart rate, pulse quality, mucous membrane color, and capillary refill time are used to assess perfusion. Tachycardia (as an example, greater than 180 beats per minute in dogs and greater than 260 beats per minute in cats) with weak, thready pulses, and pale mucous membranes indicates poor perfusion from hypovolemia, shock, or systemic inflammatory response. [Note: Cats do not have the same baroreceptor response to hypovolemia as dogs, so feline heart rates can be normal or low in the face of hypovolemia. Also, both dogs and cats will have bradycardia in the terminal stages of shock (decompensatory shock).] Either tachycardia or bradycardia with weak and/or skipped pulses may indicate a life-threatening cardiac arrhythmia that should be addressed. A prolonged capillary refill time may indicate poor cardiac output or circulation; however, caution must be used since capillary refill time can still be present in patients with no heart beat.

Respiratory rate, respiratory character and effort, and mucous membrane color help determine ventilation and oxygenation adequacy. Rapid respirations, shallow or labored breathing, and cyanotic mucous membranes are all indicators of poor oxygen exchange such as may be seen with pneumothorax, pleural effusion, pulmonary edema, pulmonary contusions, pneumonia, or pulmonary thromboembolism. Any abnormal changes in the parameters listed above warrant additional investigation and intervention as discussed later in this chapter.

Oxygenation can be assessed via the partial pressure of arterial oxygen (PaO_2) and arterial oxygen saturation of hemoglobin (SaO_2) on an arterial blood gas or, less invasively and more frequently, via pulse oximetry. Pulse oximeters display pulse rate and hemoglobin saturation; therefore, the use of pulse oximeters is limited in the presence of vasoconstriction and poorly detectable pulses. However, the detection of a weak pulse or difficulty finding a pulse may indicate impaired peripheral circulation and warrant additional investigation. If the pulse rate displayed on the pulse oximeter does not match the palpable pulse rate or auscultable heart rate, then the hemoglobin saturation reading should be considered unreliable. Pulse oximeters measure the percent hemoglobin saturation by transmitting red and infrared light through the blood and tissues. Red light is absorbed more by unsaturated hemoglobin than infrared light, whereas infrared light is more absorbed by oxygenated hemoglobin than red light. The amount of light absorbed is measured and the pulse oximeter calculates and displays the percentage of hemoglobin that is oxygenated. In the process of calculation, the pulse oximeter is able to cancel the hemoglobin in venous blood and tissues by measuring during a pulse (hence, the term *pulse* oximeter), thereby estimating the percent saturation of arterial hemoglobin (SpO_2). The SaO_2 (and thus the SpO_2) is related to the partial pressure of oxygen (PaO_2) by a sigmoidal curve known as the oxygen-hemoglobin dissociation curve. A normal PaO_2 at sea level and room temperature is from 80 to 110 mmHg, which corresponds to a pulse oximeter reading of 95% to 100%. Since 90% SaO_2 corresponds to a PaO_2 of

60 mmHg, treatment with supplemental oxygen is indicated when the SpO_2 falls below 90%.

Adequacy of ventilation can be assessed on a blood gas or via capnography. End-tidal carbon dioxide ($ETCO_2$) is measured via capnography and can be used as an estimate of the arterial partial pressure of carbon dioxide ($PaCO_2$) that is measured directly by arterial blood gas analysis. Normal $PaCO_2$ is between 35 and 45 mmHg. Since CO_2 diffuses rapidly across the pulmonary capillary endothelium and alveolar tissues, $ETCO_2$ values are similar to $PaCO_2$. An $ETCO_2$ over 60 mmHg indicates hypoventilation, while an $ETCO_2$ below 20 mmHg indicates hyperventilation.

Level of consciousness should be monitored at least hourly to make sure the patient is waking properly. When recovering from anesthesia, patients should gradually transition from sleeping to wakefulness (although some sedation is acceptable depending on the administration of analgesics or sedatives). Most patients will awaken over a period of 15–20 minutes.[1] Prolonged recoveries will be seen in critically ill, hypothermic, hypoglycemic, anemic, hypoxemic, and hypoproteinemic patients. Patients that are over-anesthetized will also take longer to return to consciousness. Dysphoric or anxious patients may require administration of a sedative (acepromazine or dexmedetomidine) to calm the patient and reduce the risk of injury. A change in consciousness to a more depressed state indicates a problem that should be investigated and corrected as soon as possible (i.e., increased intracranial pressure, hypoglycemia, sepsis, or shock secondary to hemorrhage).

Patients should also be monitored for evidence of pain and discomfort. It is no longer considered acceptable to allow a patient to remain painful because of the belief that pain will help restrict activity and, therefore, assist in healing. Both human and animal patients recover better and faster when their pain has been appropriately addressed. Pain can be difficult to assess in the veterinary patient; differentiating between pain and anxiety can be chal-lenging. Both should be addressed since pain has been shown to be increased in the anxious patient.[2] Documented painful behavior in domestic animals includes vocalization, shivering, reluctance to move, restlessness or inability to get comfortable, guarding the injured area, aggression, excessive salivation, dilated pupils, hypertension, and increased respiratory rate. Postoperative pain management is discussed in more detail in Chapter 19.

Critical cases and patients with abnormalities in the basic parameters mentioned above require additional monitoring. Blood pressure can be measured directly via an arterial catheter or indirectly using Doppler or oscillometric technology. Any patient that had prolonged hypotension while under anesthesia, significant hemorrhage, sepsis, or that may be in danger of developing a systemic inflammatory response should have blood pressure monitored. Direct arterial pressures and oscillometric indirect pressures have the benefit of providing systolic, diastolic, and mean pressures. The ideal mean arterial pressure to ensure adequate perfusion of the brain and kidneys is between 80 and 90 mmHg. Mean pressures below 60 mmHg result in inadequate blood flow to the kidneys and could result in renal damage. Also, inadequate perfusion of the kidneys may predispose to damage caused by the use of NSAIDs. Autoregulation in the brain maintains adequate cerebral blood flow as long as the mean arterial blood pressure is between 50 and 150 mmHg. If a method to obtain mean arterial pressure is not available, Doppler indirect pressure measurements are still useful. A systolic pressure greater than 100 mmHg will usually indicate adequate tissue perfusion.

Glucose should be monitored in patients whose ability to regulate blood glucose concentrations is impaired. Very young, debilitated, and septic patients (such as those with septic peritonitis), as well as those in immediately postoperative recovery from portosystemic shunt attenuation or excision of an insulinoma, should have blood or serum glucose checked immediately postoperatively and frequently thereafter, as the individual case requires, in the first 24–48 hours. Hypoglycemia (blood glucose less than 60 mg/dL) will prolong recovery from anesthesia. Other signs of hypoglycemia include lethargy, depression, tremors, weakness, ataxia, seizures, and coma. Patients at risk for hypoglycemia who are able to eat should be fed small meals every two to three hours to help maintain euglycemia. Hypoglycemic patients and patients at risk of hypoglycemia that are unable to eat should have dextrose added to their intravenous fluids (usually 2.5% or 5% dextrose in a balanced electrolyte solution) and may require a 25% dextrose bolus (1 mL/kg) to control clinical signs.

Hemorrhage is always a potential complication of surgery. Blood loss may be severe in some procedures, such as splenectomy for a ruptured splenic mass, liver lobectomy, and in cases of trauma. Measurement of packed cell volume (PCV) and total protein (TP) is a quick method to ascertain blood loss. However, in peracute hemorrhage PCV and TP will be normal (or the same as baseline) until fluid shift from the intracellular and interstitial compartments to the intravascular space occurs. A complete blood count (CBC) can also be used. Postoperative patients who have had significant blood loss or who may be hemorrhaging postoperatively should have a PCV/TP checked immediately postoperatively, and then as needed, depending on the case. Early signs of hemorrhage include light pink or pale mucous membranes, increased heart rate, weak peripheral pulses, and drop in blood pressure. Advanced signs of hemorrhage are weakness, collapse, and death. A distended abdomen or dyspnea may be noted if the bleeding occurs in the abdominal or thoracic cavity, respectively. Total protein may fall before PCV if splenic contraction occurs. Treatment includes judicious fluid therapy and blood transfusion. While rapid intravenous crystalloid or other fluid bolusing may be necessary for resuscitation of a patient in hemorrhagic shock, care must be taken not to

cause rehemorrhaging by dislodging early clots as the fluid therapy increases blood pressure. A process called hypotensive resuscitation is practiced in actively hemorrhaging cases, whereby blood pressure is monitored and fluid therapy is titrated to achieve an arterial blood pressure above that which would cause renal impairment (i.e., above a mean arterial pressure of 60 mmHg), but not as high as normal. In such cases, the targeted mean arterial blood pressure is typically 70–80 mmHg. Reoperation may be required to find and ligate bleeding vessels; however, increased intra-abdominal pressure from the accumulating abdominal fluid or from an abdominal bandage usually controls intra-abdominal hemorrhage that has resulted from surgical manipulations. Elective procedures, especially ovariohysterectomy, should be monitored for postoperative hemorrhage, just as any other operative procedure.

Central venous pressure (CVP) is used to monitor volume status in critical postoperative patients and to guide intravenous fluid therapy. Normal CVP is between 0 and 10 cm H_2O. Values less than 0 cm H_2O indicate hypovolemia and the need for increased or ongoing fluid therapy; whereas, values greater than 10 cm H_2O indicate volume overload or myocardial insufficiency, and fluid therapy should be decreased or discontinued. To measure CVP, a water manometer (or intravenous extension tubing adjacent to a centimeter ruler) is connected by means of a three-way stopcock to a central venous line, usually a jugular catheter (Figure 20.1). The manometer is placed perpendicular to the floor with the 0 cm mark located at the level of the right atrium (Figure 20.2). Sterile saline is first used to flush the jugular catheter, then the line is closed to the patient and the manometer is filled. The line is then opened to both the patient and the manometer, and pressures are allowed to equilibrate (Figure 20.3). Once the fluid level stops falling, CVP is read at the bottom of the fluid meniscus (Figure 20.3). The meniscus should oscillate up and down approximately 1 mm with each breath. A

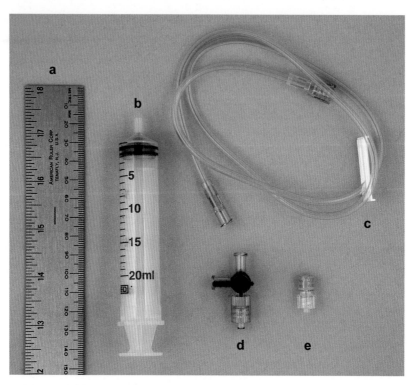

Figure 20.1   Supplies (in addition to a central venous catheter) for central venous pressure measurement: (a) ruler (or alternatively, a water manometer – not shown); (b) 20 mL syringe for sterile 0.9% sodium chloride; (c) intravenous extension tubing; (d) stopcock; and (e) intravenous catheter cap.

stationary meniscus should alert to a possible artifactual reading.

Hypoproteinemic patients often require colloid therapy to maintain intravascular volume and to prevent the formation of edema. Colloid osmotic pressure (COP), also called colloid oncotic pressure, is measured from a blood sample with an instrument called a colloid osmometer, and is used to guide colloid administration. Normal COP values are between 20 and 25 mmHg. Values less than 15 mmHg warrant intervention to maintain plasma oncotic pressure. Causes of hypoproteinemia include loss (protein-losing enteropathy, protein losing-nephropathy, abdominal effusion), lack of protein intake (anorexia), and lack of protein production (liver failure). Consequences of hypoproteinemia and low plasma oncotic

pressure include edema and delayed tissue healing.

In addition to monitoring the parameters listed above, good nursing care is essential for all patients. The purpose of nursing care is to keep the patient as comfortable as possible and in a state of optimal hygiene. Patients recovering from surgery should be kept warm, clean, and dry. The effects of hypothermia have been discussed previously. Excessive moisture on the skin is uncomfortable and can lead to maceration and infection. Urine and fecal scalding should be avoided by immediately picking up after the patient, regular checking/changing bedding in recumbent patients, using absorbent padding under patients, and gently washing a soiled patient with water or waterless shampoo. Bathing human intensive care unit patients with

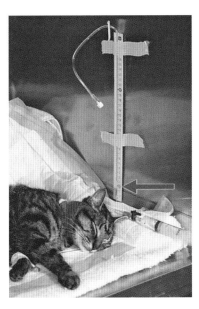

Figure 20.2   Central venous pressure setup in a postoperative feline patient. Note that the zero centimeter mark toward the bottom of the ruler (indicated by the arrow) is on a level equal to the level of the cat's right atrium with the cat in left lateral recumbence.

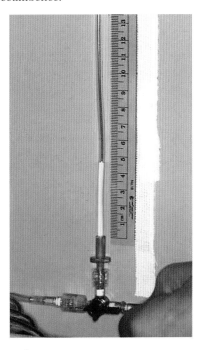

Figure 20.3   Closeup view of a central venous pressure measurement using intravenous extension tubing and ruler for a manometer. The central venous pressure should be read at the bottom of the fluid meniscus, and in this case is 4.6 cm H_2O.

chlorhexidine has been shown to decrease nosocomial infection rates; therefore, chlorhexidine should be considered for cleaning at risk veterinary patients.

All patients should be supplied with appropriate bedding. Recumbent animals require thicker bedding and should be turned from side to side every four to six hours to prevent decubital ulcers. Incisions should be monitored at least twice daily to make sure they are clean and dry with no evidence of swelling, redness, dehiscence, or discharge. Patients will become uncomfortable if they are unable to void their bladders. Ambulatory patients can be walked or carted outside. Urinary bladders should be gently expressed or emptied via a urinary catheter in nonambulatory patients who are unable to void their bladders (i.e., a dog recovering from hemilaminectomy). Retained urine can lead to urinary tract infection. Urinary catheterization and attachment to a closed urine collection system should be considered in recumbent patients for hygiene purposes and can also be used to monitor urine output.

Orthopedic patients often have a dressing or bandage placed postoperatively. Dressings, such as Bioclusive (Johnson & Johnson, Langhorne, PA) and Telfa Island Dressings (Covidien, Mansfield, MA), are placed over an incision to protect it and prevent contamination until a fibrin seal has formed. Bandages are placed to protect an incision, provide additional stabilization for a limb, and/or provide moderate pressure to decrease postoperative swelling. Bandages should be kept clean and dry at all times. They should be monitored for slipping as this can lead to constriction of the limb and interfere with circulation. Digits should be checked regularly for swelling, indicating a bandage that is too tight. Bandages should be changed if strikethrough is noted, if they become wet or soiled, or if slipping or swelling is noted.

Intravenous catheters should not be removed in healthy patients undergoing elective surgery until they are awake and body temperature has returned to normal. Intravenous catheters should be maintained in critical and debilitated patients and in patients receiving intravenous pain medications (via intermittent injections or constant rate infusion) postoperatively. The types of intravenous catheters that may be in place in a surgical patient include peripheral venous catheters (cephalic, lateral saphenous), central venous catheters (external jugular), and arterial catheters. There are some differences in maintaining each type of catheter; however, all should be monitored for patency, proper placement, and development of inflammation or infection. Unused catheters should be flushed with saline every six hours to maintain patency. Arterial catheters should be flushed and locked with heparinized saline when not in use. Alternatively, arterial lines can be maintained by connecting them to heparinized saline in a pressure bag. Heparinized saline is not necessary for venous catheters. In fact, overuse of heparinized flush can inadvertently heparinize the patient (i.e., prolong clotting times), particularly in small dogs and cats.

Since veterinary patients often move around in their cage or run, it is important to ensure that catheters remain in place. Inadvertent subcutaneous administration of fluids and medications may occur, potentially with disastrous consequences, if an intravenous catheter is dislodged or partially pulled out. An intravenous catheter should be removed once it is no longer needed, if swelling or phlebitis is noted, or if patency cannot be safely restored. At least twice daily inspection of catheter sites is necessary to detect and promptly address catheter-related problems.

Chest tubes, feeding tubes (esophagostomy, gastrostomy, jejunostomy), indwelling urinary catheters, and drains should be kept clean and patent. If a chest tube is used for intermittent evacuation of the pleural space, it is important to make sure that the clamp is in place and closed when the tube is not in use to prevent iatrogenic pneumothorax. The patient should be prevented from chewing or pulling the tubes by placing a t-shirt, stockinette, bandage, or

Elizabethan collar. The stomas around chest tubes, feeding tubes, and drains should be monitored at least twice daily for redness, swelling, leakage, and discharge. A thorough discussion of surgical tubes and drains can be found in Chapter 17.

Most surgical patients, with the exception of uncomplicated elective procedures, will be kept on intravenous fluids after surgery. Both crystalloids and colloids are used, based on the patient's needs. The most common crystalloids used postoperatively include lactated Ringer's solution, Normosol-R, Plasma-Lyte, and 0.9% sodium chloride. Potassium chloride, dextrose, and B-vitamins may be added according to the patient's individual requirements. Colloids include hetastarch, dextran, blood products, and Oxyglobin (Biopure Corporation, Cambridge, MA), although the availability of the latter has fluctuated over the years. Isotonic crystalloids are typically chosen for maintenance fluids. Calorie-based fluid maintenance is the dosage of fluids on the premise that one milliliter of water is lost for every kilocalorie of energy that is utilized. As such, the same formula as that used for calculating daily resting energy requirement can be used to calculate daily fluid maintenance (see this chapter, section on Nutritional Support). Maintenance fluid administration rates are appropriate for orthopedic patients without other complicating factors. Critical patients and patients with metabolic dysfunction, such as renal disease, require higher rates ranging from 1.5 times maintenance to shock doses (90 mL/kg) of fluids. Lower fluid rates are indicated for cardiac patients. When colloids are used, the dosage is based on the needs of the patient and the goal of the colloid, but the basic dosage for hetastarch and dextran is 20 mL/kg/day. Care should be taken when using colloids in cats, as cats are more sensitive to colloid effects than dogs. In general, give colloids to cats at lower dosages and slower rates than calculated for dogs. Fluid therapy that is too aggressive can lead to volume overload and pulmonary edema. Readers are referred to medicine, critical care, and fluid therapy textbooks for more detailed discussion of intravenous fluid therapy.

The routine use of antibiotics after surgery is not indicated. Administration of antibiotics should be reserved for known bacterial infections, preferably based on culture and susceptibility results. When perioperative antibiotics are continued postoperatively, they are discontinued within 24 hours. See Chapter 4 for a complete discussion of antibiotic use in small animal surgery.

NUTRITIONAL SUPPORT

Nutrition is essential to meet the metabolic needs of all surgical patients. When calorie intake is insufficient, the body is unable to mount an adaptive response due to the influence of catecholamines, glucocorticoids, and other products of the inflammatory process. As a result, instead of utilizing fat stores as an energy source (as a healthy animal would) the surgical patient continues to break down muscle for protein, which results in a net loss of lean body mass. Malnutrition and the concomitant loss of lean body mass decrease the patient's ability to repair tissue and resist infection with the ultimate result of increasing patient morbidity and chance of death. Oral intake of food is ideal, if the patient is able to eat. While it is recommended that nutritional intervention should take place if a patient has been anorexic or partially anorexic for five days or longer,[3] early feeding (within 24 hours of surgery) is best for surgical patients. Interventional nutrition should be employed if voluntary oral intake does not occur within 24 hours or is contraindicated.

If the gastrointestinal tract is functional, enteral feeding via a feeding tube should be considered. Preplanning for nutritional support and placement of a feeding tube during surgery when warranted (such as in patients with prolonged preoperative anorexia, severe debilitation, or extensive gastrointestinal resection) can prevent future anesthetic episodes a few days later to place a feeding tube when the patient refuses to eat. Furthermore, it is prudent to take advantage of anesthesia to place a feeding tube whenever the surgical procedure itself or the postoperative management (i.e., nausea-inducing analgesics) is prone to causing anorexia. For example, it would be a good idea to place a jejunostomy tube prior to closing the abdomen for a surgical procedure where the operative manipulations could result in nausea or anorexia. In fact, it would be better to have a jejunostomy tube in a postoperative abdominal surgery patient that does not require a feeding tube than not to have one in a similar patient who does not eat or begins vomiting.

Options for feeding tubes include nasoesophageal, esophagostomy, gastrostomy, and jejunostomy tubes. Care and maintenance of feeding tubes are discussed previously and in Chapter 17. Smaller diameter tubes, such as nasoesophageal and jejunostomy tubes, require use of a liquid diet. Larger tubes can accommodate canned foods such as Hill's Prescription Diet a/d (Hill's Pet Nutrition, Inc., Topeka, KS), Iams Veterinary Diet Maximum Calorie (The Iams Company, Dayton, OH), or Royal Canin Recovery RS (Royal Canin USA, Inc., St. Charles, MO).

In general, a veterinary diet should be used. Concurrent medical conditions may impact the choice of diet. One example would be in renal patients where a low protein diet may be desirable. The reader is referred to nutrition textbooks for detailed discussion of diet selection for various disease states. The resting energy requirement (RER) for most patients can be calculated using the equation *kcal/day = 30(weight in kg) + 70*. The RER for patients less than 2 kg and greater than 45 kg should be calculated using the equation $kcal/day = 70(weight\ in\ kg)^{0.75}$. Illness factors are no longer used in determining energy requirements of sick patients. One-quarter to 1/2 of the RER is given on day one, with an increase to 100% of the RER by the sec-

ond or third day. The total volume should be divided into four to six feedings per day, unless a jejunostomy tube is being used. Jejunostomy feeding is delivered by constant rate infusion because distention of the intestine with boluses will cause pain and may compromise absorption of the diet. Most clinicians begin jejunostomy feedings with less than the calculated calories and volume, and increase the amount daily with hopes of reaching the RER by the third day of jejunal feeding.

Potential complications of enteral feeding tubes include clogging of the tube, refeeding syndrome if a patient has been anorexic for some time and rapid reinstitution of feeding occurs, vomiting, diarrhea, premature removal by the patient, and aspiration if the tube is incorrectly placed in the nasopharynx or trachea. The amount of fluid provided via enteral feeding should be included in the calculation of the daily fluid requirement to avoid overhydration of the patient. Enteral feeding may be gradually reduced once the patient is eating at least 60% of its RER and discontinued once the patient is able to meet its energy requirements. Tubes should not be pulled until it is certain the patient will continue to eat enough to meet its daily RER. Percutaneously placed gastrostomy tubes, and jejunostomy tubes that have been applied without using the interlocking box technique, should not be removed until 10 days (gastrostomy tubes) or 5 days (jejunostomy tubes) after placement to allow sufficient adhesions to form between the stomach or jejunum and the body wall. The interlocking box method [See Chapter 17] allows for safe immediately postoperative removal of a jejunostomy tube, and this is advantageous in the event of inadvertent removal or if the patient begins eating soon after surgery and can be sent home before the fifth postoperative day.

Parenteral nutrition should be considered for any patient without a jejunostomy tube that is unable to tolerate oral or enteral feedings due to vomiting, severe pancreatitis, or an increased risk of aspiration due to the inability to protect the airway. Commercial formulations for partial parenteral nutrition (PPN) and total parenteral nutrition (TPN) are available. In general, a dedicated intravenous catheter and the ability to maintain aseptic vascular access, 24-hour nursing care, and the ability to run in-house serum chemistries for patient monitoring must be available. All catheters and lines must be handled with aseptic technique to minimize contamination. Partial parenteral nutrition is indicated for short-term use only as it does not provide for all caloric requirements. Because TPN is intended to provide for all caloric requirements and is initiated gradually over 3 days, TPN should only be used in cases that are expected to require parenteral nutrition for 3 days or longer. Worksheets are available to calculate PPN and TPN requirements.[3]

Potential complications associated with parenteral nutrition include clogging of the line or catheter, phlebitis, thromboembolism, and sepsis. Most of these complications can be avoided by careful adherence to monitoring and aseptic protocols. Serum concentrations of glucose, electrolytes, phosphorus, and magnesium should be monitored in all animals receiving parenteral nutrition. Parenteral feeding can be discontinued once the patient is consuming 60% or more of its RER. The reader is referred to nutrition textbooks for detailed information on parenteral nutrition.

PHYSICAL ACTIVITY

Physical activity should be restricted to a kennel or small room with short, controlled leash walks for dogs to eliminate for the first 10–14 days after surgery to allow the incision to heal. Most orthopedic procedures require confinement for six to eight weeks to allow for bone healing. Exceptions include young dogs (puppies) that can heal in three to four weeks and procedures such as femoral head and neck excision where early return to controlled activity is encouraged to increase range of motion at

the coxofemoral joint. In most soft tissue procedures, normal activity may be resumed once the sutures or staples are removed. A gradual return to normal activity after confirmation of adequate bone healing is recommended for orthopedic patients to strengthen muscles, ligaments, and tendons and to prevent overuse injuries of the affected limb.

Physical therapy is beneficial for patients during extended periods of enforced rest and for immobile patients. The benefits of physical therapy include prevention of muscle contracture, decreased muscle atrophy, maintenance of normal joint range of motion, improved circulation, and improved function of the affected limb. Simple forms of physical therapy include cold packing for the first 24 hours after surgery to decrease inflammation and swelling, followed by warm packing to help increase circulation and relax tissues. Warm packing also helps resolve edema and seroma. Passive range of motion exercises serve to maintain joint mobility and flexibility. Ambulatory patients can perform their own physical therapy by controlled leash walks, walking up or down inclines or stairs, and swimming. More information on physical therapy can be found in other surgical textbooks.

FOLLOWUP

Followup care is as important as perioperative care for the surgical patient. Followup care includes a combination of written instructions, recheck visits, and phone conversations. Patients should be released with written instructions for the owners to follow. Dismissal instructions should minimally include the procedure performed and instructions for activity restriction (amount and length of time), incision and/or bandage monitoring and care, prevention of licking and chewing of the surgery site, nutrition, and follow-up visits for suture removal, physical examination, laboratory monitoring, and radiographs, as is appropriate for the patient. The written instructions should also include recommendations for the owner to call if any complications arise.

Skin sutures and staples are typically removed 10–14 days postoperatively, but may be left in place longer if delayed wound healing is expected. Patients with hyperadrenocorticism or that are taking corticosteroids may require a longer time to heal. Sutures for auricular hematoma repair should be left in at least 17 days to allow for fibrosis of the cartilage layers of the pinna. Incisions over areas of high motion are subjected to large amounts of tension and, therefore, require more time to heal. The consequence of removing sutures too early is incisional dehiscence and of leaving them in too long is local irritation and formation of draining tracts. Some surgeons will close the skin of spay and castration incisions with intradermal sutures instead of skin sutures. A followup appointment at 10–14 days to check incisional healing is still advised in these cases.

Sutures are removed by grasping the ends of the suture with the fingers or an instrument such as a hemostat or thumb forceps and cutting the loop of the suture with stitch scissors (Figure 20.4). Use caution not to cut both sides of the loop to prevent retention of part of the suture and a potential foreign body reaction. Skin staples are removed using a surgical staple remover. The staple remover is placed so that the side with two "teeth" is slid under the staple. The instrument is closed so that the single "tooth" engages the cross-member of the staple and causes the staple to bend in half, straightening the legs and removing the staple from the skin (Figure 20.5). In the absence of a staple remover, a mosquito hemostatic forceps can be used to spread open the staple and remove it. Sometimes, a staple will have turned in the skin. Mosquito hemostats can be used to rotate the staple into the original position for easier removal. Manipulating skin staples with hemostatic forceps may cause patient discomfort.

Some procedures, such as parathyroidectomy or insulinoma excision, require labora-

tory followup. Patients undergoing cystotomy for urolith removal should have regular urinalyses and imaging studies performed to monitor for effectiveness of therapy and recurrence of stones. Radiographic evaluation for bone healing should be performed eight weeks postoperatively for most adult patients. Pediatric orthopedic patients can be checked at two to four weeks postoperatively since their bones heal faster. Some procedures such as repair of a mandibular fracture or placement of an external skeletal fixator for fracture repair require more time to heal. The intervals of radiographic rechecks should be adjusted accordingly.

Ensuring client compliance with followup recommendations can be difficult at times, especially in cases where the client lives a long distance from the veterinary hospital, has limited mobility, or limited funds. Referral centers with good relations with their referring veterinarians may opt to have all or most followup care take place at the referring practice. Some veterinarians do not charge for suture removal or for quick well-being rechecks in order to encourage compliant followup. Compliance can be improved by informing the owner of the importance of followup and by providing a realistic estimate of costs (such as for repeated laboratory work or radiographs).

A brief telephone call a day or two after surgery to check on the patient can go a long way in instilling confidence in the veterinarian and making the owner feel that the veterinarian cares about their pet. The telephone call may also provide opportunity to prevent complications by timely intervention if a problem is revealed. The veterinarian should also be available to take a client telephone call or to call back in a timely manner if the client perceives a problem with their pet. Prompt communication, of course, requires skill and training of the receptionist or technician answering the telephone to determine if the problem needs to be addressed immediately by having the

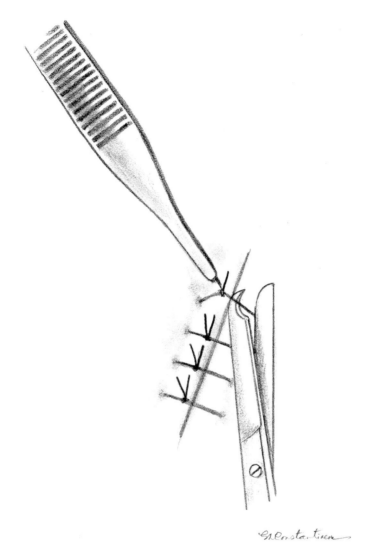

Figure 20.4   Suture removal using stitch scissors. One end of the suture is being grasped with thumb forceps while the loop of the suture is cut with stitch scissors.

patient return to the hospital, if the doctor needs to be interrupted to take the call, or if the problem can wait for a return call. Communication among the practice team members is essential.

In short, good followup care is a combination of reexamination of the patient and good communication among the veterinarian, veterinary staff, and the owner. Followup care should be tailored to the needs of each individual patient, and can include monitoring of incision healing, recovery, laboratory workup, and radiographic examination, as well as moral support of the client. Complications can be

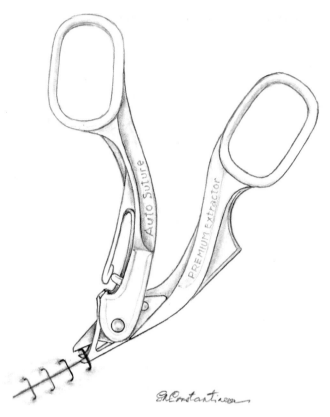

Figure 20.5 Removal of skin staples. The staple remover is placed so that the side with two "teeth" is slid under the staple. The instrument is closed so that the single "tooth" engages the cross-member of the staple and causes the staple to bend in half, straightening the legs, and thereby removing the staple from the skin.

identified and treated in a timely manner. Finally, the surgeon can ensure that the patient has healed adequately before returning to normal activity.

REFERENCES

1. Quandt JE. Postoperative patient care. In: Slatter DH, ed. *Textbook of Small Animal Surgery*, 3rd ed. Philadelphia, Pennsylvania: Saunders, 2003: 2608–2612.
2. Carroll GL. Analgesia and pain. *Vet Clin North Am Small Anim Pract* 1999; 29: 701–717.
3. Chan DL, Freeman LM. Nutrition in critical illness. *Vet Clin North Am Small Anim Pract* 2006; 36: 1225–1241.

ADDITIONAL RESOURCES

Additional information useful for patient aftercare in small animal surgery can be found in the following textbook, publication, and textbook chapters:

1. DiBartola SP, ed. *Fluid, Electrolyte and Acid-Base Disorders in Small Animal Practice*, 3rd ed. Philadelphia, Pennsylvania: Saunders, 2005.

2. Kirk CA, Bartges JW, eds. *Dietary Management and Nutrition, Veterinary Clinics of North America: Small Animal Practice.* Philadelphia, Pennsylvania: Saunders, November 2006:36(6).

3. Knap K, Johnson AL, Schulz K. Fundamentals of physical rehabilitation. In: Fossum TW, ed. *Small Animal Surgery*, 3rd ed. St. Louis, Missouri: Mosby, 2007:111–129.

4. Willard MD, Seim HB. Postoperative care of the surgical patient. In: Fossum TW, ed. *Small Animal Surgery*, 3rd ed. St. Louis, Missouri: Mosby, 2007:90–110.

INDEX

Keep up with critical fields

Would you like to receive up-to-date information on our books, journals and databases in the areas that interest you, direct to your mailbox?

Join the **Wiley e-mail service** - a convenient way to receive updates and exclusive discount offers on products from us.

Simply visit **www.wiley.com/email** and register online

We won't bombard you with emails and we'll only email you with information that's relevant to you. We will ALWAYS respect your e-mail privacy and NEVER sell, rent, or exchange your e-mail address to any outside company. Full details on our privacy policy can be found online.

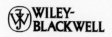
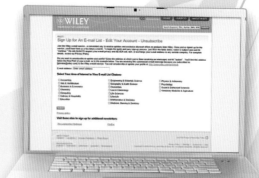

17841